Volume 10. CONCEPTS IN DRUG METABOLISM (in two parts), *edited by Peter Jenner and Bernard Testa*

Volume 11. PHARMACEUTICAL ANALYSIS: MODERN METHODS (in two parts), *edited by James W. Munson*

Volume 12. TECHNIQUES OF SOLUBILIZATION OF DRUGS, *edited by Samuel H. Yalkowsky*

Volume 13. ORPHAN DRUGS, *edited by Fred E. Karch*

Volume 14. NOVEL DRUG DELIVERY SYSTEMS: FUNDAMENTALS, DEVELOPMENTAL CONCEPTS, BIOMEDICAL ASSESSMENTS, *Yie W. Chien*

Volume 15. PHARMACOKINETICS, SECOND EDITION, REVISED AND EXPANDED, *Milo Gibaldi and Donald Perrier*

Volume 16. GOOD MANUFACTURING PRACTICES FOR PHARMACEUTICALS: A PLAN FOR TOTAL QUALITY CONTROL, SECOND EDITION, REVISED AND EXPANDED, *Sidney H. Willig, Murray M. Tuckerman, and William S. Hitchings IV*

Volume 17. FORMULATION OF VETERINARY DOSAGE FORMS, *edited by Jack Blodinger*

Volume 18. DERMATOLOGICAL FORMULATIONS: PERCUTANEOUS ABSORPTION, *Brian W. Barry*

Volume 19. THE CLINICAL RESEARCH PROCESS IN THE PHARMACEUTICAL INDUSTRY, *edited by Gary M. Matoren*

Volume 20. MICROENCAPSULATION AND RELATED DRUG PROCESSES, *Patrick B. Deasy*

Volume 21. DRUGS AND NUTRIENTS: THE INTERACTIVE EFFECTS, *edited by Daphne A. Roe and T. Colin Campbell*

Volume 22. BIOTECHNOLOGY OF INDUSTRIAL ANTIBIOTICS, *Erick J. Vandamme*

Volume 23. PHARMACEUTICAL PROCESS VALIDATION, *edited by Bernard T. Loftus and Robert A. Nash*

Volume 24. ANTICANCER AND INTERFERON AGENTS: SYNTHESIS AND PROPERTIES, *edited by Raphael M. Ottenbrite and George B. Butler*

Volume 25. PHARMACEUTICAL STATISTICS: PRACTICAL AND CLINICAL APPLICATIONS, *Sanford Bolton*

Volume 26. DRUG DYNAMICS FOR ANALYTICAL, CLINICAL, AND BIOLOGICAL CHEMISTS, *Benjamin J. Gudzinowicz, Burrows T. Younkin, Jr., and Michael J. Gudzinowicz*

Volume 27. MODERN ANALYSIS OF ANTIBIOTICS, *edited by Adjoran Aszalos*

Volume 28. SOLUBILITY AND RELATED PROPERTIES, *Kenneth C. James*

Volume 29. CONTROLLED DRUG DELIVERY: FUNDAMENTALS AND APPLICATIONS, SECOND EDITION, REVISED AND EXPANDED, *edited by Joseph R. Robinson and Vincent H. Lee*

Volume 30. NEW DRUG APPROVAL PROCESS: CLINICAL AND REGULATORY MANAGEMENT, *edited by Richard A. Guarino*

Volume 31. TRANSDERMAL CONTROLLED SYSTEMIC MEDICATIONS, *edited by Yie W. Chien*

Volume 32. DRUG DELIVERY DEVICES: FUNDAMENTALS AND APPLICATIONS, *edited by Praveen Tyle*

Volume 33. PHARMACOKINETICS: REGULATORY - INDUSTRIAL - ACADEMIC PERSPECTIVES, *edited by Peter G. Welling and Francis L. S. Tse*

Volume 34. CLINICAL DRUG TRIALS AND TRIBULATIONS, *edited by Allen E. Cato*

Volume 35. TRANSDERMAL DRUG DELIVERY: DEVELOPMENTAL ISSUES AND RESEARCH INITIATIVES, *edited by Jonathan Hadgraft and Richard H. Guy*

Volume 36. AQUEOUS POLYMERIC COATINGS FOR PHARMACEUTICAL DOSAGE FORMS, *edited by James W. McGinity*

Volume 37. PHARMACEUTICAL PELLETIZATION TECHNOLOGY, *edited by Isaac Ghebre-Sellassie*

Volume 38. GOOD LABORATORY PRACTICE REGULATIONS, *edited by Allen F. Hirsch*

Volume 39. NASAL SYSTEMIC DRUG DELIVERY, *Yie W. Chien, Kenneth S. E. Su, and Shyi-Feu Chang*

Volume 40. MODERN PHARMACEUTICS, SECOND EDITION, REVISED AND EXPANDED, *edited by Gilbert S. Banker and Christopher T. Rhodes*

Volume 41. SPECIALIZED DRUG DELIVERY SYSTEMS: MANUFACTURING AND PRODUCTION TECHNOLOGY, *edited by Praveen Tyle*

Volume 42. TOPICAL DRUG DELIVERY FORMULATIONS, *edited by David W. Osborne and Anton H. Amann*

Volume *43*. DRUG STABILITY: PRINCIPLES AND PRACTICES, *Jens T. Carstensen*

Volume 44. PHARMACEUTICAL STATISTICS: PRACTICAL AND CLINICAL APPLICATIONS, Second Edition, Revised and Expanded, *Sanford Bolton*

Volume 45. BIODEGRADABLE POLYMERS AS DRUG DELIVERY SYSTEMS, *edited by Mark Chasin and Robert Langer*

Volume 46. PRECLINICAL DRUG DISPOSITION: A LABORATORY HANDBOOK, *Francis L. S. Tse and James J. Jaffe*

Volume 47. HPLC IN THE PHARMACEUTICAL INDUSTRY, *edited by Godwin W. Fong and Stanley K. Lam*

Volume 48. PHARMACEUTICAL BIOEQUIVALENCE, *edited by Peter G. Welling, Francis L. S. Tse, and Shrikant V. Dighe*

Volume 49. PHARMACEUTICAL DISSOLUTION TESTING, *Umesh V. Banakar*

Additional Volumes in Preparation

GOOD MANUFACTURING PRACTICES FOR PHARMACEUTICALS: A PLAN FOR TOTAL QUALITY CONTROL, THIRD EDITION, *edited by Sidney H. Willig and James Stoker*

MANAGING THE CLINICAL DRUG DEVELOPMENT PROCESS, *David M. Cocchetto and Ronald V. Nardi*

Pharmaceutical Dissolution Testing

Umesh V. Banakar

with contributions by
William A. Hanson, Chetan D. Lathia, Albertha M. Paul,
Santosh J. Vetticaden, and John H. Wood

informa
healthcare

New York London

First published in 1992 by the Taylor & Francis Group, LLC.

This edition published in 2010 by Informa Healthcare, Telephone House, 69-77 Paul Street, London EC2A 4LQ, UK.

Simultaneously published in the USA by Informa Healthcare, 52 Vanderbilt Avenue, 7th Floor, New York, NY 10017, USA.

Informa Healthcare is a trading division of Informa UK Ltd. Registered Office: 37–41 Mortimer Street, London W1T 3JH, UK. Registered in England and Wales number 1072954.

A CIP record for this book is available from the British Library.

Library of Congress Cataloging-in-Publication Data available on application

ISBN-13: 9780824785673

Orders may be sent to: Informa Healthcare, Sheepen Place, Colchester, Essex CO3 3LP, UK
Telephone: +44 (0)20 7017 5540
Email: CSDhealthcarebooks@informa.com
Website: http://informahealthcarebooks.com/

For corporate sales please contact: CorporateBooksIHC@informa.com
For foreign rights please contact: RightsIHC@informa.com
For reprint permissions please contact: PermissionsIHC@informa.com

Printed and bound in India by Replika Press Pvt. Ltd.

This work is dedicated to the fond memories of my late grandmother, Aaji. I am eternally indebted to her for three virtues—patience, perseverance, and positive thinking—which were communicated to me through her approach to life and life-style itself.

Foreword

The importance of dissolution rate on clinical performance of drugs and drug delivery systems has long been recognized. It is the overwhelmingly important property of dosage forms that contributes to the rate and extent of drug availability to the body and, as such, is deserving of the effort that has been put forth to develop dissolution systems that provide fundamental information on the dissolution process of many drugs and chemicals as well as meaningful in vitro dissolution system models that can be correlated with some index of in vivo performance.

Notwithstanding the considerable efforts expended in trying to understand fundamentals and application of dissolution, great deficiencies in our database still exist. Indeed, in the applied area of attempting to model in vivo with in vitro systems, it is not yet possible to routinely correlate in vitro dissolution rate data with biological performance of sustained-release systems, i.e., in vivo data. The reason for this is simply that we do not yet understand the many biological variables that can influence the dissolution rate of dosage forms and, as such, all in vitro models are unable to realistically duplicate biological conditions.

An appreciation of the historic development of oral in vitro dissolution apparati dramatizes our general lack of the biological variables involved in dissolution. Thus, when the Stohl-Gershberg disintegration apparatus was first introduced it was run in 500 mL of fluid, because it was believed that was the volume of the resting stomach. The 32 cycles per minute of tube movement was to simulate peristaltic motion of the stomach, and no allowance was made for any form of mixing conditions. The resting stomach has closer to 30–50 mL of fluid in the fasted state and the motility pattern is divided into three separate phases of differing activity. The role of various biological solutes, in conjunction with the now-known mixing characteristics and motility pattern of the stomach, has not been fully explored. Indeed, the present official dissolution apparati bear no relationship to physiological conditions, and hence it is not possible to completely examine dissolution of drugs and drug delivery systems under simulated biological conditions nor to explore the influence of physiological conditions, e.g., pH, bile salts, enzymes, and glycoproteins, on the dissolution process.

Despite the importance of dissolution, the various publications in scientific journals and review articles, and the numerous committees formed within the Academy of Pharmaceutical Sciences and AAPS, there are surprisingly few comprehensive texts in the field and none that delineate problems in the area. The present text is badly needed and fills a void in the field. Dr. Banakar has provided a valuable service in the preparation of this text.

Joseph R. Robinson
University of Wisconsin
Madison, Wisconsin

Preface

More than 100 years ago, Bernard S. Proctor recognized that "pill" dissolution was a necessary prerequisite for drug absorption. Nevertheless, it was not until 1930 that pharmaceutical scientists attempted to relate in vitro testing to in vivo availability. Parrot et al. have stated: "The release of a drug from the primary particle and its subsequent availability to the body is governed by the dissolution rate of the particle." There is little doubt that the determination of dissolution rates is an important tool in the design, fabrication, evaluation, and quality control of solid dosage forms.

Dissolution analysis of pharmaceutical solid dosage forms has emerged as the single most important test that, when carried out appropriately, will ensure the quality of the product. Interest in dissolution standards and their significance has been mounting steadily during the past decade. Knowledge of critical operating variables for a dissolution device is important to the pharmaceutical scientist interested in product development, quality control, and research applications. Since the recognition of the fact that the dissolution rate of a drug from its dosage form can often become the rate-limiting process in the physiological availability, interest has been focused on the development of a reliable in vitro dissolution test method that can positively characterize the in vivo dissolution rate-controlled absorption of drugs.

Dissolution tests are critical and they are difficult to carry out properly. There are a variety of critical factors that influence the dissolution behavior and subsequent bioavailability characteristics of a drug and drug product(s).

With the steady accumulation of data in this discipline over the past two decades, pharmaceutical dissolution technology has become an important area of study in pharmacy schools and a vital item in the armamentarium of technical know-how of a pharmaceutical scientist. Since dissolution is extremely important in pharmaceutical systems, particularly solid dosage forms, each chapter is devoted to a specific area in dissolution technology. Each area is discussed in sufficient depth with regard to historical background and development, theoretical and practical aspects, and current status. A wide variety of examples, citing references, along with rational guidelines for potential applications in practice are provided. It is the intention of this book to present a consolidated update of and comprehensive information on dissolution technology that is not otherwise currently available as a single source, and to promote better understanding and fuller appreciation of the phenomenon.

It is hoped that *Pharmaceutical Dissolution Testing* will serve as an invaluable guide to aid the pharmacy professional, in both academia and practice (industry or otherwise), in selecting and utilizing the available means in overcoming problems in design and development of better dosage forms. It is anticipated that the collective knowledge gained hereby will result in acquisition of expertise in the field of dissolution technology.

I wish to extend my gratitude and sincere appreciation to Ms. Barbara Lorimor for her excellent technical expertise in preparing the manuscript. I also wish to acknowledge Ms. Kathleen Gardon, editorial assistant, for meticulous proofing. I appreciate the contributions by the authors of Chapters 4, 6, 10, and 11. Special appreciation is extended to Sandra Beberman and Carol Mayhew of Marcel Dekker, Inc., for their expert assistance. I owe special thanks to Dr. Joseph R. Robinson for writing the foreword to this text and for his encouragement in bringing this project to fruition. Last but not the least, I am indebted to my wife, Suneeta, and to my parents for their unending love and support.

Umesh V. Banakar

Contents

ONE

Introduction, Historical Highlights, and the Need for Dissolution Testing

INTRODUCTION

Dissolution is defined as the process by which a solid substance enters in the solvent to yield a solution. Stated simply, dissolution is the process by which a solid substance dissolves. Fundamentally, it is controlled by the affinity between the solid substance and the solvent.

Pharmaceutical solid dosage forms and solid-liquid dispersed dosage forms on administration undergo dissolution in biological media, followed by absorption of the drug entity into systemic circulation. In determining the dissolution rate of drugs from solid dosage forms under standardized conditions, one has to consider several physicochemical processes in addition to the processes involved in the dissolution of pure chemical substances. The physical characteristics of the dosage form, the wettability of the dosage unit, the penetration ability of the dissolution medium, the swelling process, the disintegration and deaggregation of the dosage form are a few of the factors that influence the dissolution characteristics of drugs. Wagner proposed the scheme depicted in Fig. 1.1 for the processes involved in the dissolution of solid dosage forms (1). This scheme was later modified to incorporate other factors that precede the dissolution process of solid dosage forms. Carstensen proposed a scheme incorporating the following sequence (2):

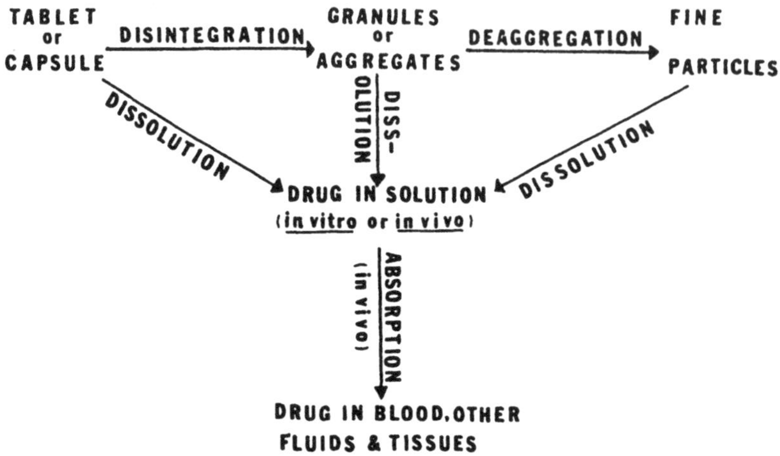

Fig. 1.1 Schematic illustration of dissolution process of solid dosage forms. (From Ref. 2.)

1. Initial mechanical lag
2. Wetting of the dosage form
3. Penetration of the dissolution medium into the dosage form
4. Disintegration
5. Deaggregation of the dosage form and dislodgment of the granules
6. Dissolution
7. Occlusion of some particles of the drug

It is apparent from Fig. 1.1 that the rate of dissolution of the drug can become the rate-limiting step before the drug appears in blood. However, when the dosage form is placed into the gastrointestinal tract in solid form, there are two possibilities for the rate-limiting step. The solid form must first dissolve and the drug in solution must then pass through the gastrointestinal membrane. Freely water-soluble drugs will tend to dissolve rapidly, making the passive diffusion of drug and/or the active transport of drug the rate-limiting step for absorption through the gastrointestinal membrane. Conversely, the rate of absorption of poorly soluble drugs will be limited by the rate of dissolution of the undissolved drug or disintegration of dosage form. Intermediate cases exist when the absorption rate is not clearly determined by one of the two steps but is affected by both of them. In such instances, neither of the steps is rate-limiting.

Dosage forms vary with regard to the rate at which they can present drug in solution to the gastrointestinal mucosa. Assuming that dissolution is rate-limiting, drugs administered orally in solution form (e.g., syrups, elixirs, and solution) are most rapid in presenting drug for absorption because the dissolution step is eliminated by the dosage form itself. Consequently, the fastest absorption for a given drug would be expected from a solution dosage form. Rank-order approximation for rate of absorption among the variety of dosage forms from fastest to slowest is presented in Fig. 1.2.

The rate of dissolution of a pure drug substance is determined by the rate at which solvent-solute forces of attraction overcome the cohesive forces present in the solid. This process is rate-limiting when the release of solute into solution is slow and the transport into bulk solution is fast. In this case dissolution is said to be *interfacially controlled*. Dissolution may also be *diffusion controlled*, where the solvent–solute interaction is fast compared to transport of solute into the bulk solution. In diffusion-controlled dissolution process, a stationary layer of solute adjacent to the solid–liquid interface is postulated and is commonly referred to as the diffusion layer. The saturation concentration of solute develops at the interface and decreases with distance across the diffusion layer. The various kinetic aspects of dissolution are discussed in detail in the following chapters. However, in order to fully understand the intricacies associated with the theories of dissolution, it is imperative to discuss the fundamentals of the dissolution process. The following sections of this chapter are devoted to the development of primary concepts associated with a mechanistic understanding of the various dissolution processes.

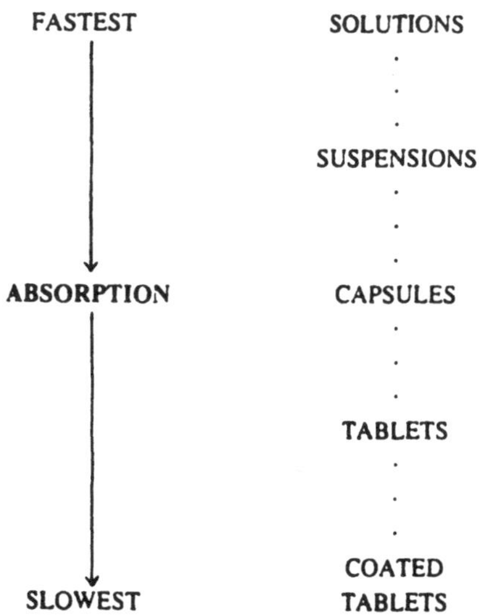

Fig. 1.2 Rank order of dissolution rates and thus absorption rates for various dosage forms.

HISTORICAL HIGHLIGHTS

The earliest reference to dissolution can probably be found in an article by Noyes and Whitney in 1897, describing "The Rate of Solution of Solid Substances in Their Own Solution." They suggested that the rate of dissolution of solid substances is determined by the rate of diffusion of a very thin layer of saturated solution that forms instantaneously around the solid particle. They even developed a mathematical expression correlating the rate of dissolution and the solubility gradient of the solid. Most modern mathematical treatments of dissolution phenomena still revolve around this basic expression. Interestingly, the work of Noyes and Whitney, together with the studies that followed in the early part of the twentieth century, were based primarily on the physicochemical aspects of dissolution as applied to chemical substances. The most prominent of these investigations that deserve recognition are those of Nernst and Brunner in 1904 for their application of Fick's law of diffusion to the Noyes–Whitney equation, and those of Hixson and Crowell in 1931 for their development of the famous cube-root law of dissolution.

During the 1950s the focus of investigations shifted from the influence of physicochemical characteristics of drugs on dissolution to an examination of the effects of dissolution behavior of drugs on the biological activity of dosage forms. In 1951, Edwards suggested that, due to its poor solubility, the analgesic activity of aspirin tablets can be controlled and/or modified by its rate of dissolution within the gastrointestinal tract. However, Edwards' suggestion was not backed by bioavailability data. In 1960 Levy and Hayes concluded that the incidence of local irritation and the absorption rate of acetyl salicylic acid are a function of its dissolution rate in its particular dosage form. In 1961, Levy correlated dissolution and absorption rates of different commercial aspirin tablets and proved that Edwards' hypothesis was correct. With the report of these findings, investigators from both industry and academia were prompted to reevaluate the various intricacies and facets of dissolution testing. In the late 1960s dissolution was awarded compendial status and dissolution testing became a mandatory U.S. pharmacopoeial requirement for several dosage forms. In the following years, various problems associated with dissolution testing surfaced, together with the numerous factors that influence the dissolution rate of drugs and dosage forms. To date, much effort is being expended to answer various questions posed by dissolution testing at large.

Dissolution is far from being understood perfectly. Despite the large success of several reported in vitro–in vivo correlation studies, dissolution is not a predictor of therapeutic efficiency. Dissolution can best be described as a qualitative tool that can provide valuable information about the biological availability of a drug product. Additionally, the precision and accuracy of the testing procedure depend to a large extent on the strict observance of many subtle parameters and detailed operational controls. These factors make dissolution testing far from a simple routine measurement. Despite these shortcomings, dissolution testing to date seems to be the most sensitive and reliable predictor of bioavailability and is one of the most important of the quality control tests performed on drugs and drug products.

INTRODUCTORY MATHEMATICS OF DISSOLUTION

It has long been recognized that the release of active drug from a drug product may be greatly influenced by the physicochemical properties of the drug as well as the dosage form (3). The availability of drug is usually determined by the rate of release of drug from the physical system (dosage form). The release of a drug from its dosage form is usually determined by the rate at which it dissolves in the surrounding medium. The rate of dissolution of a chemical or drug from the solid state is defined as the amount of drug substance that goes into solution per unit time under standardized conditions of liquid/solid interface, temperature, and solvent composition. In biopharmaceutics, *rate of dissolution* usually refers to the rate at which the drug dissolves from an intact dosage form or from fragments or particles formed from the dosage form during the test (4). The terms of solution or rate of dissolution may be used interchangeably, as done by Hixson and Crowell (5). However, most authors prefer the terms *rate of dissolution* or *dissolution rate*.

In the following sections we provide readers with the introductory mathematical concepts of dissolution of solids, focusing primarily on intrinsic dissolution-rate constants, dissolution of particulate systems, and dissolution of binary mixtures. Other complex models are discussed in greater depth in chapter 2.

Intrinsic Dissolution-Rate Constants

The rate at which a substance dissolves in a liquid to form a solution is governed by physical parameters such as the surface area of the substance at a given time during the process of dissolution, the shape of the substance, the characteristics of solid/liquid interface, and the solubility of the substance in the liquid. Hence, dissolution can be considered a specific type of certain heterogeneous reaction which results in a mass transfer as a net effect between the escape and deposition of solute molecules at a solid surface. Mathematically, this can be expressed as

$$\frac{dM}{dt} = -kA(C_s - C) \tag{1.1}$$

where M is the mass of substance remaining to be dissolved; A is the surface area exposed to the dissolution medium; C_s is the saturation concentration, commonly referred to as *solubility* in the dissolution medium; C is the amount dissolved or the concentration of drug in solution (dissolution medium) at time t; and k the intrinsic dissolution rate constant or simply the dissolution rate constant.

The equation expresses the fact that when C is small, $C < 0.15C_s$, then k is proportional to C_s, since $(C_s - C)$ is large (i.e., $C << C_s$). If this applies, then to a good approximation we may write

$$\frac{dM}{dt} = -kAC_s \tag{1.2}$$

Equation (1.2) is commonly referred to as a *sink-condition equation*, which implies that sink conditions exist during the process of dissolution. It must be noted, however, that A is not constant except initially, when only very small quantities of solute have dissolved and where there is an amount of solute far in excess of saturation.

When the process of dissolution takes place under sink conditions, a stagnant film of liquid (dissolution medium) is adsorbed onto the solid, the thickness of this film being l cm. The liquid in the film that is in direct contact with the solid is saturated with drug in solution. The concentration of the drug in solution then drops as the distance from the dissolving solid surface increases. At the end of the film, l cm from the surface, the concentration in the film is the same as that in the bulk solution, C_b. The driving force behind the movement of solute molecules through the stagnant film is the concentration gradient that exists between the saturation concentration of the solute, C_s, in the stagnant layer at the surface of the solid and its concentration on the farthest side of the stagnant film, C_b. A schematic representation of dissolution as a physicochemical phenomenon is shown in Fig. 1.3. The greater this difference in concentration, the faster the rate of dissolution.

Applying Fick's first law of diffusion to Eq. (1.2), the flux, J [defined as the rate of flow of material through 1 cm^2, i.e., $J = (dM/dt)/A$], can be expressed as

$$J = -D\left(\frac{\delta C}{\delta x}\right) \tag{1.3}$$

where D is the coefficient of diffusion and x is the distance (here from the solid surface), as shown in Fig. 1.3. If the concentration gradient, $\delta C/\delta x$, is linear, if $C = C_s$ at the surface $(x = 0)$, and if $C = C_b$ (the bulk concentration at the interface between the bulk solution and the film, where $x = 1$), then $\delta C/\delta x = (C_b - C_s)/l$. Therefore,

$$\frac{1}{A}\frac{dM}{dt} = -D(C_b - C_s)\frac{1}{l} = -k(C_s - C) \tag{1.4}$$

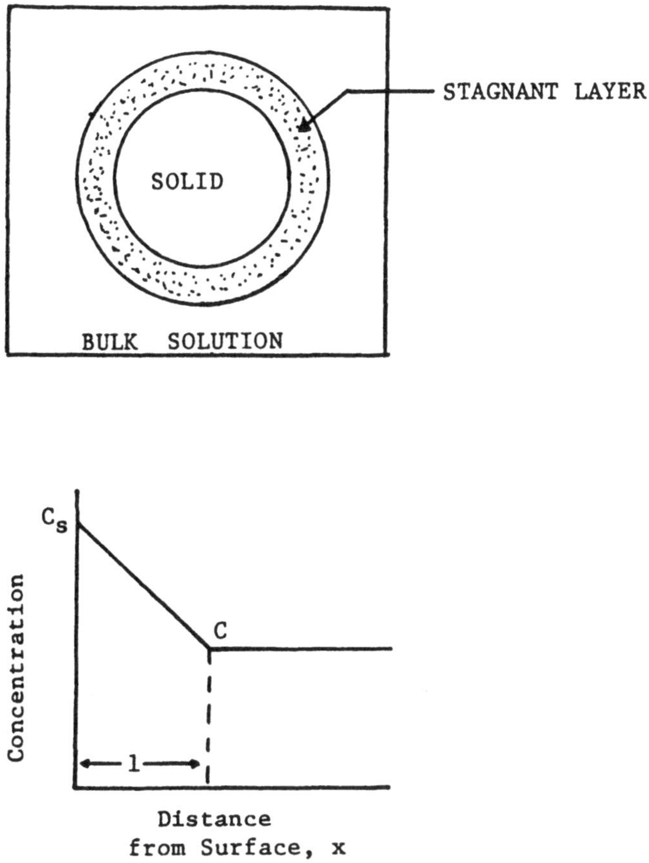

Fig. 1.3 Schematic representation of a physical model depicting a dissolution process.

or simply

$$\frac{dM}{dt} = -kA(C_s - C) \tag{1.1}$$

On a closer examination of Eq. (1.1), we can recognize that the overall dissolution rate increases with increasing intrinsic dissolution rate, intrinsic dissolution rate constant k, increased surface area A, and increased solubility C_s. It must be pointed out that the intrinsic dissolution rate constant differs from drug to drug and is a function of the diffusion coefficient D (cm^2/s), of the drug in question and the thickness of the liquid film, l (cm). The relationship that takes the above-mentioned factors into account is given as

$$k = \frac{D}{l} \text{ cm} \cdot s^{-1} \tag{1.5}$$

If the agitation intensity of a system containing suspended particles is increased, the thickness of the film will decrease progressively. Hence k is a function of the test as well. Additionally, if the product of $A(C_s - C)$ is maintained constant for many drugs tested by the same test, the relative magnitude of k values will indicate the effective ease of dissolution.

If the surface area A were to remain constant and the volume of the dissolution medium were denoted by V, then Eq. (1.1) could be integrated and rewritten as (for the amount dissolved)

$$V\left(\frac{\delta c}{\delta t}\right) = kA(C_s - C) \tag{1.6}$$

since $M = VC$. If sink conditions prevail, Eq. 1.6 can be integrated to

$$C = \frac{kAC_s}{V}t \qquad C_s - C \sim C_s \tag{1.7}$$

If sink conditions do not prevail, Eq. (1.6) can be rearranged to

$$\frac{dc}{C_s - C} = \frac{kA}{V}dt = -d\ln(C_s - C) \tag{1.8}$$

which on integration yields

$$-\ln(C_s - C) = \frac{kA}{V}t + \text{constant} \tag{1.9}$$

At $t = 0$, $C = 0$; therefore, $-\ln(C_s - 0) = 0 + \text{constant}$. The integration constant is $(-\ln C_s)$. Thus the equation that defines the intrinsic dissolution rate process under nonsink conditions will be

$$\ln(C_s - C) = \ln C_s - \frac{kA}{V} \tag{1.10}$$

or

$$C = C_s(1 - e^{-\alpha t}) \tag{1.11}$$

where $\alpha = k(A/V)$. The graphical representation of this relationship is shown in Fig. 1.4. Initially, the system confirms to sink conditions where the curve is superimposable on its own tangent and obeys Eq. (1.7). The asymptote portion of the curve represents the solubility C_s of the compound.

If we calculate the difference between the solubility and the observed concentration $(C_s - C)$ and graph it as a function of time semilogarithmically, we

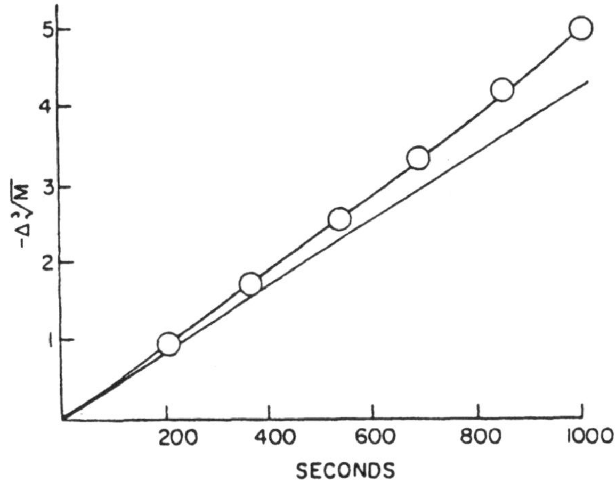

Fig. 1.4 Cube-root dissolution plot for oxalic acid tablets with $d_0/h_0 = 2.75$. [From J. T. Carstensen, *Solid Pharmaceutics: Mechanical Properties and Rate Phenomena*, Wiley, New York (1980).]

can determine the time when $C_s - C$ equals one-half the saturation concentration, $t_{0.5}$. The dissolution rate constant k can then be calculated by

$$k = 0.693 \frac{V}{At_{0.5}} \tag{1.12}$$

Dissolution of Single-Component Systems: Particulate Systems

The earlier discussion concerning intrinsic dissolution rate constants made no reference to the nature of the particles undergoing dissolution. Most of the theories developed for dissolution of particulate systems revolve around Eq. (1.1). Furthermore, it is assumed that the dissolution characteristics of all the crystal faces or of all the surfaces are identical (i.e., the particles dissolve in an isotropic fashion). Additionally, it is assumed that the particles are isometric, which takes into account the shape factor of the particle, which is given by the expression

$$\alpha = \frac{A}{V^{2/3}} \tag{1.13}$$

where A and V denote the surface area and volume of the particle, respectively. The isometric nature of the particle implies that α is independent of time during dissolution. This will be true only for spherical and cubical particles. Given N particles of density ρ (g/cm^3) and assuming sink conditions, the dissolution equation can be written as

$$\frac{dm}{dt} = N\rho\left(\frac{dv}{dt}\right) = NAC_s = Nk\alpha V^{2/3}C_s \tag{1.14}$$

where m denotes the mass dissolved at time t.

Simplification followed by integration of Eq. 1.14 gives

$$V_0^{1/3} - V^{1/3} = \frac{\alpha k C_s}{3\rho}t \tag{1.15}$$

where V_0 is the initial volume of the particle; and k, C_s, and ρ are constants that can be collectively grouped and represented as K. Multiplying both sides of Eq. (1.15) by $(M_0/V_0)^{1/3}$, where the subscript zero denotes initial conditions, gives

$$M_0^{1/3} - M^{1/3} = \left(\frac{M_0}{V_0}\right)^{1/3} K\alpha/3 \tag{1.16}$$

since $K = kC_s/\rho$.

Equation (1.16) is a slightly modified form of the Hixson–Crowell cube root law (5). Figure 1.4 illustrates the linear relationship of $(-\Delta M^{1/3})$ as a function of time. However, positive (upward) deviations from the cube-root law, particularly for monodispersed systems, have been reported (6), as shown in Fig. 1.4. These deviations can be attributed to the lack of isometry of most real particles.

If the shape factor α is time dependent, such as $\alpha(t)$, we can calculate the integrated mean value for α at any time t^* by

$$\alpha_m = \frac{1}{t^*}\cdot\int_0^{t^*}\alpha(t)\,dt \tag{1.17}$$

where m is the integrated mean value for α.

If one considers a cylinder with initial diameter d_0 and height h_0, a reduced time parameter u can be introduced, which can be expressed as

$$u = 2(kC_s/h_0\rho)t \tag{1.18}$$

Linearity of u with t implies a constant K and adherence to Eq. (1.16).

When the ratio $d_0{:}h_0 > 1$ becomes large, the shape of the cylinder will approach that of a plate. Conversely, when the ratio $h_0{:}d_0 > 1$ becomes large, the shape of the cylinder will approach that of a needle. Under such circumstances, geometrically, the percent of material dissolved at any time t will be

$$p = 100\left\{1 - \left[1 - u\left(\frac{h_0}{d_0}\right)^2\right](1-u)\right\} \tag{1.19}$$

where p is the percent of material dissolved at time t.

Equation (1.19) permits the calculation of u at any time point. There will be only one real root considering the cubic characteristics of the equation. Expressing the height and the diameter in terms of h_0, d_0, and time and hence u, we can now calculate the shape factor α from Eq. (1.13) and estimate via an equivalent of Eq. (1.17) given by

$$\alpha_m = \frac{1}{u^*}\int_0^{u^*} \alpha(u)du \tag{1.20}$$

where u^* is the reduced time parameter at t^*. Thus, the following equation results

$$\alpha_m = 3.69\left\{\frac{1}{2}\left[\frac{(d_0/h_0 - u)}{1-u}\right]^{2/3} + \left[\frac{1-u}{(d_0/h_0 - u)}\right]^{1/3}\right\} \tag{1.21}$$

A plot of α_m as a function of u is shown in Fig. 1.5, and α_m as a function of percent of material dissolved, p, is shown in Fig. 1.6. More complex situations dealing with the hydrodynamics of the system and its relation to the dissolution rate constant and with dissolution of polydispersed powders are discussed in the following chapters.

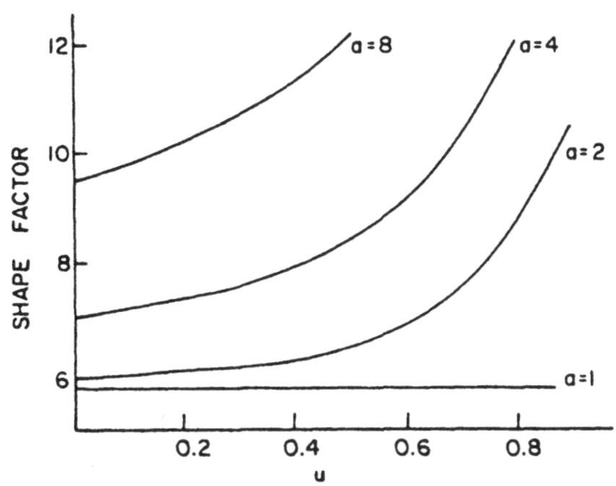

Fig. 1.5 α_m as a function of u for various values of a ($a = d_0/h_0$). [From J. T. Carstensen, *Solid Pharmaceutics: Mechanical Properties and Rate Phenomena*, Wiley, New York (1980).]

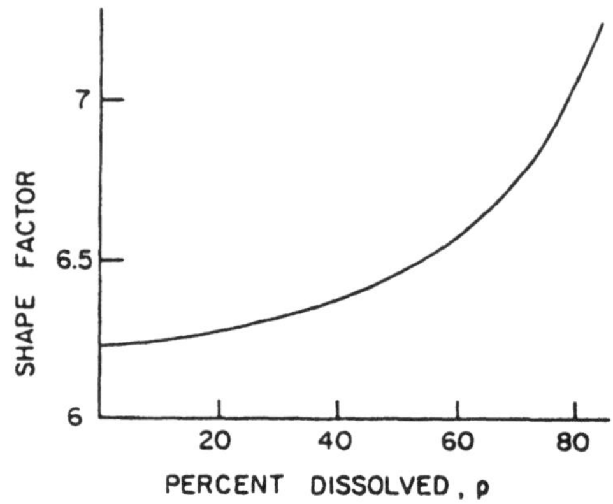

Fig. 1.6 α_m as a function of p when $d_0/h_0 = 2.75$. [From J. T. Carstensen, *Solid Pharmaceutics: Mechanical Properties and Rate Phenomena*, Wiley, New York (1980).]

Dissolution of Multicomponent Systems: Binary Mixtures

Binary mixtures are routinely confronted in pharmaceutical solid dosage forms: drug embedded in an insoluble matrix, compressed mixture of two substances, and so on. Three cases warrant discussion during the characterization of dissolution of such systems. They are

1. When one of the components dissolves more rapidly than the other
2. When both components dissolve at the same rate
3. When one of the components constitutes an insoluble matrix

In the first case, let's assume a compressed mixture of two substances, *A* and *B*, where both *A* and *B* are soluble and that *B* dissolves more rapidly than *A*. Furthermore, it is assumed that the material dissolves in a horizontal direction from a unit total surface area ($1\ \text{cm}^2$) and the dissolving surface recesses as shown in Fig 1.7. If f_A and f_B represent the fraction of substances *A* and *B*, respectively, present in the mixture and R_A and R_B their respective rates of dissolution, the following holds true:

$$f_A = 1 - f_B \tag{1.22}$$

Since *B* dissolves more rapidly, then during a specific time interval δt, a volume of δl will have dissolved. As all of *B* has dissolved in the surface, we can write the dissolution rate of *A* as

$$R_A = k_A S_A \tag{1.23}$$

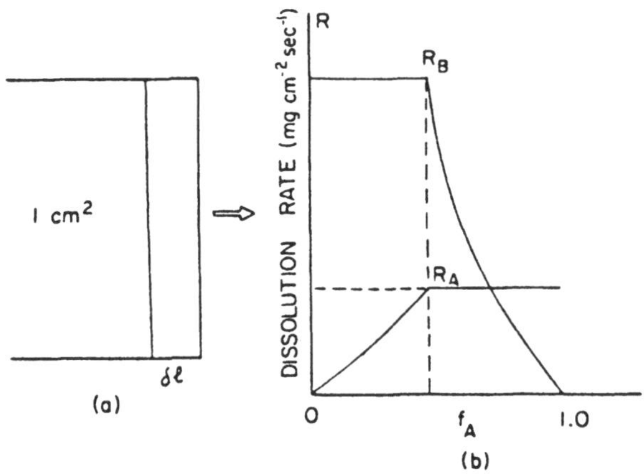

Fig. 1.7 Dissolution of binary mixtures: (a) side view of a block permitting dissolution from the end surface; (b) dissolution rates R_A and R_B of two soluble substances A and B, respectively, in a molten or compressed mixture. Dissolution rate as a function of fraction of A. [From J. T. Carstensen, *Solid Pharmaceutics: Mechanical Properties and Rate Phenomena*, Wiley, New York (1980).]

where S_A is the solubility of A in the dissolution medium. During the time interval δt, the amount of A that will be dissolved can be expressed as $R_A \delta t$. The amount of A dissolved will be the product of the fraction of A present in the mixture, f_A, and the volume dissolved, $1\delta l$, and the density, ρ_A. Hence, it follows that

$$R_A \delta t = f_A \delta_l \rho_A \tag{1.24}$$

or

$$\delta l = R_A \frac{\delta t}{f_A} \rho_A \tag{1.24a}$$

Similarly, we can calculate the amount of B dissolved at time t. Then by inserting Eq. (1.24a) in Eq. (1.23) we can obtain

$$R_B = \frac{f_B}{f_A} \left(\frac{R_A \rho_B}{\rho_A} \right) \tag{1.25}$$

Equation (1.25) implies that for a given solid composition of A:B, the dissolution rates are constant and steady-state conditions prevail. Also, given that $R_B > R_A$, R_A is independent of the composition and R_B will decrease in hyperbolic fashion with the fraction of A as exemplified in Eq. (1.25).

A similar argument will hold true for the second case, where $R_A > R_B$, leading to the same equation with A and B inverted:

$$R_A = k_A S_A \tag{1.26}$$

$$R_B = \frac{f_B}{f_A}\left[\frac{R_A \rho_B}{\rho_A}\right] \tag{1.27}$$

$$R_A = \frac{f_A}{f_B}\left[\frac{R_B \rho_A}{\rho_B}\right] \tag{1.28}$$

$$R_B = k_B S_B \tag{1.29}$$

When $R_A = R_B$, then from Eqs. (1.28) and (1.29) or (1.26) and (1.27)

$$\frac{f_B}{f_A} = \frac{k_B S_B \rho_A}{k_A S_A \rho_B} \tag{1.30}$$

In the third case, component A is soluble and is a constituent of the insoluble matrix. Higuchi has treated this situation, which is illustrated in Fig. 1.8 (7). In this case, the matrix contains a mass A per cubic centimeter of the soluble substance. Let E denote the porosity of the matrix and t the time after exposure of the matrix to the dissolution medium. Then at time t the dissolution medium will have penetrated the matrix to a finite distance l. The amount of A that has been released after time t per unit cross-sectional area A can be expressed as

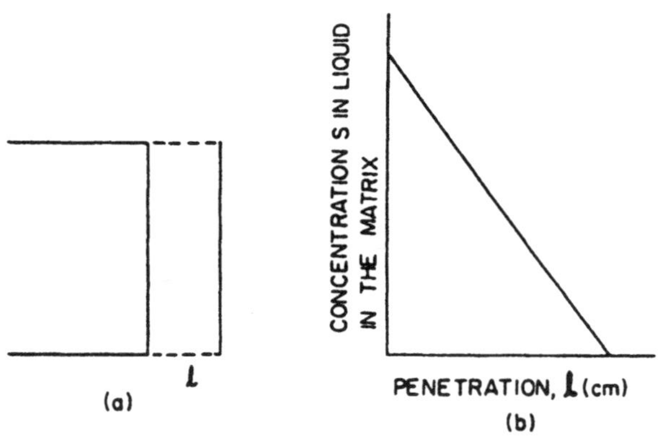

Fig. 1.8 Dissolution of binary mixtures: (a) side view of a block permitting dissolution through the right surface only (l is the level of penetration at time t); (b) concentration of the interstitial liquid as a function of distance from the exposed end of the block. [From J. T. Carstensen, *Solid Pharmaceutics: Mechanical Properties and Rate Phenomena*, Wiley, New York (1980).]

$$Q = Al - 0.5EC_s l \tag{1.31}$$

where Q is the amount of A released in the dissolution medium at time t. Differentiating Eq. (1.31) yields:

$$\frac{dQ}{dt} = (A - 0.5EC_s)\frac{dl}{dt} \tag{1.32}$$

Recalling Fick's law of diffusion, and expressing it in terms of the rate of substance released, can be stated as

$$\frac{dQ}{dt} = \frac{DEC_s}{l} \tag{1.33}$$

Combining Eqs. (1.32) and (1.33) and integrating, we arrive at

$$0.5l^2 = \left[\frac{DEC_s}{A - 0.5EC_s}\right]t \tag{1.34}$$

Combining Eq. (1.34) with Eq. (1.30) gives

$$Q = \left[2DEC_s(A - 0.5EC_s)\right]^{1/2} t^{1/2} \tag{1.35}$$

Equation (1.35) is commonly referred to as the Higuchi square-root law. There are many reports in the literature proving the validity of this expression (8–11).

THE NEED FOR DISSOLUTION TESTING

Generally, dissolution of the drug occurs not only from the fine particles of the drug ultimately produced from the physical breakdown of the dosage form, but also to a small extent from the intact dosage form itself before its disintegration and from the fragments and aggregates produced after disintegration as well. As indicated in Fig. 1.1, dissolution occurs simultaneously from several types of solids. There is adequate evidence to conclude that the rate at which a drug dissolves from its intact or fragmented dosage forms in the gastrointestinal tract, or in a parenteral injection site, often partially or completely controls the rate at which the drug appears in the systemic circulation. Additionally, adequate evidence points to the fact that in many instances the results from in vitro dissolution rate experiments can be used to explain the observed differences in in vivo availability. When the dissolution process is markedly slower than the disintegration process, deaggregation process, and absorption process, dissolution essentially completely controls the rate of absorption. There may be many cases where two or more of the processes proceed at a rate within a factor of 20 of each other, where the rate of dissolution would only partially control the rate of absorption. It should be noted, however, that the rates of the processes of disintegration, deaggregation, and dissolution all depend on the composition and method of preparation of the dosage form. The formulator can alter the formulation factors, which can be reflected in changes in the rates of these processes.

Scientific evidence has shown that dissolution testing provides the means to evaluate critical parameters such as adequate bioavailability and provides information necessary to the formulator in development of more efficacious and therapeutically optimal dosage forms. The position of the Food and Drug Administration is that bioavailability testing in which humans are used as test subjects should be minimized by development and implementation of in vitro dissolution standards that reflect in vivo drug performance (12). In vitro test requirements have been established for drugs such as digoxin and prednisone. The current edition of USP/NF requires dissolution testing for 52 drugs. To date, such in vitro dissolution tests seem to be the most sensitive and reliable predictors of in vivo availability.

When carried out appropriately, dissolution analysis of pharmaceutical dosage forms has emerged as the single most important test that will ensure the quality of a product. In several instances, the dissolution results have been correlated with the bioavailability of a product, in which case the dissolution test can also ensure the bioavailability of the product between batches that meet dissolution criteria. It follows that, knowledge of critical operating variables for a dissolution testing device is important to the pharmaceutical scientist interested in product development, quality control, and research applications.

It is quite apparent that in vitro dissolution testing of a pharmaceutical dosage form, whether in development or in circulation, is imperative not only to ensure batch-to-batch quality equivalence both in vitro and in vivo, but also to screen formulations during product development to arrive at optimally effective products. To do so, the test should be designed so as to mimic closely biological environmental conditions.

The development and use of in vitro dissolution test models to evaluate and describe dissolution and absorption in vivo serves the following purposes:

1. It is likely that the physicochemical properties existing in the model may be of significance in the in vivo process once a successful model that adequately mimics the in vivo situation has been developed. As a result, we may obtain a better understanding of the in vivo environment by the design and operation of a well-characterized in vitro model.

2. Such model systems can be used to screen potential drugs and their associated formulations for their dissolution and absorption characteristics. Meaningful quantitative screening of the effect of formulation changes and structural modifications can readily be undertaken once successful in vitro–in

vivo correlations have been established by the use of these models. Even in the absence of in vivo data or in vitro–in vivo correlation, strictly on the basis of in vitro data alone, we can predict in a relative manner which form of the drug or dosage form will result in optimization of a particular desired effect. This does not necessarily mean accelerated dissolution or complete absorption will be achieved. Frequently, a sustained effect may be desired; also, the locus of the drug action may not be systemic, in which case transport of the drug out of the lumen of the gastrointestinal tract is undesirable (13).

3. As indicated earlier, in vitro dissolution test systems can serve as quality control procedures once the form of the drug and its formulation have been finalized.

It is apparent that for in vitro dissolution systems to be of value they must represent in vivo systems very closely—to such a degree that consistent in vitro–in vivo correlations are obtained. All models do not necessarily comply with this requirement, implying that factors other than those considered in these models are operative in the in vivo environment. Also, the magnitude of a factor considered in an in vitro model may vary significantly from that existing in vivo. The various in vitro dissolution devices that have been described in the literature, and the degree to which they resemble or do not resemble that which is believed to occur in vivo, are described in Chapters 6–9.

Some investigators argue that the best dissolution test device of any system is the system itself. The validity of this statement cannot be denied. However, we must recognize the advantages in cost, labor, and convenience that can be associated with the use of a well-designed in vitro dissolution test system. Dissolution tests are difficult to carry out properly. Because dissolution of a dosage form in vivo is often the rate-limiting factor determining the physiologic availability of a drug, the measurement of the in vitro dissolution rate (or some related parameter) is more likely to offer a meaningful indication of physiological availability. The crucial test of any in vitro dissolution test model is its correlation to the in vivo situation. To date, no universal dissolution test has been devised that in every instance gives the same rank order for in vitro dissolution and in vivo availability for different formulations or batches of the same drug.

REFERENCES

1. J. G. Wagner, *Drug. Intell. Clin. Pharm.*, *4*, 32 (1970).
2. J. Carstensen, in *Proc. 2nd Wisconsin Update Conf., Dissolution-State of the Art, 1982*, University of Wisconsin, Madison (1982).
3. A. B. Morrison and J. A. Campbell, *J. Pharm. Sci.*, *54*, 1 (1965).
4. J. G. Wagner, in *Biopharmaceutics and Relevant Pharmacokinetics*, Drug Intelligence Publications, Hamilton, IL (1971), pp. 190–196.

5. A. Hixon and J. Crowell, *Ind. Eng. Chem.*, *23*, 923 (1931).
6. J. E. Goyan, *J. Pharm. Sci.*, *54*, 645 (1965).
7. T. Higuchi, *J. Pharm. Sci.*, *52*, 1145 (1963).
8. T. J. Roseman and W. I. Higuchi, *J. Pharm. Sci.*, *59*, 353 (1970).
9. T. J. Roseman, *J. Pharm. Sci.*, *64*, 1721 (1975).
10. H. Fessi, J. P. Marty, F. Puisieux, and J. T. Carstensen, *Int. J. Pharm.*, *1*, 265 (1978).
11. Y. W. Chien, H. J. Lambert, and D. E. Grant, *J. Pharm. Sci.*, *63*, 365 (1974).
12. U. V. Banakar and L. H. Block, *Pharm. Technol.*, *7*, 107 (1983).
13. J. Swarbrick, in *Current Concepts in Pharmaceutical Sciences: Biopharmaceutics*, J. Swarbrick, ed., Lea & Febiger, Philadelphia (1970), pp. 265–296.

TWO

Theories of Dissolution

INTRODUCTION

Over the last couple of decades, knowledge in the area of dissolution methodology, in both theory and practice, has grown enormously. Numerous diversified attempts have been made to explain various intricacies associated with the process of dissolution and their implications in rational design of drug-dosage form. In most cases, these attempts have resulted in establishment of new and/or modified theories of dissolution, commonly referred to as *models* in the literature. In this chapter we review various pioneering approaches (theories) put forth by various investigators in the field of dissolution testing to explain the process of dissolution. In most cases, attention is given to situations in which physical models have been applied, in contrast to those where empirical or arbitrary mathematical kinetic models have been employed.

HISTORICAL

It is well known that for dissolution of a solid to occur, solute molecules must first escape from the surface of the solid and then undergo some form of transport process away from the surface into the bulk of the solvent (1). Depending on the relative significance of these two processes and the means by which the transport is effected, it is possible to set up physical models to account for the resulting dissolution behavior. From the standpoint of dissolution-rate mechanisms involving pure substances, there are basically three processes that have been accessible to the physical model treatment (2–4). These have been employed alone or in combinations in setting up models to describe dissolution-rate mechanisms.

Case 1: Diffusion Layer Model. This model, the simplest of the three, assumes a static liquid film adjacent to the solid surface. The model was probably suggested initially by Nernst and Brunner (5,6). It is assumed that there exists in a liquid film of thickness l, a negative velocity component in the direction perpendicular to the surface. The reaction at the solid–liquid film interface is assumed to be rapid. Once the solute molecules pass the liquid film–bulk film interface, rapid mixing occurs and the concentration gradient is destroyed. Then the rate of the solute movement, and therefore the dissolution rate, are determined entirely by Brownian motion diffusion of the molecules in the liquid film. Case 1 is depicted schematically in Fig. 2.1.

Case 2: Interfacial Barrier Model. This model assumes that the reaction at the solid surface, and thus the diffusion across the interface, is not much slower than diffusion across the liquid film. As a result, solid–solution equilibrium may not be assumed, and this consideration must be accounted for in the model. The process at the solid–liquid interface now becomes rate limiting with respect to the transport process. This model is illustrated in Fig. 2.2, where the relatively rapid transport process now occurs by diffusion through a static liquid film.

Case 3: Danckwerts' Model. This model assumes that transport of solute away from the solid surface is achieved by means of macroscopic packets of solvent reaching the solid–liquid interface by eddy diffusion in a random fashion. These solvent packets attach themselves to the surface. During their residence at the interface, the packets are able to absorb solute according to

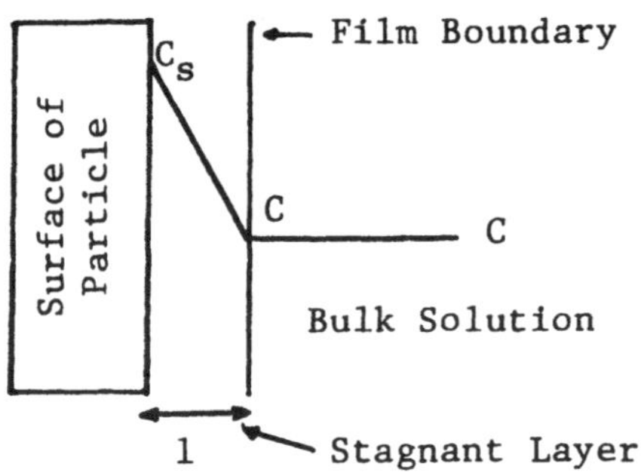

Fig. 2.1 Diffusion layer model (From Ref. 1.)

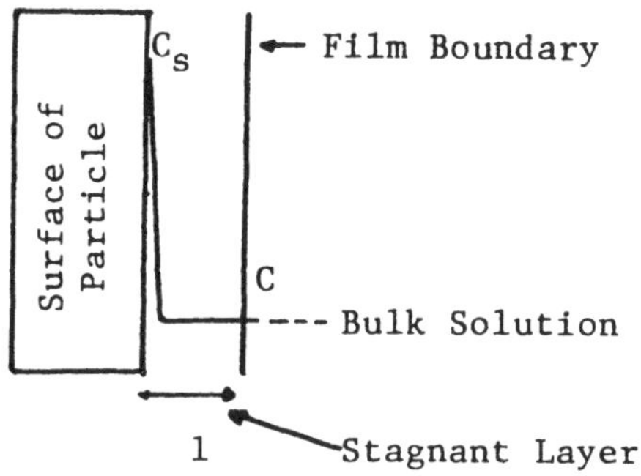

Fig. 2.2 Interfacial layer model. (From Ref. 1.)

the usual laws of diffusion and are then replaced by fresh packets of solvent. Assuming the solid surface reaction to be instantaneous, this surface renewal process may then be related to the solute transport rate and hence dissolution. Figure 2.3 illustrates this phenomenon as suggested by Danckwerts (7).

SINGLE-PARTICULATE SYSTEMS

Dissolution of particles, powders in particular, has been studied extensively. The simplest form of model for dissolution of a solid into a dissolution medium is that of a single spherical particle in a large volume of fluid. On somewhat the same order of simplicity is the dissolution of monodispersed powder sample in a large volume of fluid. Dissolution of monodispersed powder sample in a small volume of liquid is more complicated, as is the dissolution characterization of dissolution of monodispersed nonspherical particles. Essentially, these phenomena follow one or a combination of two or three of the prevailing theories.

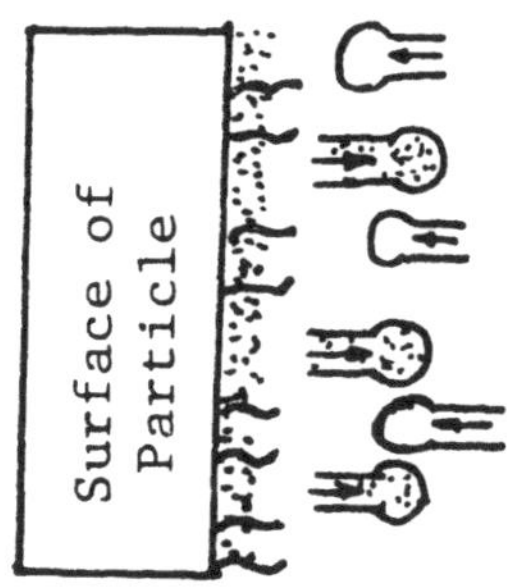

Fig. 2.3 Danckwerts' model. (From Ref. 1.)

Film Theory

In 1904, Nernst (5) proposed the film theory, which demonstrates some basic principles concerning the dissolution of single particulate systems and is less complicated than the other theories. When a solid particle is immersed in an agitated liquid and allowed to dissolve, the bulk liquid will continuously be exposed to the solid surface with a certain velocity. At any given instant, during the process of solubilization or dissolution, a stagnant layer or film surrounds the particle. Called the *Nernst–Brunner thickness layer*, this l-cm layer need not be hydrodynamically stagnant but behaves as such, so that a linear concentration gradient is developed within it (6,8,9). Additionally, it is assumed that this concentration gradient imparts a concentration C at the boundary between the film and the bulk solution and that the concentration at the surface is the saturation concentration, C_s. It is further assumed that the thickness of this boundary is independent of the particle size. This phenomenon is similar to that exhibited in Fig. 2.1. Assuming steady state, *Fick's first law of diffusion* can be employed, which states that

$$J = -D\frac{\delta C}{\delta x} \tag{2.1}$$

where $J\,(\mathrm{mg}\cdot\mathrm{cm}^2\cdot\mathrm{s}^{-1})$ is the amount of substance passing perpendicularly through a unit surface area per unit time, D is the diffusion coefficient, and $\delta C/\delta x$ the concentration gradient, which is considered constant by virtue of its being the slope of the line, as shown in Fig. 2.1. For a mass of substance dissolved in a given volume V of dissolution medium with a surface area A of dissolving solid particle, Eq. (2.1) can be written as

$$\frac{V}{A}\frac{dC}{dt} = \frac{-D(C - C_s)}{l} \tag{2.2}$$

Simplistically, the mass of the solid dissolved, m, with respect to time can be given by

$$\frac{dm}{dt} = \frac{DA(C_s - C)}{l} \tag{2.3}$$

or

$$\frac{dm}{dt} = kA(C_s - C) \tag{2.3a}$$

where k is called the dissolution-rate constant. This result is similar to the one observed during the determination of intrinsic dissolution rate as discussed in Chapter 1. However, it does not account for the boundary conditions.

Equation (2.3) may be integrated and subjected to boundary conditions, yielding (5)

$$\ln(1 - m/m_\infty) = \ln(1 - C/C_s) = \frac{DA}{Vl}t = k\frac{A}{V}t \tag{2.4}$$

where m_∞ is the mass of substance dissolved at $t = \infty$. Under sink conditions, where $C << C_s$, Eq. (2.4) becomes

$$C = \frac{DAC_s}{lV}t = \frac{kAC_s}{V}t \tag{2.5}$$

It must be noted, however, that the surface area A is assumed to remain constant. This assumption is not always true when powders dissolve. To determine values of the dissolution-rate constant k, which are independent of surface area and dependent on species, attempts have been made to design experimental setups where the area of the dissolving surface can be held constant. Several such attempts have been made and reported in the literature (10–12). However, the apparatus described by Wood et al. (10) has gained maximum prominence and is being widely used. Interested readers are directed to the corresponding references.

The change in surface area during dissolution can be explained by employing the Hixson–Crowell treatment (13), which can be simplified by using *Noyes–Whitney approximation* (14). Under sink conditions, such a dissolution process can be defined by

$$\frac{dc}{dt} = \frac{kA}{V}C_s \tag{2.6}$$

If the dissolving solid substance is assumed monodisperse and spherical, then n such particles of density ρ and of radius r_0 initially and r at time t will contribute a concentration C given by

$$C = \alpha(r_0^3 - r^3) \tag{2.7}$$

where

$$\alpha = \frac{n\rho}{V}\frac{4\pi}{3}$$

Since $A_{\text{sphere}} = n \cdot 4\pi r^2$, then differentiating Eq. (2.7) with respect to t, followed by equating the results with Eq. (2.6), yields

$$\frac{dc}{dt} = \frac{k}{V}(n \cdot 4\pi r^2)C_s \tag{2.8}$$

Considering the fact that the radius of the particle reduces as dissolution proceeds, Eq. (2.8) may be written as

$$-\frac{dr}{dt} = \frac{kC_s}{\rho} \tag{2.9}$$

or

$$r_0 - r = \left[\frac{kC_s}{\rho}\right]t \tag{2.10}$$

Multiplying both sides of the equation by the volume factor for a sphere $(n \cdot 4\pi\rho/3)^{1/3}$, we can express the dissolution of monodispersed spherical particles in terms of mass as

$$m_0^{1/3} - M^{1/3} = kt \tag{2.11}$$

where m_0 is the initial mass of spherical particles dissolved at $t = 0$, M is the total mass of spherical particles undergoing dissolution, and the overall rate constant K can be expressed as

$$K = \frac{2kC_s}{\rho}\left[n\frac{\pi}{6}\rho\right]^{1/3} = \frac{kC_s m_0^{1/3}}{\rho r_0} \tag{2.12}$$

Niebergall and Goyan (15) extended the Hixson–Crowell equation to the situation where the amount under investigation (m_0) equals the amount needed to saturate the solution (M_s). Recalling the Noyes–Whitney equation (1.1), we can state

$$\frac{dM}{dt} = kA(C_s - C) \tag{1.1}$$

The concentration C can be expressed as $(m_0 - M)/V$, and the saturation concentration C_s can be expressed as M_s/V. Hence, Eq. (2.3a) becomes

$$V\left[\frac{dM}{dt}\right] = kA[M_s - (m_0 - M)] \tag{2.13}$$

For N particles undergoing dissolution, their surface area (A) and weights can be given by

$$A = N\pi d^2 \tag{2.14}$$

$$M = \frac{N\pi d^3\rho}{6} \tag{2.15}$$

so that

$$AM^{-2/3} = N^{1/3}\left[\frac{6}{(\pi - \rho)}\right]^{2/3}\pi = N^{1/3}\left[\frac{6 \cdot \sqrt{\pi}}{\rho}\right]^{2/3} = N^{1/3} \cdot \Gamma \tag{2.16}$$

where the shape factor $\Gamma = (6\sqrt{\pi}/\rho)^{2/3}$. Inserting Eq. (2.16) in Eq. (2.13) yields

$$V\frac{dM}{dt} = kN^{1/3}\Gamma M^{2/3}(M_s - m_0 + M) \tag{2.17}$$

When $m_0 = M_s$, Eq. (2.17) reduces to

$$\frac{dM}{M^{5/3}} = \left(\frac{kN^{1/3}\Gamma}{V}\right) dt \tag{2.18}$$

which can be integrated and subjected to initial conditions to give

$$M^{-2/3} - m_0^{-2/3} = \frac{2kN^{1/3}\Gamma}{3V} t \tag{2.19}$$

or

$$M^{-2/3} - m_0^{-2/3} = \beta t \tag{2.19a}$$

where the proportionality constant $\beta = kN^{1/3}\Gamma/V$. Equation (2.19a) is commonly referred to as the *negative-two-thirds law*. Niebergall and Goyan employed salicylamide and benzoic acid as test substances and showed that the negative-two-thirds law holds good only up to approximately 30% of saturation (15).

The Hixson–Crowell treatment has been extended to nonsink conditions by several workers. The noteworthy treatments were reported by Short and coworkers (16) and by Pothisiri and Carstensen (17). It is not always experimentally convenient to arrange $M_s = m_0$. Consequently, under nonsink conditions, M_s is different from m_0. The modification required for the case $M_s > m_0$ is given below.

For convenience, Eq. (2.3a) can be written as

$$\frac{dM}{dt} = -k\Gamma M^{2/3}(M_s - m_0 - M) \tag{2.20}$$

where $M = m_0 - C$ is the mass of solid remaining to be dissolved at time t. By considering $M = u^3$ and $M_s - m_0 = F^3$, Eq. (2.20) can be written as

$$\frac{du}{dt} = -k(u^3 - F^3) \tag{2.21}$$

By employing Dwight's standard integral to Eq. (2.21) (18)

$$-\Gamma k(t_2 - t_1) = 3\int_{u(t_1)}^{u(t_2)} \frac{1}{u^3 + F^3} du \tag{2.22}$$

$$= \left[\frac{1}{2}F^{-2} \ln \frac{(u + F)^2}{F^2 + u^2 - Fu} + \frac{\sqrt{3}}{F^2} \arctan \frac{2u - F}{F^3}\right]_{t=t_1}^{t=t_2} \tag{2.22a}$$

$$= [I\{u(t)\}]_{t=t_1}^{t=t_2} \tag{2.22b}$$

for any two times, t_1 and t_2.

Therefore,

$$k = \frac{1}{t_2 - t_1}[IM^{1/3}(t_2) - IM^{1/3}(t_1)] \tag{2.23}$$

By calculating the shape factor Γ ($\Gamma = [6 \cdot \sqrt{\pi}/\rho]^{2/3}$) and determining $M = m_0 - C$ experimentally at different times t_1 and t_2, I, and thus k, the dissolution rate, can be determined from Eq. (2.23).

Pothisiri and Carstensen developed a similar model under nonsink conditions. If sphericity is assumed, as in case of Hixson–Crowell treatment, C_s is assumed to be independent of the radius of the particle r, and sink conditions are not invoked. In such a situation, we have the following expression for the concentration of solute in the medium at time t:

$$C = \frac{n\rho}{V}\frac{4\pi}{3}[r_0^3 - r^3] = \alpha \cdot [r_0^3 - r^3] \tag{2.24}$$

where n is the number of particles and $\alpha = n\rho/V\frac{4\pi}{3}$. Combining the expression for Fick's law of diffusion and Eq. (2.24) yields

$$\begin{aligned} dc &= k(n^4\pi r^2)[C_s - \alpha \cdot (r_0^3 - r^3)]dt \\ &= -\frac{n\rho}{V}\frac{4\pi}{3}3r^2dr \end{aligned} \tag{2.25}$$

or

$$-\frac{\rho}{V}dr = k(\beta + \alpha r^3)dt \tag{2.25a}$$

where $\beta = C_s - (m_0/V)$ is positive when $m_0 < C_sV$. It is assumed that the amount of solute used is insufficient to saturate the dissolution medium completely. Since the term $(\beta + \alpha r^3)$ is positive, Eq. (2.25a) may be written as

$$\frac{dr}{\beta + \alpha r^3} = \frac{-kV}{\rho}dt \tag{2.26}$$

The integral of the left-hand side is

$$\Phi(r) = \frac{q}{6\beta}\ln\frac{(r+q)^2}{r^2 - qr + q^2} + \frac{q}{\beta\sqrt{3}}\arctan\frac{2r - q}{q\sqrt{3}} \tag{2.27}$$

where $q = (\beta/\alpha)^{1/3}$. When integrated and subjected to initial conditions, Eq. (2.26) will take the form

$$\Phi(r) = \Phi(r_0) - \frac{kV}{\rho}t \tag{2.28}$$

The authors showed that Eq. (2.27) holds good up to 65% of saturation, unlike the treatment offered by Niebergall and Goyan (15) where Eq. (2.19a) is reliable up to 35% saturation of the dissolution medium. Although the simple film theory should fail on many counts (19,20), it gives surprisingly excellent correlation with experimental values.

Despite the fact that film theory is based on severe assumptions, Patel and Carstensen (21) have proved it to be a good working model. The Niebergall–Goyan equation, the Short–Sharkey–Rhodes equation, and the Pothisiri–Carstensen equations are shown to hold through 80–90% of the dissolution process for $p-$hydroxybenzoic acid and sodium chloride, at values both below and above the amount necessary to saturate the dissolution medium. Deviations are attributed to experimental difficulties and improper definition of monodisperseness rather than the assumptions made in the theory.

Convective-Diffusion Theory

The most widely accepted theory for dissolution rates is that reported by Noyes and Whitney, which was subsequently modified to include the stagnant or unstirred diffusion layer concept reported by Nernst and Brunner. It is apparent from these theories that the three variables controlling the dissolution rate, viz. the surface area exposed for dissolution and the diffusivity and the solubility of the dissolving substance, can be determined by independent measurements, whereas the effective diffusion layer thickness is a model-independent parameter. Its significance and utility outside the confines of the model are necessarily limited.

Nelson and Shah (22) state that transport-controlled dissolution in a stirred liquid involves two fundamental processes: molecular diffusion and forced convection as a result of fluid flow. They developed a model based on mathematical expressions for mass transport by diffusion and convection, which were combined to give a "convective-diffusion" differential equation. Hence this involves selecting appropriate boundary conditions and solving the differential equation utilizing these boundary conditions.

The convective diffusion equation given by Levich (23) is

$$\frac{\delta c}{\delta t} = (D \text{ div grad } c) - (V \text{ grad } c) \tag{2.29}$$

where D is the diffusivity of solute, V is the velocity component, and c is the concentration of the solute at time t. The first term on the right-hand side of Eq. (2.29) is the diffusion contribution, whereas the second term arises from convection. For steady state, the change in concentration with time is zero, so that the first term equals the second term.

The physical working model can be developed on the basis of the following assumptions. The liquid flowing past the dissolving surface is in the x direction, and convective flow in the y and z directions is nonexistent. The solid is dissolving by diffusion in the z direction, which is normal to the surface of the dissolving solid. With these assumptions, under steady-state conditions Eq. (2.29) becomes

$$D\frac{\delta^2 c}{\delta z^2} = Vx\frac{dc}{dx} \tag{2.30}$$

where x, y, and z are cartesian coordinates and V_x is the liquid velocity in x direction.

It must be noted that in cases where a solid plane is positioned parallel to the unidirectional, frictionless flow, a parabolic laminar hydrodynamic boundary layer develops on the solid (24). Additionally, if the solid undergoes dissolution, the diffusion boundary layer is well characterized. In most dissolution testing equipment, the fluid flow regime is turbulent to ensure efficient mixing, in which case parabolic boundary layers do not develop. However, under turbulent circumstances, it is customary to consider the fluid layer immediately adjacent to a solid wall as having a laminar nature (25). Furthermore, assuming that laminar flow may be described by a linear velocity profile, the liquid velocity V_x can be given by

$$V_x = \alpha z \tag{2.31}$$

where α is the rate of shear in the boundary layer. A schematic representation of the convective diffusion model is shown in Fig. 2.4.

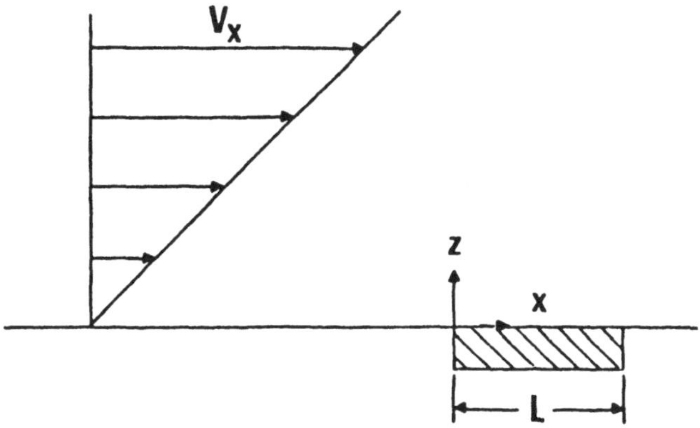

Fig. 2.4 Convective diffusion model. (From Ref. 22.)

Substituting Eq. (2.31) in Eq. (2.30) with boundary conditions

$$C = C_0 \qquad \text{for } 0 < x < \mathrm{L},\ z = 0 \tag{2.32a}$$

$$C = 0 \qquad \text{for } z = \infty \tag{2.32b}$$

$$C = 0 \qquad \text{for } x = 0 \tag{2.32c}$$

yields Eq. (2.33):

$$D\frac{\delta^2 c}{\delta z^2} = \alpha z \frac{\delta c}{\delta x} \tag{2.33}$$

The prerequisite for Eq. (2.32a), the first boundary value, is that a saturated layer always exists at the solid–liquid interface and that any interfacial barrier or reaction is insignificant. The second and third boundary conditions, as expressed in Eqs. (2.32b) and (2.32c), respectively, relate to sink conditions.

The mathematical solution to Eq. (2.33) is

$$C = \frac{C_0 \beta \int_0^\infty e^{-\beta^3} d\beta}{4/3\Gamma} \tag{2.34}$$

where $\beta = z\left(\dfrac{\alpha}{qD_x}\right)^{1/3}$ and Γ is the gamma function or more commonly recognized as the shape factor. Hence, the initial rate of dissolution is

$$k = -D\left(\frac{\delta c}{\delta z}\right)_{z=0} \tag{2.35}$$

On substitution of Eq. (2.34) into Eq. (2.35) and after the necessary differentiation is performed, Eq. (2.35) can be integrated over one surface of a rectangular tablet of length L (in the direction of flow) and width b to obtain

$$k = 0.808 D^{2/3} C_0 \alpha^{1/3} b L^{2/3} \tag{2.36}$$

If Eq. (2.35) is integrated over one surface of a circular tablet of radius r, then

$$k = 2.157 D^{2/3} C_0 \alpha^{1/3} r^{5/3} \tag{2.37}$$

Equations (2.36) and (2.37) describe the initial dissolution rates from the surface of a rectangular tablet and a disk, respectively, provided that the boundary conditions are met and the assumptions in their derivations are valid.

Nelson and Shah (22) conducted experiments employing rectangular and circular surfaces of compressed compacts of homologous series of p-aminobenzoate esters with respect to solubility, geometry, and agitation conditions. The correlation between experimental results and theory was reasonably good considering that the test conditions were somewhat less than ideal.

Surface Renewal Theory

The supposition of the existence of a stagnant layer is not usually observed. Instead, it is visualized that turbulence extends to the surface and that there is no boundary layer. In its place, it is supposed that the surface is continually being replaced with fresh dissolution medium. Additionally, it can be viewed that molecules must dissolve or, more technically, "solvate," and that the diffusion of solvent from bulk through the layer of thickness l to the surface is the rate-limiting step. Hence, from Danckwerts' model

$$\frac{dm}{dt} = A(\gamma D)^{1/2}(C_s - C_b) \tag{2.38}$$

where γ is the interfacial tension and C_b is the concentration of the solute in the bulk medium. This equation can be employed to determine the rate of production of fresh surface. For small particles

$$\frac{dm}{dt} = A\frac{D}{r} + (rD)^{1/2}(C_s - C_b) \tag{2.39}$$

When γ approaches 0 or r approaches 0, Eq. (2.39) takes the form of Eq. (2.38) wherein it is noted that r approaches unity.

It must be pointed out that the film and penetration theories are not separate unrelated concepts. It can be argued that the transfer to younger parts of a surface would be by the theory of penetration because the outer edge of the elements has not yet been reached. However, the transfer into the older parts follows the stagnant layer theory since steady-state conditions exist.

Limited-Solvation Theory

Theories describing the actual mechanism of dissolution or solvation of the solid have, by necessity, been derived from studies of solute mass transfer. While the theories of mass transport differ somewhat, they are based on the assumptions that solid–solution equilibrium or saturation concentration exists at the solid–liquid interface and that mass transfer is the slow step in the dissolution process and thereby controls the rate of dissolution.

Dissolution can be considered a complex process composed of the solvent–solid interaction leading to solvation of the molecule followed by movement of the solvated molecule to the bulk of the dissolution medium. In general, dissolution may be described by two rate processes (26):

1. The rate of the interfacial or solid–solvent reaction
2. The rate associated with the diffusional or transport process

Langenbucher (27) pointed out that the dissolution behavior of solid drug substances involves modifications of the beaker or stirred-tank model (10), where the drug is dissolved in a fixed volume of solvent and the agitation is accomplished by means of a stirrer or some rocking or shaking action. In such methods, the drug concentration in the dissolution medium increases from zero up to either the saturation limit or concentration corresponding to complete dissolution of the available drug mass. This concentration buildup is different from the in vivo process, in which the dissolved drug is removed continuously from the liquid by absorption. Consequently, Langenbucher proposed a theory based on the mass transfer in a fixed bed of drug material traversed by a continuous flow of solvent (dissolution medium) in a vertical-exchange column. This column-confined dissolution can follow either ascending dissolution or descending dissolution, depending on the direction of the flow of dissolution medium with respect to the dissolving material in the column, as shown in Fig. 2.5.

When the dissolution of a solid is diffusion controlled, Fick's second law of diffusion, where

$$\frac{\delta c}{\delta t} = \frac{\delta}{\delta x}\left[D(C) \cdot \frac{\delta c}{\delta x}\right] \tag{2.40}$$

may be utilized to calculate the concentration profile for a static system. Solving Eq. (2.40) under suitable initial and boundary conditions permits calcula-

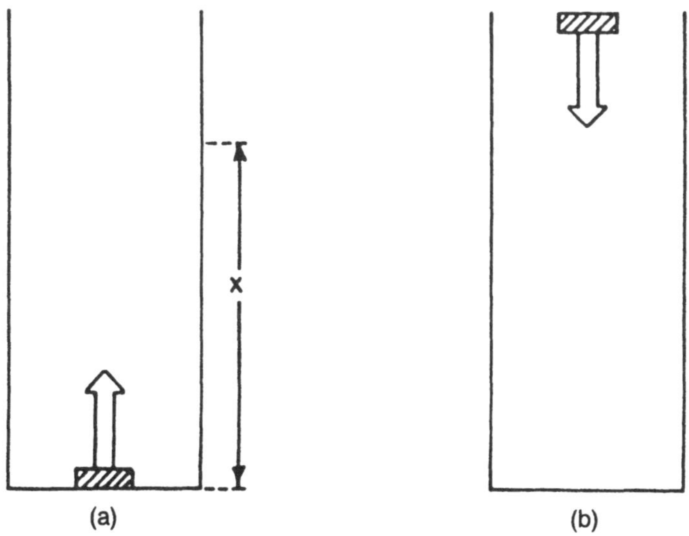

Fig. 2.5 Column dissolution: ascending type (a) and descending type (b). (From Ref. 26.)

tion of the theoretical concentration at any time and point in space. The following conditions apply for this type of model, where steady state is not assumed:

$$\text{Boundary conditions:}\quad C = C_s \qquad \text{for } x = 0 \text{ and } t > 0 \tag{2.41a}$$

$$\text{Initial conditions:}\quad C = 0 \qquad \text{for } x > 0 \text{ and } t = 0 \tag{2.41b}$$

The solution of Eq. (2.40) under the conditions of Eqs. (2.41a) and (2.41b) was given by Boltaks (28) as

$$C_{(x,t)} = C_s \left[1 - \frac{\int_0^x \frac{1}{D} e^{-\frac{1}{2t}\int_0^x \frac{1}{D} x\, dx}}{\int_0^\infty \frac{1}{D} e^{-\frac{1}{2t}\int_0^x \frac{1}{D} x\, dx}} \right] \tag{2.42}$$

Equation (2.42) may be evaluated by the iterative procedure using the solution of Eq. (2.40) for constant D, which yields

$$C = C_s \left(\frac{1 - \operatorname{erf}(x)}{2\sqrt{Dt}} \right) \tag{2.43}$$

where erf denotes the Gassian error function. Theoretical concentration profiles are shown in Figs. 2.6 and 2.7.

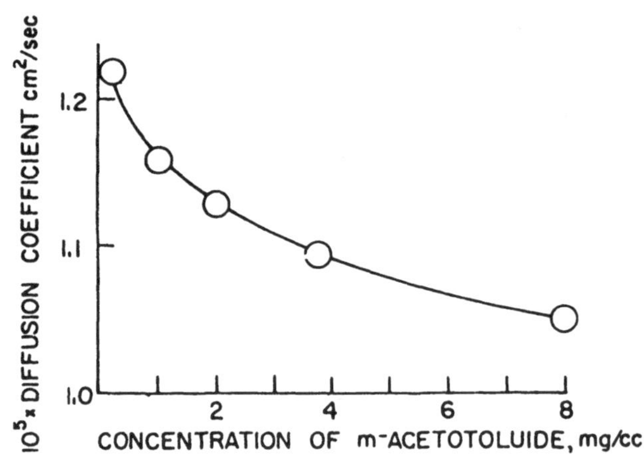

Fig. 2.6 Diffusion coefficient as a function of concentration of *m*-acetotoluide (refer to the text for details). (From Ref. 26.)

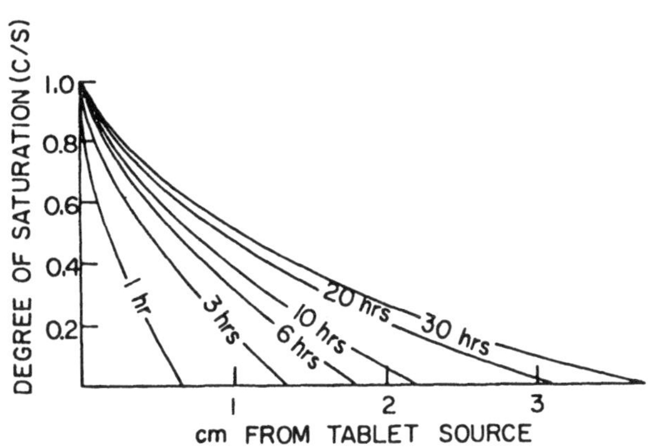

Fig. 2.7 Degree of saturation as a function of distance from tablet source. (From Ref. 26.)

It must be noted that several factors affect the dissolution rates in column-confined dissolution. The column length, the nature of flow (ascending or descending), the configuration and physical dimensions of the column, the type of flow (laminar or otherwise), and characteristics of the dissolving substance are some of the crucial factors that influence the dissolution rates.

Carstensen and Dhupar (29) extended the concept of column-confined dissolution and applied to monodisperse system dissolving in a column at low liquid velocities. Employing the following methodology, they derived equations for dissolution of a soluble solid in a column into a liquid stream.

Consider a column of solid powder of length l cm and cross-section σ cm^2 (Fig. 2.8). The surface area of the amount of powder (b g) in 1 cm length column is denoted as A (square centimeter/centimeter). The liquid enters from the bottom of the column at a flow rate of V_i cm^3/s. It dissolves solid from the column and exits with a rate of V'cm^3/s, where V' includes increase rate due to dissolved solid. If V denotes the average of V_i and V' and if E is the porosity of the powder, the magnitude of the average linear velocity denoted by $\bar{v}$ is given by (30)

$$\bar{v} = \frac{V}{\sigma E} \tag{2.44}$$

Under the condition where the liquid is always close to saturation, S(g/mL), upon exit and if one denotes the exit concentration S_q, where q, the degree of saturation, is close to unity, then the following holds: in t s, VtmL will have passed through the column and will have saturated to a degree of S_q, i.e., will have dissolved $VtS(q - f)$ g, if the incoming liquid is of a degree of saturation

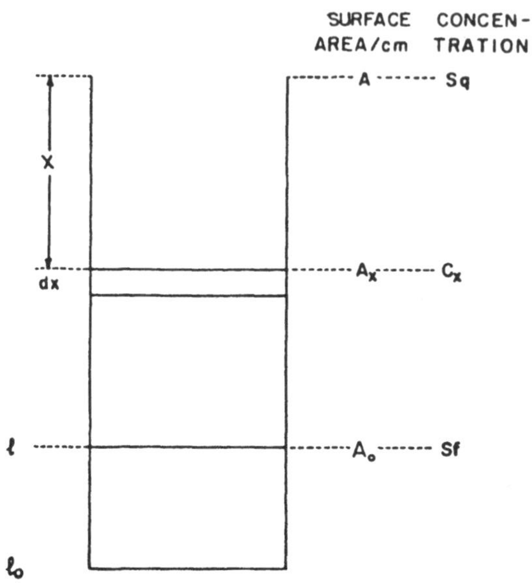

Fig. 2.8 Column-confined dissolution. A, surface area per centimeter of column length; x, distance from top of column; l length of column at time t; S, saturation concentration; f, degree of saturation of feed; q, degree of saturation of efflux; C_x, concentration at point x in the column. (From Ref. 29.)

of f. Since there is b g of solid powder per linear column centimeter, $VtS(q - f)/b$ will have disappeared, i.e.

$$l = l_0 - \frac{VtS(q - f)t}{b} = l_0 - \alpha t \tag{2.45}$$

so that the column length should decrease linearly in time.

When referring to Fig. 2.8 and employing the terminology of this figure, it is noted that a volume element dx, which is x cm from the top of the column, contains solid with a surface area of $A_x d_x$, so that the dissolution rate in this volume element would be $k\,Ax\,dx\,(S - C_x)$, where k is the intrinsic dissolution rate constant in cm/s. Hence the dissolution rate over the entire column at time t, when the length is l cm, is

$$\frac{dm}{dt} = \int_0^l kAx(S - C_x)dx \tag{2.46}$$

It appears that A_x is high at the bottom of the solid column and then rapidly drops to a constant value (refer to Fig. 2.9). This is expected. This drop in A_x occurs over a length of less than 3 cm (i.e., $< 10\%$ of the length of the column). Therefore, A_x is given by

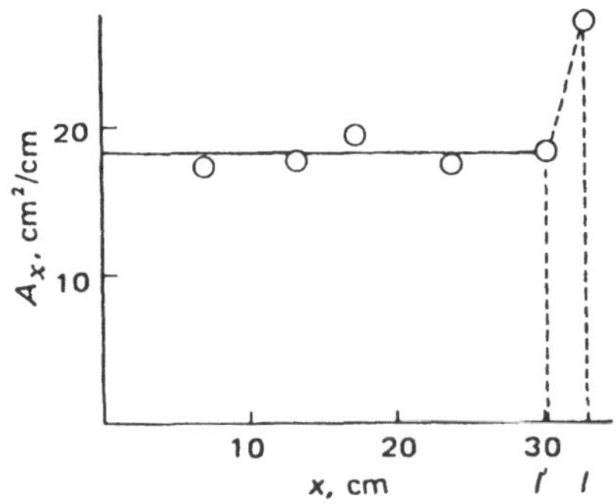

Fig. 2.9 Surface area per column length after dissolution experimentation. A_x as a function of x for 10/20-mesh

$$A_x = A_0 \qquad x < l' \tag{2.47a}$$

$$A_x = A_0 + \Phi(x - l') \qquad l' < l \tag{2.47b}$$

where Φ is the slope of the nonlnear portion of Fig. 2.9 and where l' denotes the point where A_x starts increasing and is close to l, the total length of the column. Hence, accounting for this factor in Eq. (2.46) then yields

$$-\frac{dm}{dt} = kA_0 \int_0^l (S - C_x)dx + k \int_{l'}^l \Phi(x - l')(S - C_x)dx \tag{2.48}$$

The shape of the resultant curve (29) suggests that with real particles in real packaging as opposed to hypothetical spheres with theoretical porosities, the concentration C_x is a function of x given by

$$\ln \left[\frac{S - C_x}{S - C_l} \right] = gx + j \tag{2.49}$$

Since, $x = l$ implies that the left-hand-side of Eq. (2.49) is zero, it follows that $0 = gl + j$, i.e., $j = -gl$, so

$$S - C_x = (S - C_l)e^{g(x-l)} \tag{2.50}$$

When $x = 0$, $C_x = S_q$; and since $C_1 = S_f$, it follows that

$$e^{gl} = \frac{1 - f}{1 - q} \tag{2.51}$$

Introducing Eqn. (2.50) in Eqn. (2.48) yields

$$-\frac{dm}{dt} = kA_0 \int_0^l S(1 - f)e^{g(x-l)}dx + k \int_{l'}^l \Phi(x - l')S(1 - f)e^{g(x-l)}dx \tag{2.52}$$

Under the assumption that $l \sim l'$, Eq. (2.52) can be simplified to

$$\frac{-dm}{dt} = \frac{kA_0 Sl(q - f)}{\ln[(1 - f)/(1 - q)]} \tag{2.53}$$

Carstensen and Yonezawa (31) recently presented a self-consistent model for open-ended column dissolution. It is shown that when the concentration of the efflux stream from the column is plotted as a function of time, the resulting dissolution profile is fairly level at first and then drops rapidly in the form of an inverse sigmoid profile. The model, which assumes that the particles are isometric and adhere to a Levich-type particle dissolution, is based on plug flow with a given residence time (32). Good consistency was found between predicted and experimental values.

Dissolution from columns has been treated extensively by other investigators, both theoretically and experimentally (26,27,29,31,33–37). Reports investigating the influence of types of fluid flow, nature and shape of dissolving particles, length of columns, solvent flow patterns, and so on, on the dissolution rate have been published.

In summary, it can be stated that dissolution can be essentially described by two rate processes: the rate of the interfacial or solid–solvent reaction and the rate associated with the diffusional or transport process. The solution concentration at any point in the dissolution column depends on which of the two rates is faster. For the ascending dissolution model, the experimental concentration is much less than the theoretical concentration predicted by Fick's equation, based on a saturated layer model, if the interfacial rate is slow compared to the rate of diffusion. If, however, the interfacial rate is fast compared to the diffusional rate, the experimental concentration is equal to the theoretical concentration predicted by the presence of a saturation concentration at the interface.

DISSOLUTION OF MULTIPARTICULATE SYSTEMS

A number of theories have been put forth that can satisfactorily describe the dissolution of a single particle. However, the systems frequently encountered can seldom be adequately described by single-particle dissolution kinetics for monodispersed systems. Pharmaceutical scientists are interested in real pharmaceutical solid systems that can be comminuted, mixed, filled into capsules, or tableted into dosage forms that will disintegrate, resulting in a state that will permit the drug to dissolve in the gastrointestinal tract or some other biological fluid and then be absorbed through the biological membrane. Currently, there is scarcity of literature on multiparticulate dissolution of pharmaceutical systems and thus we can make few accurate predictions. However, review of some of the underlying theories of the dissolution of multiparticulate system will assist us in developing a basis for improving our ability to predict how a particular dosage form will dissolve in a biological dissolution medium.

Most pharmaceutical dosage forms are polydisperse systems. Many investigators have shown that particles prepared by procedures such as milling, precipitation, and so on, produce skewed particle size distribution functions as opposed to normal distribution function (38–41). These skewed distribution functions closely resemble log-normal particle-size distribution.

Higuchi and co-workers (42,43) first studied the dissolution of polydispersed powders exhibiting log-normal particle size distribution. They approximated log-normal frequency function as given in Eq. (2.54):

$$f(\log x) = \frac{1}{\sqrt{2}\pi(\sigma)} \exp \frac{(\log x - \log Dg)^2}{2\sigma^2} \tag{2.54}$$

where x is the particle diameter, Dg geometric mean diameter and σ is the standard deviation of the distribution. When expressed as a cumulative oversize distribution by the cumulative function, Eq. (2.54) will be

$$g(x) = \frac{K}{x^4} \tag{2.55}$$

where K is the frequency coefficient for the function.

Later, Carstensen and Musa (44) generated log-normal distributions by computer and traced the dissolution, using the following set of assumptions: (a) all particles are isometric and dissolve isotropically, (b) the film thickness l of the diffusion barrier around each particle is constant, (c) there exist no particle-size solubility effects, and (d) sink conditions exist. They found that the dissolution patterns could be approximated by a cube-root law up to a critical time t_c when the smallest particles of diameter a_0 would be completely dissolved. Beyond the critical time t_c, changes in slope of the cube-root plot are observed. Equation (2.56) defines the relationship observed in the cube-root plot prior to reaching t_c:

$$m_0^{1/3} - M^{1/3} = \frac{1.84kC_s m_0^{1/3}}{\sigma^{0.02} D_g \rho} t \tag{2.56}$$

It should be noted, however, that the computer-generated distributions were truncated at + and -3σ. There are two major limitations for this expression. First, Eq. (2.56) holds true only over the limited range of values tested. Second, the slope tends toward infinity when σ approaches zero.

Employing the same assumptions, Brooke (45,46) extended the treatment to nontruncated log-normal, particle-size-distributed powder and arrived at an exact expression of their dissolution rate profile. Brooke also showed that a cube-root relationship could be explained theoretically and suggested the following equation (46):

$$m_0^{1/3} - M^{1/3} = \exp(-2.54\sigma_D)\frac{2kC_s(m_0)^{1/3}}{D_g\rho} \tag{2.57}$$

where $\sigma_D = 2.3\sigma$. It can be seen from this expression that Eq. (2.57) depends on density, mean diameter, initial weight, and solubility of the solute particles, as well as the dissolution rate constant k, as expressed by Carstensen and Musa (44). However, the dependence on standard deviation is different in Eq. (2.57) due to the fact that it does not suffer from the limitations with which Eq. (2.56) is afflicted.

Real powders do not obey the assumptions commonly employed. They do not contain spherical particles and may not necessarily follow the cube-root law. Carstensen and Patel (47) studied the dissolution of oxalic acid crystals of log-normal particle-size distribution in 0.1 N HCl. They reported deviation from the classical cube-root law. A biphasic cube-root dependence was found as seen in Fig. 2.10. The slopes of the initial cube-root plots were consistent with the theory based on the dissolution of isometric, isotropic particles where the assumptions employed were those listed earlier. The dependency of the slopes of the cube-root plots on the mean particle diameter and on the particle weight fit Carstensen–Musa theory (44). Additionally, the dependence of the slopes of the cube-root plots on the standard deviation of the powder distribution obeys Brooke's treatment.

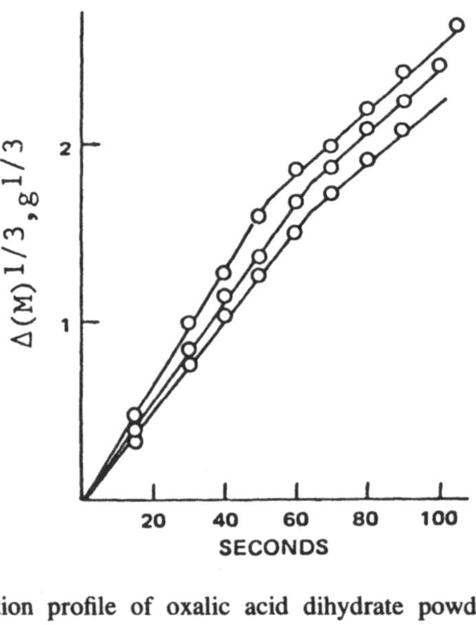

Fig. 2.10 Dissolution profile of oxalic acid dihydrate powder of geometric mean 1500 m and SD 0.108 (top), 0.129 (middle), and 0.155 (bottom). (From Ref. 47.)

DISSOLUTION OF MULTICOMPONENT POLYPHASE SYSTEMS

It is essential to characterize the dissolution-rate behavior of polyphase mixtures. These mixtures consist of more than one component. In practice, systems such as solid dispersions consist of more than one component. Drug release from such systems involves various aspects, such as simultaneous dissolution of more than one phase and differing dissolution rates within phases. These factors could affect the overall dissolution rate of the system. Hence, it is imperative to characterize the dissolution behavior of such systems under two conditions: noninteracting systems, where the components do not interact in any way with each other, and interacting systems, where the components interact to form complexes in solution. The following discussion is limited to physical modeling and subsequent mathematical analysis of two- or three-component systems.

Noninteracting Systems

For a two-phase mixture in which the two components, *A* and *B*, do not interact in any way with each other, one can describe the model in the following manner. Upon exposure to solvent, both components of the mixture should tend to dissolve at rates proportional to their solubilities and their diffusion coefficients. After some time, usually one of the phases would become depleted at the solid–liquid interface region since N_A/N_B may not be equal to $(D_A C_{SA}/D_B C_{SB}$, where N_A and N_B are the original amounts of *A* and *B* in the mixtures, D_A and D_B are the diffusion coefficients, and C_{SA} and C_{SB} are the respective solubilities. As a result, a surface layer is formed that is composed of only one of the phases. The three possible situations after zero time are illustrated in Fig. 2.11 for the one-dimensional, two-phase mixture.

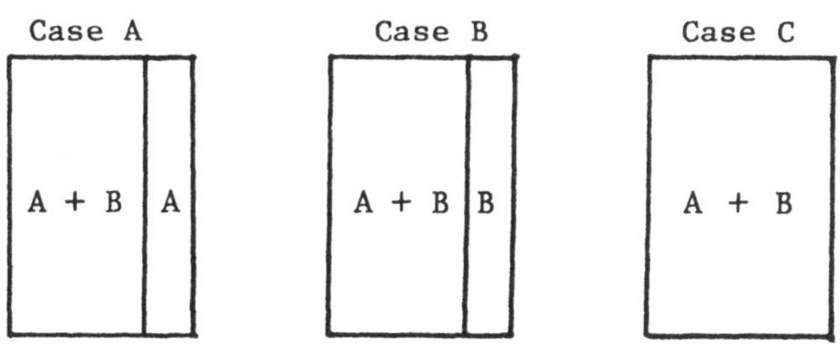

Fig. 2.11 Dissolution behavior of two-phase mixture of *A* and *B*. Case A: Phase *B* dissolves fast enough to leave a layer of pure *A* behind; case B: the reverse is true; case C: the dissolution rates of *A* and *B* are proportional to their relative amounts in the mixture. (From Ref. 1.)

Dissolution-rate equations based on this model employing the Nernst–Brunner concept for each situation given in Fig. 2.11 can be stated as follows: When

$$\frac{N_A}{N_B} > \frac{D_A C_{SA}}{D_B C_{SB}} \tag{2.58}$$

$$G_A = \frac{D_A C_{SA}}{l} \tag{2.58a}$$

and

$$G_B = \frac{D_B C_{SB}}{l} \tag{2.58b}$$

when

$$\frac{N_A}{N_B} < \frac{D_A C_{SA}}{D_B C_{SB}} \tag{2.59}$$

$$G_B = \frac{D_B C_{SB}}{l} \tag{2.59a}$$

and

$$G_A = \frac{N_A}{N_B} G_B \tag{2.59b}$$

where G_A and G_B are the dissolution rates of components *A* and *B*, respectively. Finally, at the critical mixture ratio, i.e., when $N_A/N_B = (D_A C_{SA})/(D_B C_{SB})$, both components coexist at all times at the solid–liquid interface and dissolution profiles are linear under sink conditions. However, at all other weight ratios, one or the other component forms a porous layer at the surface, which represents an additional barrier retarding dissolution of the receding phase and resulting in a curved dissolution profile for the receding component.

Excellent agreement between data and theory was observed when Higuchi et al. (48) investigated the dissolution behavior of benzoic acid–salicylic acid tablet mixtures dissolving in water. Such a physical model involving simultaneous diffusion and rapid equilibria was later tested by Shah and Parrott (49), who confirmed the hypothesis.

It must be noted that while the diffusion layer theory was employed to express the dissolution rate behavior of the surface phases in Eqs. (2.58a) and (2.59b), Danckwerts' theory could have been used instead. Additionally, the above equations have a restriction in that they are quantitatively applicable in the steady state only. This requires that the C_{SA} and C_{SB} values do not differ too greatly (say, no more than a factor of 100) if, for example, the tablet thickness is on the order of millimeters.

If one of the components is very much less soluble than the other, i.e., if either $C_{SA}/C_{SB} \rightarrow 0$ or ∞, then the problem reduces to that of solute release from an inert matrix. In such cases, one of the components acts as a carrier of the other. In such instances, the range of weight fractions over which dissolution is controlled by the carrier is very small and occurs only at the higher carrier weight fractions, as shown in Fig. 2.12. This model also predicts that the release rate of either component in the system is never greater than that of the pure component above. In addition, no dissolution advantage is predicted for eutectic mixtures, a conclusion also arrived at by Goldberg et al. (50). Therefore, where increases in dissolution rate are observed, disintegration or complex formation is likely to be involved.

Three-component systems are more complicated, there being 13 different possibilities at the solid–liquid interface, as shown in Fig. 2.13 (51).

Interacting Systems

Systems containing more than one component can interact in different ways, which can influence the dissolution behavior. Physical models have been developed describing such systems. These models address three major kinds of interacting systems.

1. Solid complex formation
2. Solid state changes
3. Coacervate formation

Soluble Complex Formation

The models for noninteracting systems can be extended to situations where the components interact in solution to form a soluble complex (48,51). Many carrier materials readily form soluble complexes with drugs, thereby enhancing or reducing the drugs' apparent solubility, as the need may be (52,53). When two such components are present in a system, such as a solid dispersion, dissolution of each component is enhanced or retarded by the contribution from the diffusing complex. Dissolution rates above those of the individual pure components are observed, as shown in Fig. 2.14. The maximum rates occur at the critical mixture ratio, which is given by (54)

$$\frac{N_A}{N_B} = \frac{D_A C_{SA} + D_{AB} K C_{SA} C_{SB}}{D_B C_{SB} + D_{AB} K C_{SA} C_{SB}} \tag{2.60}$$

where K is the binding constant and D_{AB} the diffusion coefficient of the complex. In practice, A or B could be the carrier, with the other component being the drug entity.

The magnitudes of the dissolution rates of each component, G_{max}, at the critical mixture ratio are

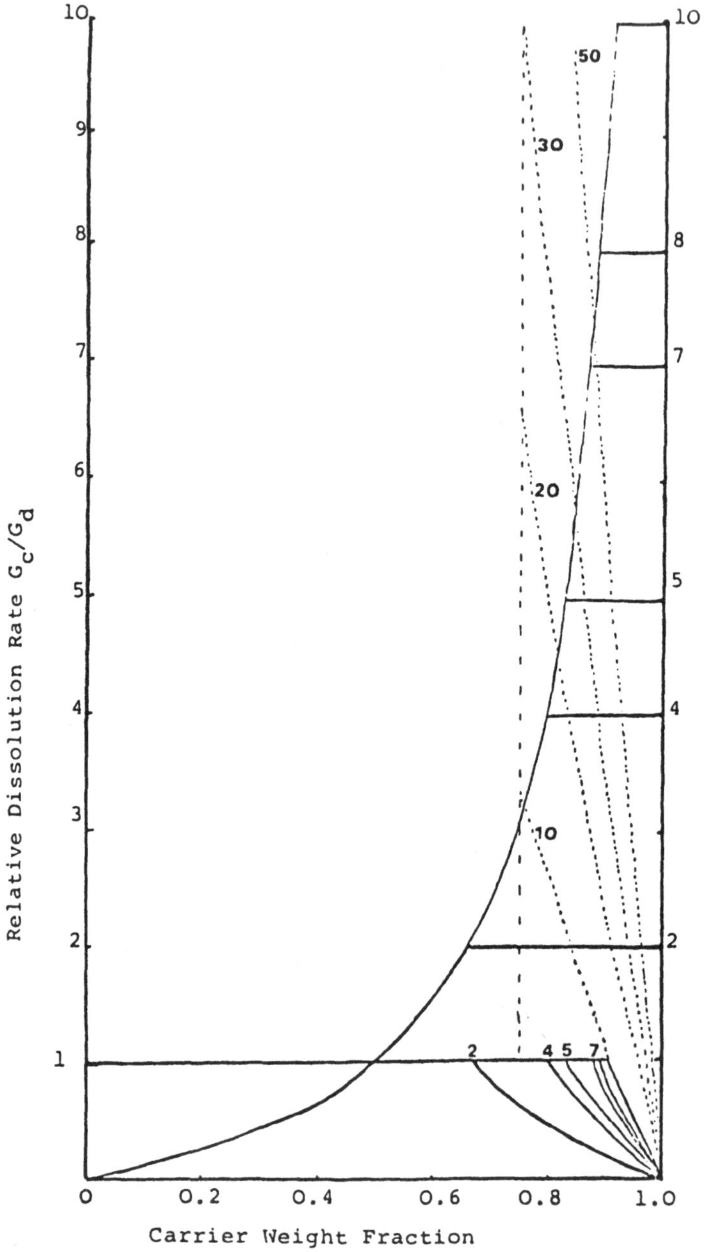

Fig. 2.12 Theoretical change in relative dissolution rates of drug and carrier with increasing carrier weight fraction for two noninteracting fractions. (From Ref. 58.)

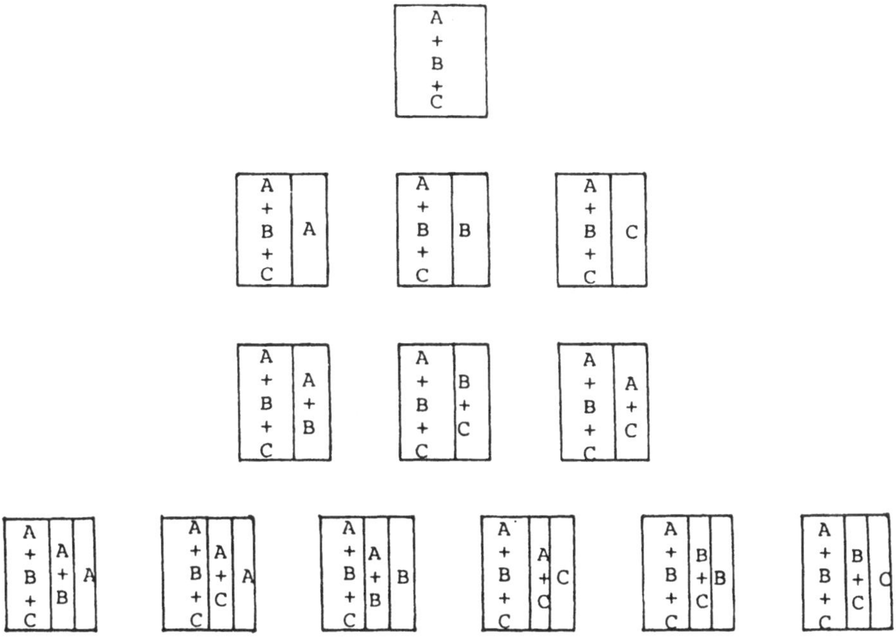

Fig. 2.13 Possible dissolution behavior of a three-component system. (From Ref. 58.)

$$G_{A,\max} = \frac{D_A C_{SA} + D_{AB} K C_{SA} C_{SB}}{l} \tag{2.61a}$$

$$G_{B,\max} = \frac{D_B C_{SB} + D_{AB} K C_{SB} C_{SA}}{l} \tag{2.61b}$$

Equations for the limiting rates at other weight fractions have also been derived (48). It should be noted that the absolute magnitude of the increase in dissolution rate at the critical mixture ratio employing Eqs. (2.61a) and (2.61b) is the same for each component, $D_{AB}KC_{SA}C_{SB}$. Hence, the relative maximum increase in dissolution rate is greatest for the less soluble component. The relative increase in drug dissolution rate is given by

$$\frac{G_{A,\max}}{G_i} = 1 + \frac{D_{AB} C_{SB} K}{D_A} \tag{2.62}$$

where G_i is the intrinsic dissolution rate of the drug. Dissolution rates of each component decline rapidly as the weight fraction deviates from the critical mixture ratio. A *soluble complex model* has been rigorously evaluated as to the release rates of both dissolving species. Good agreement with theory has been

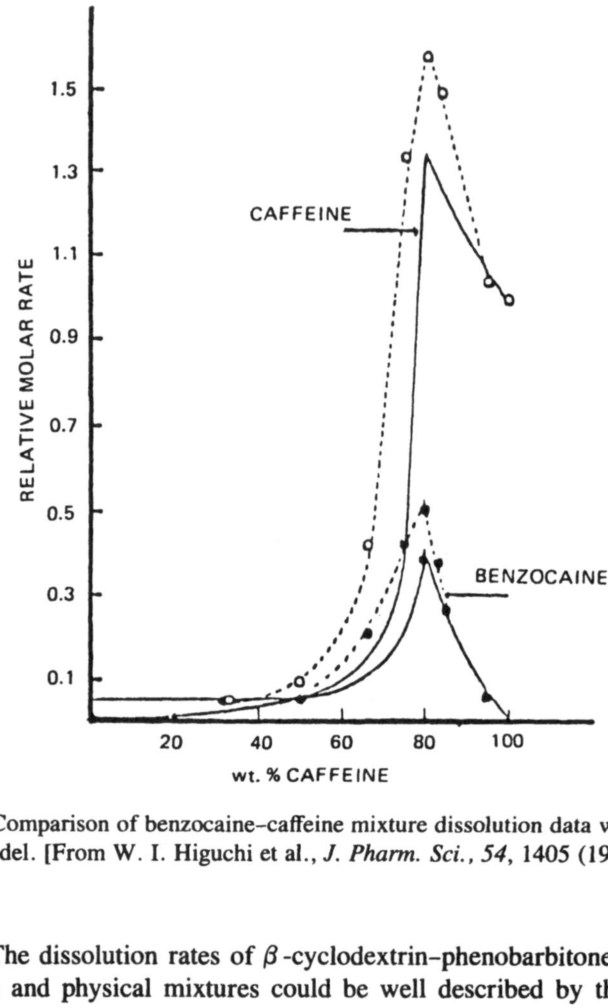

Fig. 2.14 Comparison of benzocaine–caffeine mixture dissolution data with the soluble complex model. [From W. I. Higuchi et al., *J. Pharm. Sci.*, *54*, 1405 (1965).]

reported. The dissolution rates of β-cyclodextrin–phenobarbitone freeze-dried dispersions and physical mixtures could be well described by this model, as shown in Fig. 2.15 (55). In other systems, where the release of one component (the drug) had been monitored over a range of weight fractions, qualitative agreement with theory was observed (56).

If solid-state changes do not occur in the components, drug and/or carrier, during the formation of such systems, then in theory, the dissolution rates of the multicomponent system and physical mixtures of similar composition should not differ. In practice, dispersed systems (multicomponent systems) tend to give more reproducible results, due to more intimate contact between the components. Where significant differences occur, they suggest solid-state changes during formation of the system (57).

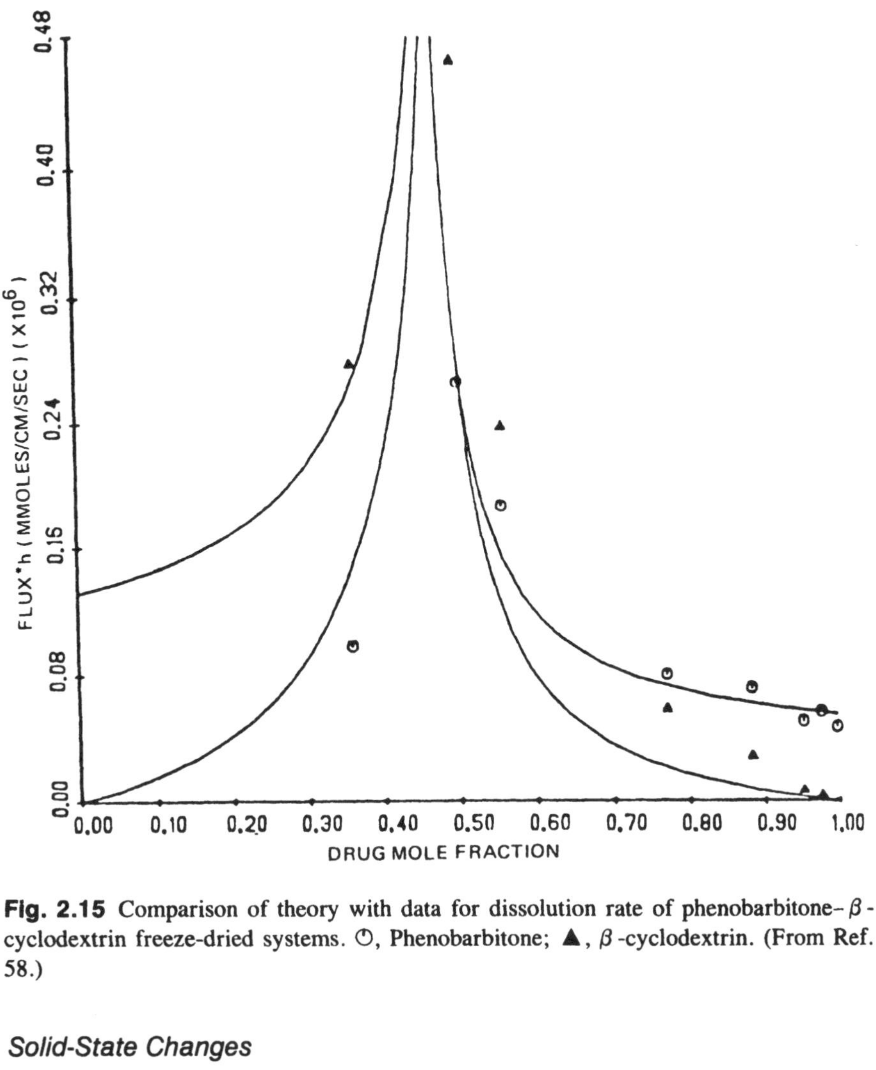

Fig. 2.15 Comparison of theory with data for dissolution rate of phenobarbitone–β-cyclodextrin freeze-dried systems. ⦶, Phenobarbitone; ▲, β-cyclodextrin. (From Ref. 58.)

Solid-State Changes

During the process of forming a multicomponent system, such as a solid dispersion, the individual components may precipitate in different solid phases from those present in a similar physical mixture (i.e., as polymorphs—solvated or amorphous phases). The physical forms produced are a function of the procedural technique, the solvent medium, the specific drug carrier system, and the relative proportion of the components present. A griseofulvin–PVP system prepared from chloroform results in precipitation as the crystalline chloroform solvate. However, spray drying of the same system yields amorphous product

(58,59). Several examples reported in the literature exhibit differing dissolution characteristics due to solid-state changes (58–64). If the new phases produced in the system have a higher solubility, remain stable in the system, and do not rapidly revert to the less soluble form on contact with the dissolution medium, enhanced dissolution from the system over the mechanical mixture can be expected. The nature of the carrier, one of the components, plays an important role in maintaining the stability of many high-energy phases.

In the sulfathiazole–PVP systems, Simonelli et al. (61) found the dissolution rates in qualitative agreement with the soluble complex model, as shown in Fig. 2.16. The enhanced dissolution rates, above those observed for mechani-

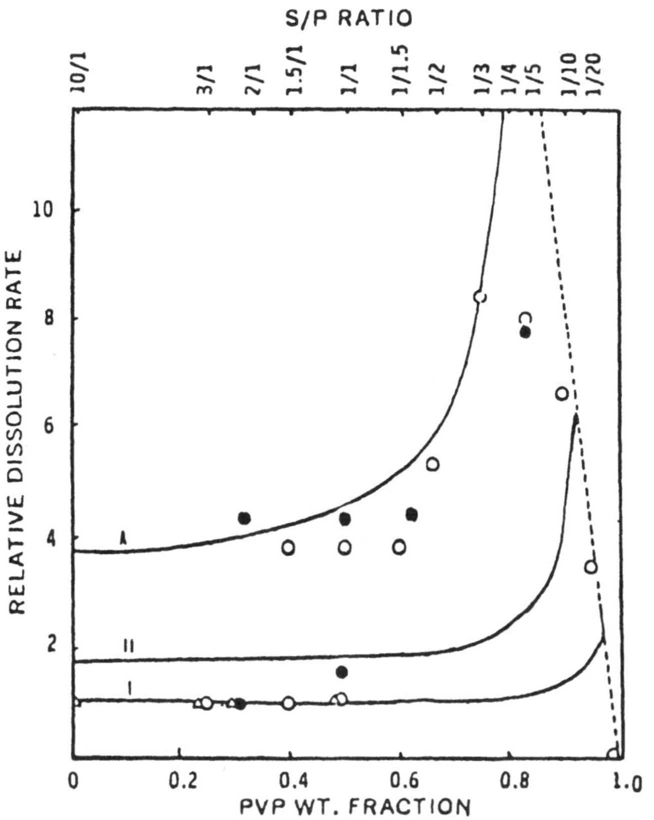

Fig. 2.16 Comparison of theoretical and experimental dissolution rates of sulfathiazole as a Function of polyvinylpyrrolidine (PVP) weight fraction. Theoretical profiles for controlling layers: I, sulfathiazole form I; II, sulfathiazole form II; A, amorphous sulfathiazole. (From Ref. 61.)

cal mixtures, in the weight fraction range where drug is expected to be the surface layer controlling the dissolution, were attributed to the formation of a high-energy amorphous phase of one of the components (the drug). This observation was supported by x-ray diffraction, dissolution, and extensive solubility data (65). Several other examples reported in the literature conform to this phenomenon (66–70).

It has been shown that considerable enhancement of dissolution rates is obtained in the region of the critical mixture ratio when the formation of a high-energy drug form is coupled with complexation. The nature of the high-energy drug phases present in such multicomponent systems is subject to some debate. It has been possible to separate the contributions from free drug and soluble complex form using dissolution, solubility, and membrane transport methodologies (71). A better understanding of the nature of these high-energy drug forms in these systems is necessary to enable prediction of their activity, dissolution behavior, and stability.

The diffusion models describing dissolution from multicomponent solids seem to adequately describe drug dissolution from systems such as solid dispersions at the lower weight fractions where the drug is expected to control dissolution.

Coacervate Formation

An alternative dissolution model proposed by Sekikawa et al. (72) envisages formation of a coacervate at the solid–liquid interface. These authors suggest that the faster drug release observed from lower-molecular-weight PVP coprecipitates supports their view, and so does the PVP–sulfathiazole system (73).

General Model for *n*-Component Systems

Early studies on dissolution rates involving multicomponent solids have been reported. Diffusion models were also suggested for the dissolution of nondisintegrating multicomponent mixtures containing noninteracting components and complexing components. Shah and Parrott (49) applied the model to the dissolution of four two-component solids. However, Carmichael et al. (52) were the first to develop a general model for the dissolution rate of a nondisintegrating sphere containing any number of components. The model was developed from the viewpoint of mass transfer and was applied to two- and three-component solids, two-component interacting solids, and three-component solids with two components interacting.

This theory is structured on assumptions similar to those for film theory. Additionally, it assumes that the effective particle shape approximates a sphere and the initial solid composed of n components is homogeneous.

From the viewpoint of mass transfer, if multicomponent diffusion effects are ignored, the change in mass with time, dM_i/dt, of a noninteracting component in a solid can be expressed as

$$\frac{dM_i}{dt} = -k_i A_i (C_i^* - C_i) \tag{2.63}$$

where k_i is the liquid phase mass transfer coefficient, A_i is the surface area available for mass transfer, and C_i^* and C_i the interfacial and bulk mass concentrations of species in the liquid phase (dissolution medium), respectively, for components $i = 1$ to n. Since, the area of sphere A is $4\pi r^2$,

$$\frac{dM_i}{dt} = -k_i 4 r_i^2 (C_i^* - C_i) \tag{2.64}$$

Since $M_i = (4/3)\pi r_i^3 X_i \rho$, where X_i and ρ are the mass fraction and bulk density, respectively, and if X_i is not time dependent, Eq. (2.64) can be written as

$$-\frac{dr_i}{dt} = \frac{D_i (C_i^* - C_i)}{l X_i \rho} \tag{2.65}$$

where for diffusion-controlled dissolution in which there is no chemical reaction, the liquid phase mass transfer coefficients are expressed in terms of diffusion coefficients D_i and the film thickness l.

As dissolution proceeds, the more soluble components dissolve faster and are depleted near the solid–liquid interface, resulting in a surface layer composed of the least soluble component. At any time the solid can be conceptualized as consisting of a homogeneous core with the initial composition, an outer shell of the least soluble component, and between them, $n - 2$ concentric layers comprised of components of intermediate solubilities. If the nth component is the least soluble component, Eq. (2.65) can be written as

$$-\frac{dr_n}{dt} = \frac{D_n}{X_n l \rho} (C_n^* - C_n) \tag{2.66}$$

and

$$-\frac{dr_i}{dt} = \frac{D_i}{(l + r_n + r_i) X_n \rho} (C_i^* - C_i) \tag{2.67}$$

where l is the film thickness and $(l + r_n - r_i)$ incorporates an internal diffusion thickness (or resistance) of $r_n - r_i$.

Equations (2.64), (2.66), and (2.67) can be employed to calculate the dissolution rates of n-component solid systems. The fluxes, J_i, can be determined employing the following equations:

$$J_i = \frac{1}{A_n} \frac{dM_i}{dt} = -k \frac{A_i}{A_n} (C_i^* - C_i) \tag{2.68}$$

and

$$J_n = \frac{1}{A_n}\frac{dMn}{dt} = -k(C_n^* - C_n) \tag{2.69}$$

where the fluxes are normalized in terms of the external surface area A_n of the solid.

These equations can be employed to model the dissolution of two- and three-component solids. In addition, these equations can be modified to include cases with interaction between the components. Interested readers are advised to refer to the original work reported by Carmichael and co-workers for details concerning such systems (52).

FINAL COMMENTS

A rigorous review of the theories and theoretical principles associated with dissolution testing is a necessity for a research scientist. However, it may be inappropriate for a person concerned primarily with various dissolution devices and with concepts of physical chemistry concerning the interaction of solids and liquids that might cause inconsistencies in test results. For such a test with broader interests, detailed discussions are presented of the various theoretical concepts in dissolution testing recognizing the basic dynamics. Some of the useful theoretical concepts are given below.

It must be recognized that the rate-limiting factor in dissolution is complex because the transfer of solid active ingredient from its corresponding system can involve a sequence of processes. Each process may require a different percentage of total time for the active ingredient to be dissolved. Second, the status of the solid–liquid interface is the key parameter for dissolution. It is the point at which fresh dissolution medium comes into contact with the surface of the solid to be dissolved. Additionally, the surface area of the dissolving substance will vary under all circumstances. As the test proceeds, the surface area decreases with nondisintegrating systems and increases with a disintegrating system. From a practical standpoint, the rate of passage of fresh dissolution medium over the dissolving substance's surface area should be kept constant, or is at least controllable and repeatable. When the particles become small, however, that becomes more difficult.

REFERENCES

1. W. I. Higuchi, *J. Pharm. Sci.*, *56*, 315 (1967).
2. D. E. Wurster and P. W. Taylor, *J. Pharm. Sci.*, *54*, 169 (1965).
3. L. Leeson and J. T. Carstensen, eds., *Dissolution Technology*, Industrial Pharmaceuticals Technology Section, APhA, Washington, D.C. (1974), pp. 1–57.
4. H. P. Koch, *Pharm. Acta Helv.*, *59*, 130 (1986).

5. W. Nernst, *Z. Phys. Chem.*, *47*, 52 (1904).
6. E. Brunner, *Z. Phys. Chem.*, *47*, 56 (1904).
7. P. V. Danckwerts, *Ind. Eng. Chem.*, *43*, 1460 (1951).
8. M. L. Brunner and St. Tolloczko, *Z. Anorg. Allg. Chem.*, *28*, 314 (1901).
9. M. L. Brunner and St. Tolloczko, *Z. Anorg. Allg. Chem.*, *56*, 58 (1907).
10. J. H. Wood, J. E. Syarto, and H. Letterman, *J. Pharm. Sci.*, *64*, 1068 (1965).
11. J. Piccolo and R. Tawashi, *J. Pharm. Sci.*, *60*, 59, 1818 (1971).
12. S. Bisaillon and R. Tawashi, *J. Pharm. Sci.*, *60*, 1874 (1971).
13. A. Hixson and J. Crowell, *Ind. Eng. Chem.*, *23*, 923 (1931).
14. A. Noyes and J. Whitney, *J. Am. Chem. Soc.*, *19*, 930 (1897).
15. P. J. Niebergall and J. E. Goyan, *J. Pharm. Sci.*, *52*, 29 (1963).
16. M. P. Short, P. Sharkey, and C. T. Rhodes, *J. Pharm. Sci.*, *61*, 1733 (1972).
17. P. Pothisiri and J. T. Carstensen, *J. Pharm. Sci.*, *62*, 1468 (1973).
18. H. B. Dwight, *Table of Integrals*, Macmillan, London (1961).
19. K. G. Nelson and A. C. Shah, *Abstracts of the APhA/APS*, Washington D.C., paper 70 (1974).
20. A. C. Shah and K. G. Nelson, *Abstracts of the APhA/APS*, Washington, D.C., paper 71 (1974).
21. M. Patel and J. T. Carstensen, *J. Pharm. Sci.*, *64*, 1651 (1975).
22. K. G. Nelson and A. C. Shah, *J. Pharm. Sci.*, *64*, 610 (1975).
23. V. G. Levich, *Physico-Chemical Hydrodynamics*, Prentice-Hall, Englewood Cliffs, N.J. (1962).
24. S. Schlichting, *Boundary Layer Theory*, 6th ed., McGraw-Hill, New York (1968).
25. R. B. Bird, W. E. Stewart, and E. N. Lightfoot, *Transport Phenomena*, Wiley, New York (1960).
26. R. L. Nedich and D. O. Kildsig, *J. Pharm. Sci.*, *61*, 214 (1972).
27. F. Langenbucher, *J. Pharm. Sci.*, *58*, 1265 (1969).
28. B. I. Boltaks, *Diffusion of Semiconductors*, Academic Press, New York, (1963), Ch. 4.
29. J. T. Carstensen and K. Dhupar, *J. Pharm. Sci.* *65*, 1634 (1976).
30. W. A. Gray, *The Packing of Solid Particles*, Chapman & Hall, London (1968), p. 129.
31. J. T. Carstensen and Y. Yonezawa, *J. Pharm. Sci.*, *75*, 764 (1986).
32. V. G. Levich, *Physico-Chemical Hydrodynamics*, Prentice-Hall, Englewood Cliffs, N.J. (1962), p. 183.
33. J. Tingstad, J. Pudzinski, L. Lachman, and E. Shami, *J. Pharm. Sci.*, *62*, 1527 (1973).
34. F. Langenbucher, *J. Pharm. Sci.*, *62*, 1737 (1973).
35. P. D. Krause and D. O. Kildsig, *J. Pharm. Sci.*, *61*, 281 (1972).
36. C. F. Lerk and K. Zuurman, *J. Pharm. Pharmacol.*, *22*, 319 (1970).
37. J. T. Carstensen, *Labo-Pharm. Probl. Tech.*, *31*, 10 (1983).
38. T. Hatch and S. P. Choate, *J. Franklin Inst.*, *207*, 369 (1929).
39. H. Haywood, *J. Pharm. Pharmacol.*, *15*, 56T (1963).
40. T. Allen, *Particle Size Measurement*, 3rd ed., Chapman & Hall, London (1981).
41. E. L. Parrott, *Pharm. Manuf.*, *2*, 31 (1985).

42. W. I. Higuchi and E. N. Hiestand, *J. Pharm. Sci.*, *52*, 67 (1963).
43. W. I. Higuchi, E. L. Rowe, and E. N. Hiestand, *J. Pharm. Sci.*, *52*, 162 (1963).
44. J. T. Carstensen and N. M. Musa, *J. Pharm. Sci.*, *61*, 223 (1972).
45. D. Brooke, *J. Pharm. Sci.*, *62*, 795 (1973).
46. D. Brooke, *J. Pharm. Sci.*, *63*, 344 (1974).
47. J. T. Carstensen and M. Patel, *J. Pharm. Sci.*, *64*, 1770 (1975).
48. W. I. Higuchi, N. A. Miz, and S. J. Desai, *J. Pharm. Sci.*, *54*, 1405 (1965).
49. S. A. Shah and E. L. Parrott, *J. Pharm. Sci.*, *65*, 1784 (1976).
50. A. H. Goldberg, M. Gibaldi, and J. L. Kanig, *J. Pharm. Sci.*, *55*, 482 (1966).
51. E. L. Parrott, M. Simpson, and D. R. Flanagan, *J. Pharm. Sci.*, *72*, 765 (1983).
52. G. R. Carmichael, S. A. Shah, and E. L. Parrott, *J. Pharm. Sci.*, *70*, 1331 (1981).
53. W. L. Chiou and S. Riegelman, *J. Pharm. Sci.*, *60*, 1281 (1971).
54. T. Higuchi and K. A. Connors, *Adv. Anal. Chem. Instrum.*, *4*, 117 (1965).
55. O. I. Corrigan and C. T. Stanley, *J. Pharm. Pharmacol.*, *34*, 621 (1981).
56. O. I. Corrigan and C. T. Stanley, *Pharm. Acta Helv.*, *56*, 204 (1981).
57. O. I. Corrigan and R. F. Timoney, *Pharm. Acta Helv.*, *51*, 268 (1976).
58. O. I. Corrigan, *Drug Dev. Ind. Pharm.*, *11*(2/3), 697 (1985).
59. H. Junginger, *Pharm. Ind.*, *39*, 383 (1977).
60. H. Junginger, *Pharm. Ind.*, *39*, 498 (1977).
61. A. P. Simonelli, S. C. Mehta, and W. I. Higuchi, *J. Pharm. Sci.*, *58*, 538 (1969).
62. O. I. Corrigan and R. F. Timoney, *J. Pharm. Pharmacol.*, *26*, 838 (1974).
63. O. I. Corrigan and R. F. Timoney, *J. Pharm. Pharmacol.*, *27*, 759 (1975).
64. O. I. Corrigan, K. Sabra, and E. M. Holohan, *Drug Dev. Ind. Pharm.*, *9*, 1 (1983).
65. O. I. Corrigan and E. M. Holohan, *J. Pharm. Pharmacol.*, *36*, 00 (1984).
66. A. P. Simonelli, S. C. Mehta, and W. I. Higuchi, *J. Pharm. Sci.*, *65*, 355 (1976).
67. H. Sekikawa, R. Hori, T. Arita, K. Ito, and M. Nakano, *Chem. Pharm. Bull.*, *26*, 2489 (1978).
68. H. Sekikawa, M. Nakano, and T. Arita, *Chem. Pharm. Bull.*, *26*, 118 (1978).
69. A. R. Ebian, M. A. Monstafa, S. A. Khalil, and M. M. Motawi, *J. Pharm. Pharmacol.*, *25*, 13 (1973).
70. A. P. Simonelli, S. C. Mehta, and W. I. Higuchi, *J. Pharm. Sci.*, *59*, 633 (1970).
71. E. I. Stupak, H. A. Rosenberg, and T. R. Bates, *J. Pharmacokinet. Biopharm.*, *2*, 525 (1974).
72. H. Sekikawa, M. Nakano, and T. Arita, *Chem. Pharm. Bull.*, *27*, 1223 (1979).
73. A. A. Badawi and A. A. El Sayed, *J. Pharm. Sci.*, *69*, 492 (1980).

ADDITIONAL READING

Bettinetti, G. P., P. Mura, and A. Liguori, *Farmaco Ed. Prat*, *43*, 331 (1988).
Canal, T., M. Lovrecich, and F. Rubessa, *Pharmazie*, *44*, 619 (1989).
Janabi II, Al., *Drug Dev. Ind. Pharm.*, *16*, 347 (1990).
Kuu, W. Y., M. R. Prisco, R. W. Wood et al., *Int. J. Pharm.*, *55*, 77 (1989).

THREE

Dissolution Testing Devices

INTRODUCTION

Approximately two decades ago, problems in biological availability of drugs were brought to the attention of regulatory agencies and compendial standards groups. The problems centered around routine investigation of identical competitive products by a pharmaceutical manufacturer. Substantial differences in bioavailability were observed during testing of the in vivo performance of the two items, which were otherwise pharmaceutically identical according to all then-existing tests for physical properties.

This triggered a study of various dissolution test methods. At that time, the major concern was over lifesaving drugs, particularly those with a narrow therapeutic index. The perfect example would be digoxin, since it is necessary for the physician to establish effective but nontoxic dosage levels for each patient in a titered dosage. Should the patient switch brands of this medication, it is imperative that the second brand closely approximate the first in its ability to sustain blood levels. It was then suggested, following investigations, that such ability could, to some degree, be correlated with dissolution-rate characteristics.

Coordination of the studies was assigned to the then director of the Drug Standards Laboratories in Washington, which operated alongside the compendial groups. Extensive and exhaustive evaluation of various methods was conducted and followed by the selection of a new and official test procedure affecting all major disciplines in pharmacy, including pharmaceutical and medical professions, regulatory agencies, and drug manufacturers. Each device was tested for its ability to discriminate between subtle variations in dissolution characteristics, reproducibility from test to test, and its adaptability as completely as possible to existing apparatus. Dissolution research continued for over 10 years, during which time the variables affecting consistent and repeatable results were studied.

The first dissolution test procedure was published in NF XIII in 1970 (1). Dissolution test methods were made a part of the specification for five drugs: indomethacin capsules, and acetohexamide, methandrostenalone, methylprednisone, and sulfamethoxyzole tablets. Method 3 was introduced for indomethacin capsules, due to a preestablished data base. This method used a modification of the existing disintegration equipment and has not been extended to other drugs.

The very first dissolution test device included a rotating basket, with the same dimensions as used now. Additionally, the device featured a 0.25-in. shaft, a water bath maintained at 37°C, and a standard 1-L resin flask with a flat or concave indentation at the apex of the bottom. A stirring device capable of maintaining a speed of 100 ±4% rpm could be employed, although other speeds were permitted.

With the establishment of an official dissolution test procedure, a series of collaborative tests were conducted by different laboratories for a variety of drugs. The resulting relative standard deviation and coefficient of variation between laboratories turned out to be wider than had been expected. This initiated the need for the development of dissolution testing standards.

Interlaboratory variability, as well as deviation from regulatory agency reports, can give rise to serious problems. In such situations, where two laboratories are within ±5 percentage points but are above or below the limits, precise definition and control of all equipment and analytical variables is necessary. Accordingly, during the 1970s, a vast amount of research was performed to determine the effect of outside variables. The literature is full of reports and summaries on these investigations (2–4).

The results of these studies provided a foundation for defining and controlling input variables in the current dissolution protocol (5). Additionally, these results stimulated more extensive research into dissolution technique and instrumentation. The compendial and regulatory authorities added restrictions on factors such as vibration, dissolved gas, statistical evaluation of test results, and so on, that influence the dissolution performance of dosage forms. The phenomenon of dissolution of dosage forms is still far from being understood completely. Although we have made significant progress in evaluation techniques, as well as in understanding dissolution, more changes will be implemented in the future to assist in a fuller and more complete understanding of in vitro dissolution behavior.

In Vitro Dissolution Testing

It has long been recognized that solid drugs administered orally are not immediately available to the biological system since they are normally absorbed only from solution (6,7). During development of the dosage form, the in vitro test serves as a guide in estimating the amount of drug released per unit time in a given dissolution medium. The physiological availability of drug dosage forms cannot normally be ascertained by a simple in vitro disintegration test (8). To date, in vitro dissolution tests seem to be the most sensitive and reliable predictors of in vivo performance. Since the dissolution of a dosage form is often the rate-limiting factor determining the physiologic availability of a drug, measurement of the in vitro dissolution rate (or a related parameter) is more likely to offer a meaningful indication of physiological availability (9).

Many devices have been reported for determination of the dissolution rate. The procedures differ in degree rather than in basic principle. The conditions common to most in vitro release tests are:

1. The use of simulated gastric and intestinal fluids at 37°C
2. The use of a device for agitating the element and product at a fixed speed
3. The use of a screen for separating disintegrated particles from the bulk of the product

The time intervals, composition of the fluids, type of agitator, and mesh size of the screen are the usual variants in the methods. Assay for the drug content is performed on the dissolution medium in some procedures; in others, the product is assayed.

All methods involve the concept of providing a renewable solid-liquid interface between the dosage form and the dissolution medium that can be defined and controlled and is thus reproducible. However, it is often difficult to do so in practice. The controlled flow of fluid over a solid makes it necessary to maintain the surface of the solid in a position exposed to a nonaccelerating flow. Often, this requirement is not met, especially for a dosage form, such as a tablet, that migrates above due to the similarity of its density to that of the liquid. The same is observed for a tablet that disintegrates into various buoyant particles that float in the stream.

Most variations in dissolution methods have been devised to address such variables and bring them under control. Unfortunately, some of the methods are applicable only to individual and unique dosage forms and thus are unsatisfactory for others. Additionally, in pursuit of the development of procedures for testing the in vitro release of drug from dosage forms, numerous and diverse attempts have been made to fabricate a dissolution device mimicking the environment offered by the biological system. To date, no in vitro dissolution testing device has been developed that can generally be applied to testing the release rate of various solid dosage forms. The technological development of the various dissolution systems focusing on design and construction is the subject of this chapter. As stated well by Hersey (8): "The number of dissolution rate methods described in the literature is almost equal to the number of workers in the field, where each research team appears to develop its own preferred method." Over 200 different dissolution devices have been reported in the literature in the last two decades. The agencies responsible for setting standards have the task of selecting one, or perhaps two, of these methods for the control of drug dissolution rate from unit solid dosage forms. The purpose of this chapter is to review selected devices representative of the many described in the literature and to report on their relative merits.

CLASSIFICATION OF DISSOLUTION TESTING DEVICES

Dissolution-rate methods may be classified according to a variety of factors. Where the surface area of a pure drug is held constant, the intrinsic dissolution rate of the drug is measured in terms of amount of drug released per unit area and per unit time. With some procedures only intrinsic dissolution rate can be measured, whereas procedures evolved to measure total or apparent dissolution rate in terms of amount of drug released per unit time can normally be modified to measure intrinsic dissolution rate as well.

The agitation intensity offers another alternative for classification, since alteration of the stationary film thickness surrounding the dissolution particles is reflected in a change in the dissolution-rate constant. Thus the methods may be classified depending on the nature of flow of the dissolution medium with respect to the dissolving substrate. Accordingly, the classification will be as follows:

1. Methods exhibiting natural-convection flow characteristics
2. Methods exhibiting forced-convection streamline-flow characteristics
3. Methods exhibiting forced-convection turbulent-flow characteristics

The major difficulty associated with such a classification, however, is that a variety of agitation intensities are available for a single device. Additionally, it must be noted that it is difficult to evaluate the velocity of the dissolving medium relative to the particulate system. Consequently, distinctions between streamline and turbulent flow can best be made by visual observation in the majority of these devices.

Another method of classification is made on the basis of a gradual increase in concentration in the dissolution medium, commonly referred to as a *nonsink condition*, or alternatively, the concentration may be maintained constant or at a low level. The latter method is referred to as a *sink condition*.

Table 3.1 lists and classifies selected dissolution devices currently in use or employed in the past. It should be noted at the outset that dissolution systems

Table 3.1 Classification of In Vitro Dissolution Devices According to the Conditions Offered

Conditions offered	References
Natural-convection nonsink methods	
Klein solvometer method (1932)	10
Nelson hanging pellet method (1958)	12
Levy static disk method (1963)	13
Forced-convection nonsink methods	
Tumbling method (1930)	14
Beaker method+ (1961)	18
Rotating disk method (1962)	26
Particle size method (1965)	25
Oscillating tube method (1966)	24
USP rotating basket[a] (1969)	36
Magnetic basket apparatus (1972)	41
Modified USP basket[a] (1973)	43
Rotating filter stationary basket+ (1973–1974)	44, 45
USP paddle apparatus[a] (1978)	37
Forced-convection sink devices[b]	
Wurster–Polli adsorption method (1961, 1964)	82
Partition method (1967)	86
Dialysis method (1967–1968)	51, 88, 89
Rotating flask apparatus (1970)	50, 90
Continuous-flow/flow-through methods	
Pernaroweski et al. (1968)	93
Langenbucher method (1969)[c]	105
Baun and Walker (1969)	56
Tingstad and Riegelman (1970)	59
Modified column apparatus (1972)[c]	62
Cakiryildiz et al. (1975)	75
Takenaka et al. (1980)	115
Deutsche Arzneimittel Codex (DAC) method (1984)	106
Special methods	
Tape method (1965)	123
Pressure-controlled apparatus (1979)	128
Perturbed augular correlations (1981)	129

[a] Official methods.

[b] In addition to those listed, apparatus listed under "forced-convection nonsink methods" marked with (+) could be included in this category with minor modifications.

[c] These methods can also be included in continuous-flow apparatus.

that are minor modifications of the ones listed are excluded from Table 3.1. Unquestionably, some dissolution devices can be categorized in more than one class.

NATURAL-CONVECTION NONSINK DEVICES

The dosage form in natural-convection methods is positioned in such a manner that the surrounding dissolution medium is continuously replaced by fresh medium, due to density differences. The following three methods can be classified in this category.

Klein Solvometer Method (1932)

This method employs an instrument called a solvometer, consisting essentially of a carrier device (boat) immersed in a dissolution medium and surmounted by a float. This technique was originally developed by Klein (10) and later employed by Elliott (11). A measuring bar extends from the float above the surface into a calibrated scale. When the dosage form is placed in the "boat," the scale bar moves downward to its lowest position initially. As the dosage form dissolves, it rises gradually. Consequently, the loss in weight of the dosage form can be monitored continuously by reading the scale directly. A schematic representation of this device is shown in Fig. 3.1.

Although the scientific rationale for this method is intriguing, this device suffers from two major disadvantages. First, this technique does not permit evaluation of dosage form that disintegrates. Second, the effects of concentration of drug dissolved on both rate of dissolution and on the measuring system are not accounted for.

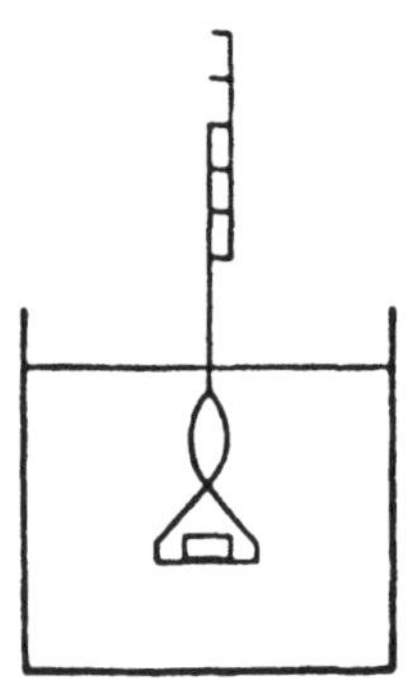

Fig. 3.1 Schematic illustration of a natural-convection dissolution testing method: solvometer device.

Nelson Hanging Pellet Method (1958)

This method, developed by Nelson (12), consists of mounting the dosage form on an aluminum strip. This assembly is, in turn, mounted on an arm of a balance that is maintained perfectly still during the dissolution process. The dosage form is positioned on the aluminum strip by applying wax on the strip. This results in restricting dissolution to one face of the dosage form. Consequently, this method can be employed for the determination of intrinsic dissolution rate of the dosage form. To do so, it is necessary to compress the dosage form, such as a tablet, under extreme pressures (e.g., 50,000 psi on a 0.5-in.-diameter tablet) to prevent disintegration and maintain a constant surface area by reducing the permeability of the compact. A representative diagram of this device is presented in Fig. 3.2.

The entire assembly is maintained at a constant temperature. Additionally, to negate the effect of the increasing concentration of the solute, only the loss of the first 30 to 40 mg from the dosage form (tablet) is measured, employing a large volume of dissolution medium. This method has serious practical limitations.

Levy Static Disk Method (1963)

This device, developed by Levy, consists of an acrylic holder over which the dosage form is mounted (13). This assembly is inserted through a rubber stopper into a known volume of dissolution medium, normally 25 mL of simulated gastric fluid (0.1 *N* HCl). The inverted vial is then placed in an incubator at 37°C, the vials removed, and the solution (dissolved drug in dissolution medium) analyzed at specified time intervals. A schematic diagram of this method is given in Fig. 3.3. It must be noted that this method is the static version of the rotating disk method, which will be discussed in forthcoming sections.

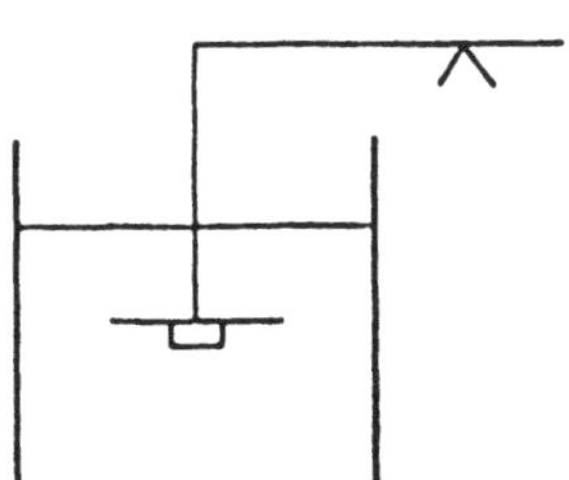

Fig. 3.2 Schematic illustration of a natural-convection dissolution testing method: hanging pellet device.

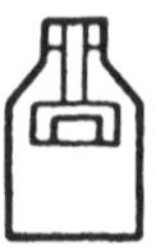

Fig. 3.3 Schematic illustration of a natural-convection dissolution testing method: static disk device.

This method is amenable to measurement of the intrinsic dissolution rate of the dosage form provided that it is positioned such that only one surface is exposed to the dissolution medium. The effect of the concentration on the dissolution rate [see Eq. (1.1)] is ignored. Additionally, it is assumed that the surface area of the dissolving surface is constant, despite some evidence of jolting that is occasionally observed (13).

FORCED-CONVECTION NONSINK DEVICES

These devices incorporate various forms of agitating assemblies that induce relative motion, such as stirring, rotation, or oscillation, between the dissolving particulate system and the dissolving medium. Over a dozen such devices can be included in this category. However, a few such devices representing this class are described in the following sections.

Tumbling Method (1930)

As early as 1930, Wruble (14) employed test tubes containing the dosage form (tablet) in the dissolution medium clamped to a revolving drum rotated at 6 to 12 rpm in a water bath at 37°C. The tubes were removed at various time intervals and the solution assayed for drug content. Figure 3.4 illustrates the schematics of this device. Souder and Ellenbogen (15) used a similar procedure (as described later) in which 90-mL bottles containing the tablet in 60 mL of dissolution medium were rotated at 40 rpm at 37°C. In a similar technique employed by Higuchi and co-workers (16,17), the rotational speed was maintained at 6 rpm.

Levy Method or Beaker Method (1961)

Levy and Hayes (18) applied to tablets the apparatus first used by Parrott et al. (19) for determination of the dissolution rate of pure benzoic acid spheres. The dissolution assembly consists of a 400-mL beaker immersed in a constant-temperature bath adjusted to 37±0.1°C. A three-blade 5-cm-diameter polyethylene stirrer is accurately centered and rotated at 59 rpm, as shown in Fig. 3.5. The tablet is gently dropped down the side of the beaker and samples

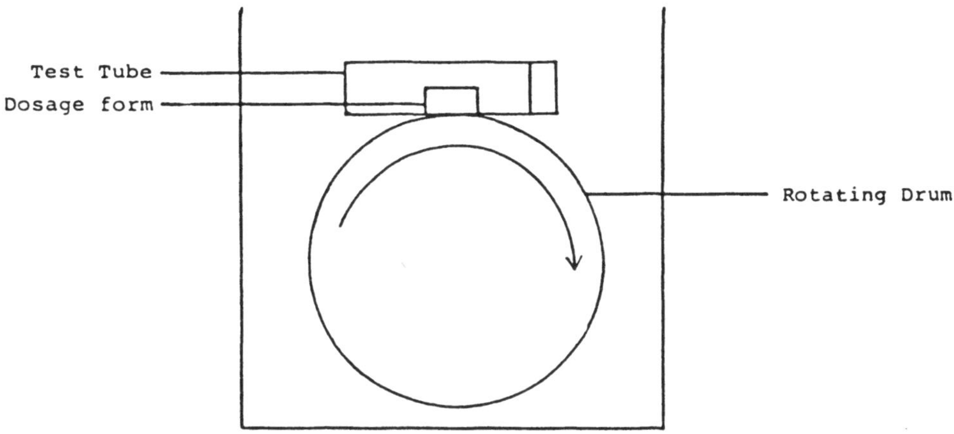

Fig. 3.4 Schematic illustration of a forced-convection nonsink dissolution testing method: tumbling device.

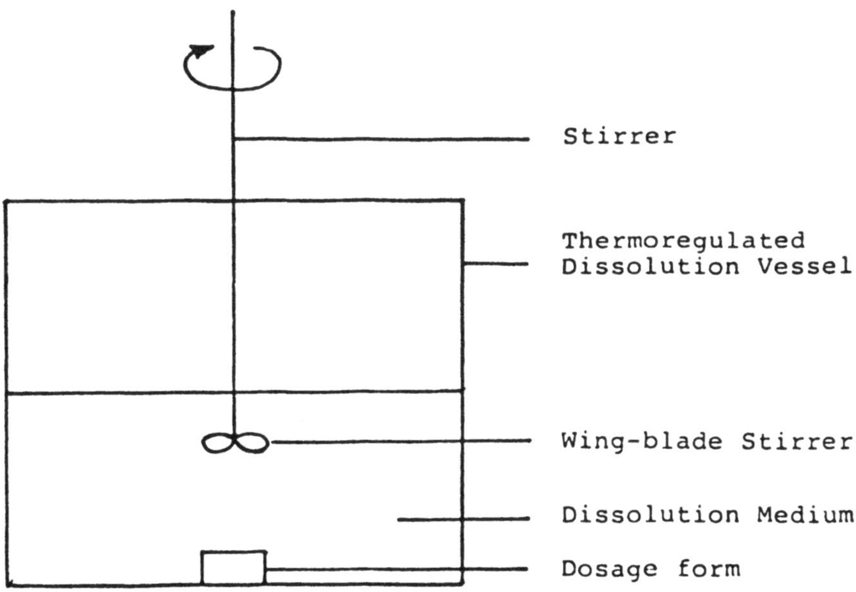

Fig. 3.5 Schematic illustration of a forced-convection nonsink dissolution testing method: Levy apparatus or beaker device.

of the solution are withdrawn for analysis. The dimensions of the beaker, stirrer, and immersion are carefully controlled so that the solution quickly equilibrates without disturbing the tablet, which upon disintegration covers an area of 1 to 2 cm^2 at the base of the beaker. This method has been adopted by various investigators (20–22) for intrinsic dissolution rate determinations. Sheffer and Higuchi (23) employed an Erlenmeyer flask and a magnetic stirrer. Broadbent et al. (24) used a shaker for stirring, and Edmundson and Lees (25) have determined dissolution by measuring particle size changes. These systems are described later in the chapter.

The inherent simplicity in the design of the apparatus and the ease of control of experimental conditions lead to its wide use in the determination of dissolution rates. However, the system does not lend itself to characterization of intrinsic dissolution rates of dosage forms per se.

Rotating Disk Method (1962)

One of the more accurate of the earlier methodologies used to determine the intrinsic dissolution rate of a solid dosage form is the rotating disk method. Levy and Sahli (26) have described the use of plexiglass holders that expose a single surface of the tablet to the dissolution medium. The studies of variation in intrinsic dissolution rate with media, temperature, and so on, are most conveniently performed from surfaces whose areas remain constant (27).

Flat-faced, 1/2-inch-diameter tablets of pure drug were prepared by means of a specially modified hydraulic press and mounted on plexiglass holders. The holder is attached to a metal shaft whose stirring speed is precisely controlled. The plexiglass holder is immersed in 500 mL of dissolution medium maintained at 37 $\pm$ 1°C. The holder is immersed into a depth of 1 in. in the dissolution medium and rotated at a speed of 555 rpm. A schematic diagram of this device is depicted in Fig. 3.6. The volume of the dissolution medium is kept constant and the tablet in the holder is weighed before and after the assay.

It is frequently desirable to measure dissolution rates of a given drug at different rates of agitation in order to fully characterize the drug's dissolution behavior and to elucidate the mechanism governing the rate of dissolution (28). Using a special assembly, Levy and Tanski (29) demonstrated nonvariability in dissolution rate at low speeds of rotation. Dissolution-rate experiments at speeds as low as 4 rpm and of 6 h duration can be carried out without measurable variation in rotational speed. This assembly offers precision speed control, a wide range of rotation rates, shaft concentricity, and constant speed over prolonged periods of time. The assembly is particularly useful for dissolution rate studies at very low rates of rotation. Furthermore, this apparatus is useful for the determination of intrinsic dissolution rates, which may be

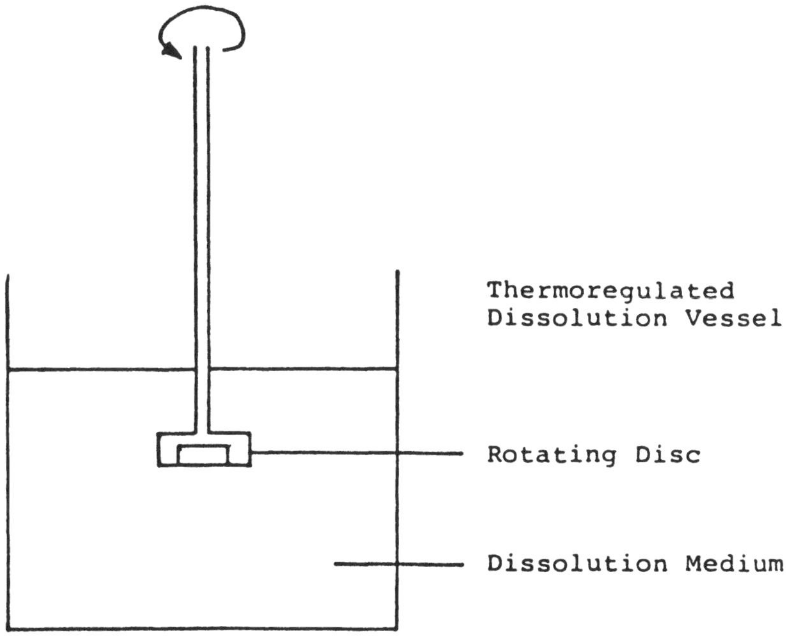

Fig. 3.6 Schematic illustration of a forced-convection nonsink dissolution testing method: rotating disk device.

insufficient in itself as regards its multiple use in dissolution-rate measurements.

Particle-Size Method (1965)

Edmundson and Lees (25) modified the beaker-type method to induce vigorous agitation to suspend the particles that were undergoing dissolution. They measured the changes in particle size employing a Coulter counter during the dissolution of crystalline hydrocortisone acetate. A correction factor was introduced in the Noyes–Whitney equation [see Eq. (1.1)] to calculate the amount of dissolved drug. This parameter, coupled with knowledge of the surface area from the particle-size data, enabled complete evaluation of the dissolution-rate constant. A representative sketch of this device is shown in Fig. 3.7.

The utility of particle-size data or surface area measurement for complete elucidation of kinetics of dissolution—for disintegrating dosage forms in particular—cannot be denied. However, for routine dissolution studies, the advantages of chemical analysis outweigh those of particle-size analysis. Additionally, this method is not suitable for dosage forms.

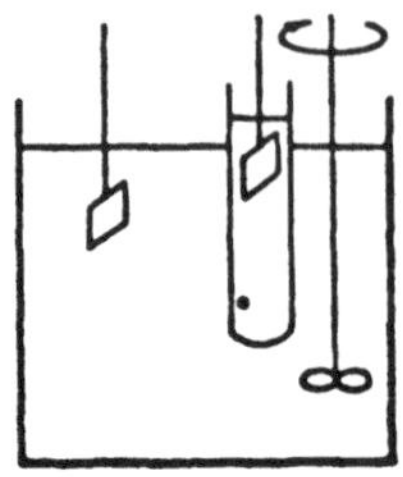

Fig. 3.7 Schematic illustration of a forced-convection nonsink dissolution testing method: Edmunson and Lees device.

Oscillating Tube Method (1966)

Broadbent et al. (24) report that use of an oscillating tube for dissolution-rate studies is a logical step from the official disintegration test. They employed the BP (*British Pharmacopoeia*) disintegration apparatus for determination of dissolution. One tablet was used in place of the usual five and the dissolution medium was 200 mL of 0.1 *N* HCl. When this volume was reduced to 140 mL, a considerable increase in agitation intensity was observed, resulting in an increase in dissolution rates. A schematic diagram of this apparatus is shown in Fig. 3.8. Various investigators have employed this method with minor modifications (30–34).

The major advantage of this method is that it offers simultaneous measurement of disintegration time and dissolution rate. Additionally, it employs readily available apparatus. However, Schroeter and Wagner (35) suggested that employment of this apparatus yields results that can raise serious doubt about the validity of a uniform disintegration test.

It must be noted that this method is useful only for determination of total dissolution rate, since the extreme agitation and abrasion caused by the mesh do not enable maintenance of a constant surface area. Additional limitations

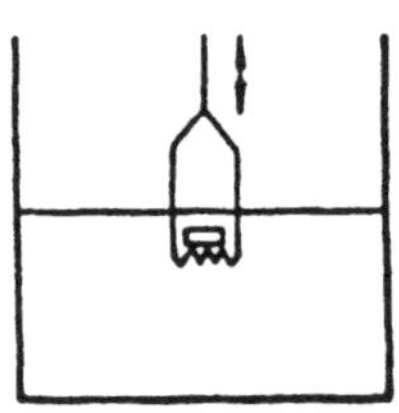

Fig. 3.8 Schematic illustration of a forced-convection nonsink dissolution testing method: oscillating tube device.

are the increasing solute concentration, lack of reproducibility and constancy of the oscillations, and the effect of dissolution medium volume and container dimensions in the intensity of agitation.

USP Rotating Basket Apparatus (1969)

Figure 3.9 illustrates the USP rotating basket apparatus, originally reported by Richter et al. (36) and standardized further by Cox et al. (37). USP lists the specifications of various parts used in its construction. The basket is centered within 2 mm of the centerline of the vessel. The rotating basket is made of 10-mesh stainless steel approximately 2.2 cm in diameter and 2.8 cm high. A lid with a center porthole and other portholes is placed over the vessel. The rotation of the shaft is maintained at 100 rpm. The temperature of the medium is maintained at 37 ±0.5°C. Aliquots should be withdrawn midway between the surface of the dissolution medium and the bottom of the vessel and midway between the cylindrical edge of the basket and the wall of the vessel. This specification was set up by the National Center for Drug Analysis in consideration of nonconformance of the specifications set by the USP. Modifications of this apparatus have been the subject of intensive study by the Joint USP–NF Panel on Physiological Availability and is designated as method I in the compendia.

Cook et al. (38) designed a stainless-steel wire basket in a Lucite frame. The basket was cylindrical in shape, 2.5 cm in diameter, and 6.5 cm long. The basket was positioned in a jar containing 2 L of dissolution medium and stirred by a T-shaped glass stirrer rotated at 150 rpm. This apparatus was also studied by the Joint USP–NF Panel; however, due to a lack of reproducibility, this method was not considered further.

Basket wobble can be created by a wobbling shaft, a bent shaft, or by the basket bottom being out of line with the top of the basket. The shaft or basket should be replaced if the wobbling is significant. Baskets with burrs or defects should not be used. Each basket must be individually set to a position 2.5 cm from the bottom of its vessel and the vessel should be marked to reproduce the positioning of the basket.

USP specifies the use of six baskets at a time (39). Depending on the type of apparatus, either one basket is lowered in the specified dissolution medium at one time or all six baskets are lowered simultaneously. The basket should remain in motion while the analyst is withdrawing aliquots at specific intervals for the measurement of drug content until the end of the dissolution period. The sampling intervals are initiated from the time of lowering of the basket in the medium.

The location of the dosage form in the stainless-steel woven basket should be noted immediately when the test is begun. Tablets should be at the bottom

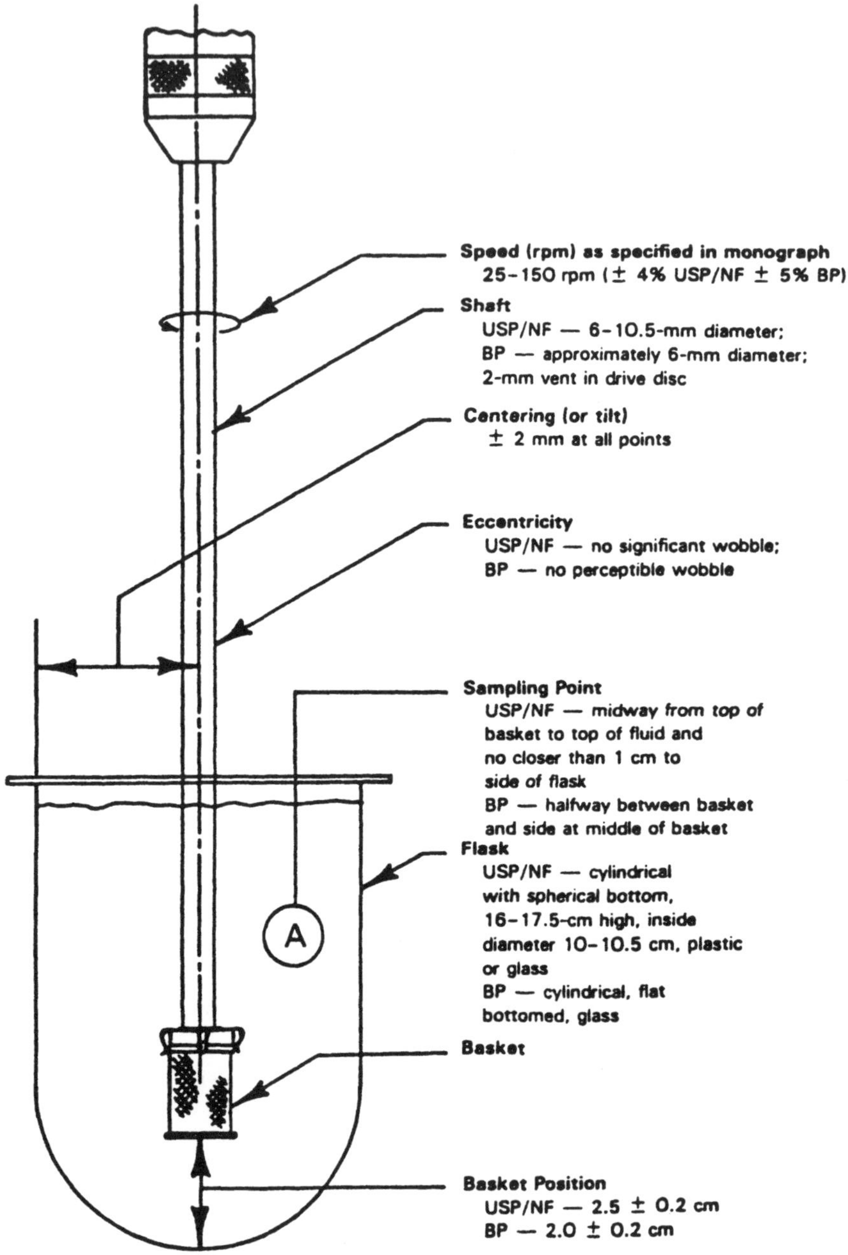

Fig. 3.9 Schematic illustration of a forced-convection nonsink dissolution testing method: USP rotating basket apparatus or USP dissolution test method I.

of the basket; capsules should be near the top of the basket. Variability in the location of the dosage form in the basket in repetitive tests may lead to erroneous results. It has been observed, for example, that a tablet may occasionally be suspended on an air bubble directly under the disk by which the basket is dipped. Results for such suspended tablets are usually considerably lower than those for the tablets located at the bottom of the basket.

Magnetic Basket Dissolution Apparatus (1972)

Different dissolution rates from different dosage forms (e.g., tablets and capsules of the same strength) are a probability even when emanating from the same manufacturer (40). A modified Levy beaker apparatus is constructed as shown in Fig. 3.10 (41,42). It consists of a 800-mL beaker with an apparatus that provides for reproducible and precise placement of the dosage form (tablet or capsule). Exact placement of the basket is ensured by attaching a magnetic bar to the outer bottom of the beaker and affixing a second magnet to the cylindrical basket. The second magnet, with attached basket, orients itself with exact reproducibility. The stainless-steel wire basket is 50 mm long and has an

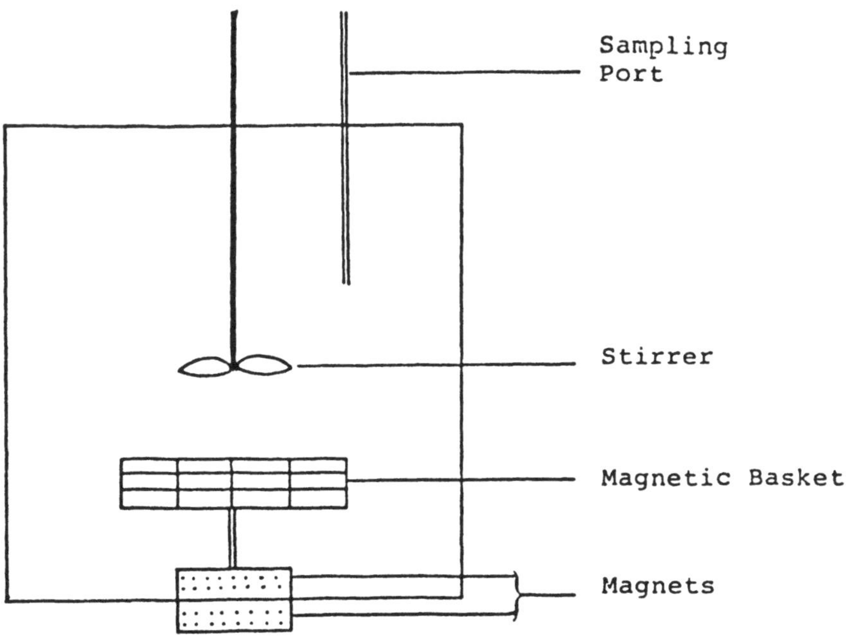

Fig. 3.10 Schematic illustration of a forced-convection nonsink dissolution testing method: magnetic basket dissolution device.

inner diameter of 11 mm for capsules and 15 mm for tablets. An epoxy resin and hardener, inert in acidic and basic environment, is used in construction of the magnetic basket. Each cylindrical basket is equipped with 8-mesh hinged door openings at the ends of the cylinder. The dosage form under investigation is placed in the dry basket and the basket, together with the magnetic assembly, is placed in the dissolution medium. The rate of stirring is electronically controlled at 60 rpm by a constant-speed, torque-controlled unit coupled to a servomotor generator. A three-bladed propeller, having a stirring diameter of 51 mm, with blades set at a 60° angle to each other and 45° from vertical orientation, provides agitation. The blades have a diameter of 18 mm and are attached to a shaft 7 mm in diameter.

The dissolution container, containing 600 mL of dissolution medium, is immersed in a constant-temperature jar at 37 ±0.05° C and allowed to equilibrate. During each run the propeller is centered in the basket and immersed to a depth of 41 mm. Electrodes are immersed to a depth of 27 mm and are 7 mm away from the wall of the beaker. On equilibration, the contents of the dissolution container adjusted to the required pH are introduced, following which the magnetic basket, together with the dosage form to be examined, is immersed.

The magnetic basket allows reproducible positioning of either a capsule or tablet in a hydrodynamic system such that the dissolution of the two different dosage forms can be studied employing the same parameters. This modification eliminates the possibility of "floating" capsules. However, the larger inner diameter of the basket does not give reproducible results for capsules, simply because they can assume more than one position within a larger basket. This assembly lends itself to an automated analysis system as well as to manual sampling. With certain reservations, the system can be used to differentiate dissolution rates between products.

Modified USP Basket Apparatus (1973)

The purpose of the basket in the USP–NF apparatus presumably is to hold the tablet or capsule in a fixed position during the disintegration process. In essence, the distance of the tablet from the center of rotation is fixed within small limits. Usually, disintegration of a tablet is involved during the dissolution test. The flow of solvent through the basket must be sufficient to disperse the tablet components and sweep them through the openings in the basket screen.

Consequently, a configurational change was introduced in the standard USP–NF rotating basket apparatus. It has been reported to exhibit better flow of the solvent through the basket (43). The stainless-steel stirring rod of the apparatus is bent at a 90° angle just above the basket to yield an L-shaped configuration, as shown in Fig. 3.11. This modification gave a maximum stirring radius of 6.1 cm for a tablet. Later, a holder of Teflon was designed for the tablet. A cylinder of 24-mesh stainless-steel screen is seam welded to fit tightly over the Teflon holder. This device ensures that the tablet is held at a fixed distance from the center of rotation. Unquestionably, the increase in dissolution rate can be attributed to the greater flow of dissolution fluid over the tablet. The major disadvantage of this modified USP–NF basket or bent basket is the wandering of the dosage form within the basket at a lower stirring speed of 60 rpm. However, inexpensive and simple construction of this device, in addition to the dual functionability of the holder (i.e., holding the dosage form and stirring), are major advantages of this apparatus.

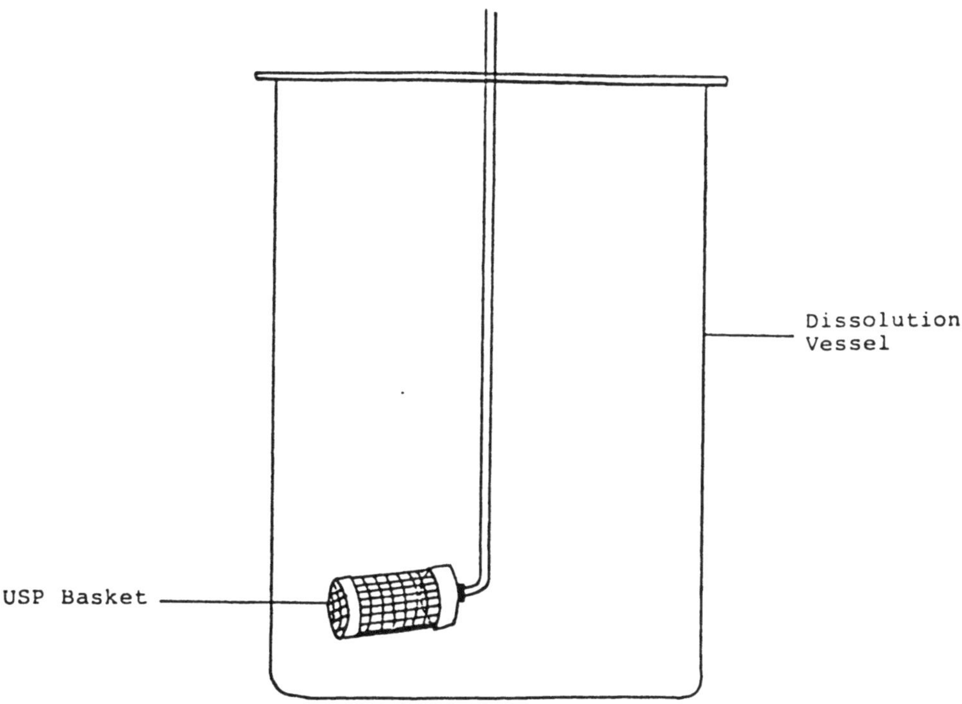

Fig. 3.11 Schematic illustration of a forced-convection nonsink dissolution testing method: modified USP basket apparatus.

Rotating Filter–Stationary Basket Apparatus (1973–1974)

The basic design of the rotating filter–stationary basket apparatus includes a stationary sample basket, a large-volume fluid container, and a rotating filter assembly with an external variable-speed magnetic stirrer (44). The thermo-jacketed glass flask has a volume capacity of 1.5 L of dissolution medium and a removable plexiglass cover. It has several ports: one port for the sample, one for the glass tube meant for withdrawal of the aliquot from the rotating filter, another for the return of dissolution fluid from the spectrophotometer flow cell, and a fourth for the thermometer.

The basket has a 12-mesh screen, in contrast to a 40-mesh screen. It is kept stationary, in contrast to the official method. The basket is held at the same position during each dissolution run, due to the positioning by the plexiglass cover. The basket is held at 2 to 5 cm from the bottom of the flask.

The solid dosage form is introduced in the basket at the start of dissolution. This assembly is centered in the dissolution flask. The level of this assembly can be varied by changing the position of the glass tube. Basically, the assembly consists of a filter head, bottom flange, cylindrical filter with flexible gasket, and dynamic seal (Fig. 3.12).

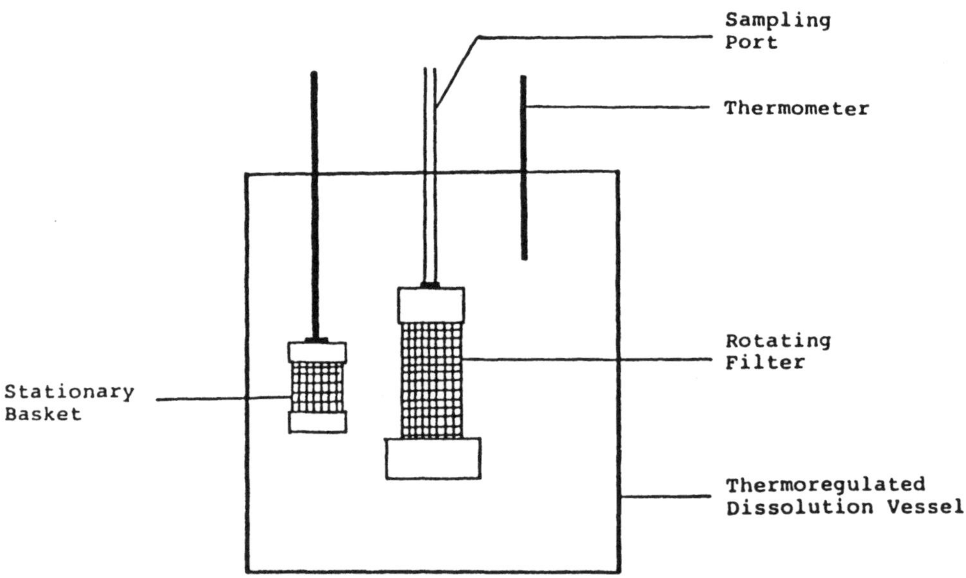

Fig. 3.12 Schematic illustration of a forced-convection nonsink dissolution testing method: rotating filter–stationary basket device.

Rotation of the filter provides variable intensity of mild laminar liquid agitation. It permits continuous filtration of the samples of dissolution fluid and rotates at a fixed speed throughout the experiment. The test is performed by suspending the solid dosage form in the basket and introducing it into the dissolution medium. Filtered fluid samples to be analyzed are continuously withdrawn through the glass tube at a flow rate of 40 mL/min.

A continuous-flow system to maintain sink conditions has been reported for the rotating filter–stationary basket method (45). Powdered drugs are tested by dispersing a weighed amount of the sample in a small volume of dissolution medium and then transferring it to the bulk medium. This assembly prevents excessive abrasion and wear of the sample due to mechanical impacts, which are common to the official method.

This assembly serves as a liquid agitation device as well as an efficient fluid sampling system. The rotation of filter prevents hydrodynamic plugging. Its relatively mild agitation conditions, retainment of the microenvironment of the sample, and accurate positioning of the sample are added advantages.

USP Paddle Method (1978)

Another official method is the USP paddle method (30). The paddle methodology specifies that the paddle shaft be centered within 0.2 cm of the centerline of the vessel. The shaft should rotate without discernible wobble, and the bottom of the paddle should be 2.5 ±0.2 cm from the bottom of the vessel (Fig. 3.13). There should be a minimal movement of the solid dosage form under the paddle until disintegration occurs. A cover plate with a center porthole and other holes is used. Shaft rotation is often maintained at 100 rpm and the temperature is maintained at 37 ±0.5°C. Aliquots should be drawn from a point midway between the upper edge of the paddle and the surface of the medium and midway between the wall of the vessel and the stirrer shaft. The point of sampling changes if the volume of the dissolution medium in the vessel is decreased. The geometry of the container and shaft must satisfy the compendial requirements. The paddle shaft should be vertically centered in the vessel, which should, in turn, be on a horizontal plane. It is imperative to employ apparatus that avoids paddle wobble.

Ideally, the lower portion of each vessel should be hemispherical. Vessels should be uniform with respect to their weight, inside diameter, and inside curvature. Statistically significant differences in dissolution rates have been reported when the same product was tested in different vessels.

The introduction of solid dosage units in the dissolution medium is staggered at 1- or 2-min intervals. Thus, sufficient time is allowed for withdrawal of the aliquot, filtration, and the replacement of the fresh media. On the other hand, all the paddles must be introduced in the dissolution simultaneously. USP specifies the use of six pieces of apparatus at a time.

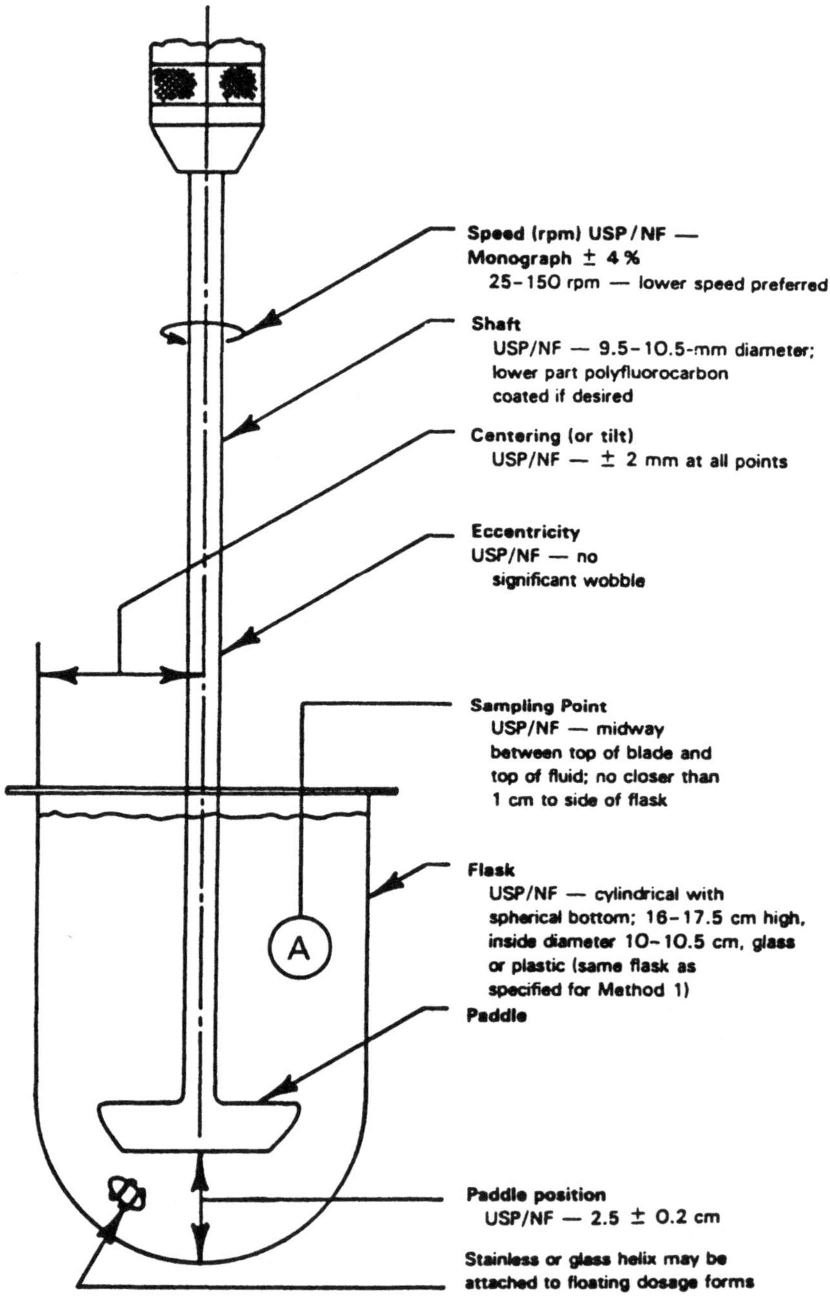

Fig. 3.13 Schematic illustration of a forced-convection nonsink dissolution testing method: USP paddle apparatus or USP dissolution test method II.

In this official method, the sample container itself serves as a liquid stirring device. Under these conditions, there can be excessive abrasion and wear of the sample due to mechanical impacts with the container surface. This adversely affects its microenvironment. Although this assembly is simple in itself, the aforementioned aspect should not be overlooked.

FORCED-CONVECTION SINK DEVICES

In the design of a reliable in vitro dissolution test model that can positively characterize the role of the dissolution process in the bioavailability of drug, it is essential that the model be capable of simulating test conditions that are likely to prevail during the in vivo dissolution process. One such condition is the maintenance of nearly perfect sink conditions during in vitro dissolution-rate determinations (i.e., the drug concentration in the dissolution medium does not exceed 10 to 20% of its solubility). This condition is required since in a dissolution rate-limited absorption process, there is no appreciable buildup of drug concentration in gastrointestinal fluids. They act as an infinite sink. Consequently, it has been suggested that unless similar sink conditions are embodied in the in vitro dissolution test model, in vitro results will bear little relation, if any at all, to the in vivo observations (46,47).

The types of systems employed for maintaining sink conditions during the dissolution process are (45) (a) fixed fluid volume, (b) multiple phase, and (c) continuous fluid flow. In a fixed fluid volume system, dissolution studies are performed in a finite volume of aqueous dissolution medium, a volume sufficient to maintain solution concentration below 10 to 20% of drug solubility.

Simplicity in the design and operation of such systems has probably favored its extensive use in a number of dissolution test methods (18,35,48–54), including those recognized by the official compendia (39). These systems, however, are unsuitable for relatively insoluble and/or high-dosage drugs, due to the practical limits up to which large fluid volumes can be conveniently used in a dissolution test.

Upon dissolution into an aqueous medium in a multiple-phase system, the drug is either partitioned into a water-immiscible organic phase or adsorbed onto a solid adsorbent. Both approaches may be employed in the dissolution-rate determinations of all drugs regardless of their solubility and dosage strength, since they provide sink conditions by constant removal of dissolved drug from the dissolution medium. Additional parameters, such as rate of partitioning and adsorption, selection of proper organic phase or adsorbent, and miscibility, often complicate these systems. The importance of selecting the proper type of organic phase in a multiphase dissolution test method has been pointed out (55).

A continuous fluid flow system provides a relatively simple and convenient test system applicable for the determination of dissolution rates of all drugs under sink conditions, regardless of their solubility and dosage strength. The sink conditions can be maintained by constant removal of the dissolved drug from the dissolution medium, facilitated by continuous elimination of the filtered dissolution medium from the dissolution chamber and simultaneous addition of fresh solvent into the chamber. Continuous filtration of effluent dissolution medium is performed by wire mesh screen or other similar static filter elements. Filtration through such a static filter may introduce analytical errors in the dissolution-rate results, due to the occurrence of filter clogging, retarding fluid flow rate and escape of solid particles into the filtrate. During the past several years, numerous continuous-flow methods, with or without cumulating reservoirs, have been reported (56–81).

Wurster-Polli Adsorption Method (1961, 1964)

Wurster and Polli (82,83) described methods for measuring dissolution rates identical to that described by Parrott et al. (84). However, they employed Norite A charcoal or bentonite in the dissolution medium to adsorb the dissolved drug, such as benzoic acid. This method can pose problems if the adsorbent modifies the viscosity, since the diffusion-controlled dissolution process is influenced by changes in viscosity (85). A diagrammatic representation of the apparatus they employed is shown in Fig. 3.14.

Partition Method (1967)

Gibaldi and Feldman (86) were able to remove solute from the dissolution medium continuously by employing an organic phase into which the drug under investigation would almost completely partition. Essentially, this method consists of a beaker and stirrer assembly, with a less dense layer of organic phase above the dissolution medium, as shown in Fig. 3.15. As pointed out earlier, to employ this method successfully, it is crucial to select the right type of organic phase.

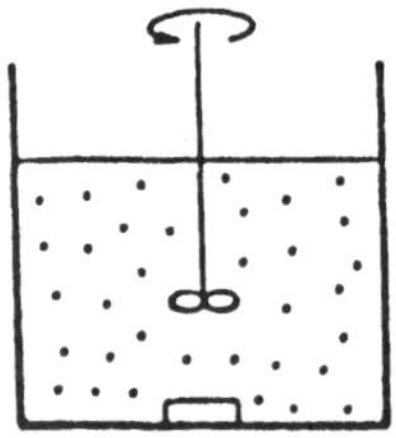

Fig. 3.14 Schematic illustration of a forced-convection sink dissolution testing method: adsorption device by Wurster and Polli.

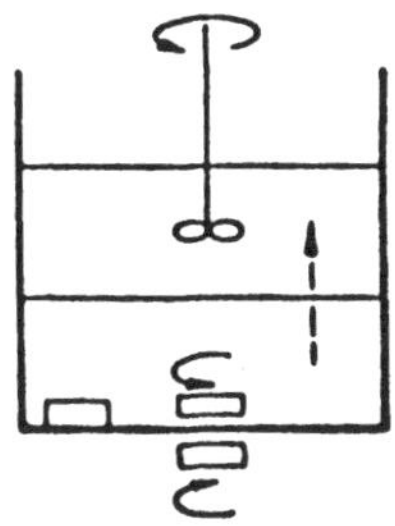

Fig. 3.15 Schematic illustration of a forced-convection sink dissolution testing method: partition method by Gibaldi and Feldman.

Dialysis Method (1968)

The use of dialysis membrane has been advocated by several workers as a device for obtaining the solute concentration without disturbing the dissolution process or the dissolution medium. Depending on the apparatus employed, it is possible to carry out dissolution studies under sink conditions. The choice of the membrane is important, for it must have a short equilibrium time and adequate physical strength and retain solid particles. It is apparent that the rate at which material appears on the distal surface of the dialysis membrane should not be a function of dialysis rate, but of dissolution rate. Simplistically, within such an in vitro model, dissolution must be the rate-limiting step. However, this point appears to have been avoided or gone unrecognized by some investigators.

Marlowe and Shangraw (87) employed a dialysis cell that consisted of dissolution medium on one side of the dialysis membrane and the dosage form on the other. This assembly was rotated at 15 rpm and samples were withdrawn from the distal end at appropriate intervals. The disadvantages inherent in the unusual, discontinuous operation of the cell were overcome by Barzilay and Hersey (88), who developed an automated dialysis method.

The method described by Ferrari and Khoury (51) involves the use of a baffled rotating round-bottomed flask at 37°C to provide a "sloshing" action similar, it is claimed, to the agitation received by the dosage form in the stomach. The filtered contents of the flask are continuously circulated through a dialyzer maintained at 37°C. The recipient stream is continuously analyzed for the amount of drug content, while the donor stream is returned to the dissolution flask. Since the pH of the recipient stream may be different from that of the donor stream, gradual pH changes may be effected. The recipient stream could also consist of an organic phase. By employing these modifications, this device could approximate physiological conditions.

Krogerus et al. (89) employed a disintegration type of assembly but replaced the disintegration cell with an oscillating dialysis cell. Samples are removed from the bath into which the cell oscillates, for assay at appropriate time intervals. Common to most dialysis cell methods, the changing diffusion gradients make interpretation of the dialysis process difficult. These different types of dialysis methods used for dissolution testing of dosage forms are illustrated in Figs. 3.16.

Rotating Flask Apparatus (1970)

Several researchers have described methods that depend, either in whole or in part, on an alternative approach to the stirring of the dissolution fluid. The principle of a slowly rotating container has been utilized by other workers. Ferrari and Khoury (51) employed an inclined flask, the walls of which were indented in a regular manner. As the flask is slowly rotated, as described earlier, the dissolution medium is subjected to a "sloshing" action, supposedly similar to that to which fluids in the gastrointestinal (GI) tract are subjected.

Gibaldi and Weintraub (50) described a rotating flask apparatus in early 1970 and later published a paper emphasizing what they claim to be the advantages of this method (90). This method uses a spherical glass flask fitted with a sampling port and capable of being rotated about its horizontal axis. This assembly is suspended in a water bath maintained at 37°C. The philosophy underlying the development of this apparatus is best described by the authors. For tablets and other solid dosage forms, low intensities of agitation are highly desirable and more likely to allow distinguishing formulations and products and correlating results with in vivo data. The method effectively precludes

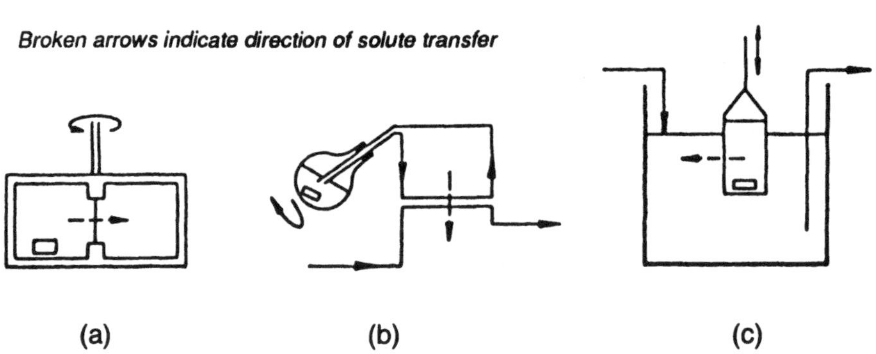

Fig. 3.16 Schematic illustration of a forced-convection sink dissolution testing method: dialysis devices using (a) rotating cell, (b) rotating flask and external dialysis, and (c) oscillating cell.

aggregation of particles at the bottom of the container (mound formation), which is considered to be physiologically unrealistic.

One of the primary disadvantages of this method is that its design makes sampling and automation somewhat difficult. As a result, this apparatus cannot be employed for routine control tests. Various designs of the rotating flask method operating on essentially the same principle are shown in Fig. 3.17.

FLOW-THROUGH DEVICES

There are obvious and insurmountable limitations to the official dissolution testing apparatus (the rotating basket and paddle methods) concerning maintenance of sink conditions for drugs that saturate rapidly in large volumes of medium. For slightly soluble drugs, the limited volume of 1000 mL becomes critical with regard to the sink requirements; hence larger dissolution containers have been proposed (e.g., 4000 mL) (91). A solution would be the continuous replacement of fluid, as originally proposed by Munzel (92) as the "half-change" method and by Pernarowski et al. (93) and Shah and Ochs (45) in their "continuous-flow" design (continuous-flow designs are discussed later in this chapter). However, these are complicated procedures, and the interpretation of a dissolution system with large flow and large holdup volume is rather complex (94).

The model character of the test requires, at least in special cases, a change of pH (i.e., a change of fluid). This presents problems with all so-called "basket" methods. Another problem is associated with dissolution testing of other dosage forms. Although the USP apparatus was adapted for testing of suppositories (45,95,96), even conventional hard-gelatin capsules present problems due to clogging (97,98). The inhomogeneity of the solution in the rotating basket (99,100) and poor reproducibility (74, 101, 102) led to enhanced use of

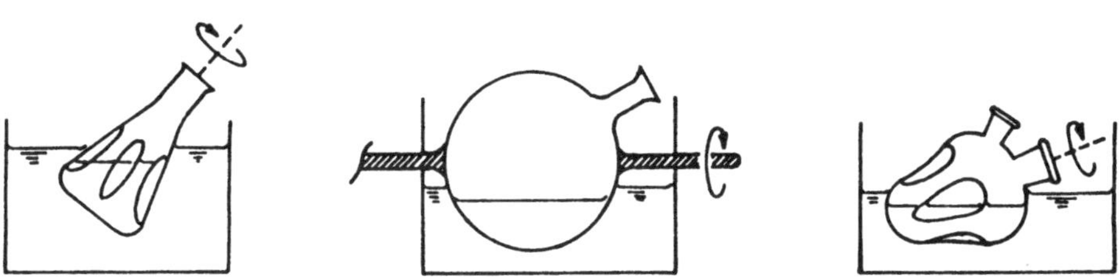

(a) (b) (c)

Fig. 3.17 Schematic illustration of a forced-convection sink dissolution testing method: rotating flask devices by (a) Ferrari and Khoury, (b) Gibaldi and Weintraub, and (c) Koch.

the paddle apparatus for testing tablets and capsules. With the paddle apparatus, "sinkers" are necessary to avoid initial floating, but no agreement on a suitable design could be achieved and poor reproducibility still exists (103,104).

The flow-through model of a dissolution system effectively solves the problem of nonsink conditions by supplying an unlimited quantity of fresh dissolution medium. The flow-through dissolution testing model has been proposed by many, but has been studied most extensively by Langenbucher (105). This method, which is designed to test the dissolution characteristics of a wide range of dosage forms, is becoming more accepted by the pharmaceutical hierarchy. It has already been incorporated into the Deutsche Arzneimittel Codex (DAC) (106). The system has not been used extensively in the United States, but its obvious advantages, particularly for drugs with low solubility, suggests that it may be used universally in the future.

In principle it works as follows: A sample is restrained in a small-volume cell and subjected to a stream of dissolution media. The special pulsating movement of the piston pump obviates the need for further stirring and/or shaking elements. The flow-through system caters not only to the determination of the dissolution rate of tablets and sugar-coated tablets, but also for suppositories, soft-gelatin capsules, powders, and granules.

In addition to the maintenance of sink conditions, flow-through systems offer distinct advantages, particularly in comparison with the more conventional USP paddle method:

1. The method permits the convenience of changing pH during dissolution testing.
2. There are only a small number of apparatus parameters that affect the test and have to be standardized.
3. The method has built-in filtration.
4. The method eliminates most of the problems of sample position in the stream of the dissolution medium.
5. The method offers ideal hydrodynamic conditions for mild agitation, homogeneity, and a mathematically definable solvent (dissolution medium) flow pattern.
6. The test can be run as either an open or a closed system.

In its typical form, the flow-through model is characterized by a vertical cylindrical cell of small dimension and volume. The dissolution medium flows through the cell from bottom to top of the cell, achieved by means of an external pump. A filtration device at the top of the cell quantitatively retains all undissolved material and provides a clear solution for subsequent assay. Additional devices for temperature control, positioning of the specimen in the cell, and eventual adjusting of liquid agitation are incorporated at various points in the design. Depending on whether the effluent returns to the source or not decides the nature of the system, open or closed. The flow-through system can be made to approximate the closed stirring system by returning the effluent to the source and maintaining the source volume at a constant level. Schematics of both open and closed flow-through systems are illustrated in Fig. 3.18, which includes the recommended basic design of a flow-through cell.

An examination of the literature reveals that numerous such devices have been described earlier by different authors. Flow-through dissolution units or "cells" of almost any kind have been proposed. There are simple cylindrical columns (56,59,61,62,72,76,80,81), either empty or filled with glass beads or glass wool (72,74,79,81,105), cells with the shape of a separatory funnel (58), rectangular cells (77), spherical cells (75,107), conical cells (57,71,79), an exponentially shaped horn (78), and so on. Even multicompartmental flow-through cells are reported (66).

The units are adjusted either horizontally (76,108,109) or vertically and the dissolution medium passing through the latter in either the ascending or descending mode, respectively. Furthermore, the dissolution fluid is pumped through the cells either in a continuous stream or in a pulsating manner (110,111), in a laminar flow (76,108), or simply in a dropwise falling manner.

The positioning of the dosage form, wherever critical, was obtained by using a pin (112) or by holding in the arms of a folded wire cross (76). The majority of workers allow their dosage form to move freely within the dissolution chamber. However, it may result in discontinuous extraction of the dosage form. Temperature control is often problematic in most units described. Jacketed cells have been employed, but such devices are extremely fragile and are expensive (108,113).

In the forthcoming sections, a few of the more prominent continuous-flow devices—more correctly designated as flow-through methods—are described. An attempt is made to point out their relative merits as well.

Continuous-Flow Apparatus by Pernarowski et al. (1968)

A schematic diagram of continuous-flow apparatus employed by Pernarowski et al. (93) is shown in Fig. 3.19. The apparatus constitutes primarily a stainless-steel basket stirrer assembly equipped with an adjustable stirrer. Ten-mesh stainless steel is used in the construction of the basket. This dissolution container is a 1-L three-necked flask. The main neck is 33 mm in diameter and the secondary necks are 20 mm in diameter. The total volume of the container is slightly greater than 1 L.

If fluid flow or changeover is necessary, the container is connected to a peristaltic pump. Flow rates up to 70 mL/min can be used. Test fluids may be pumped directly to a collection container. Alternatively, tubing lengths are kept to a minimum.

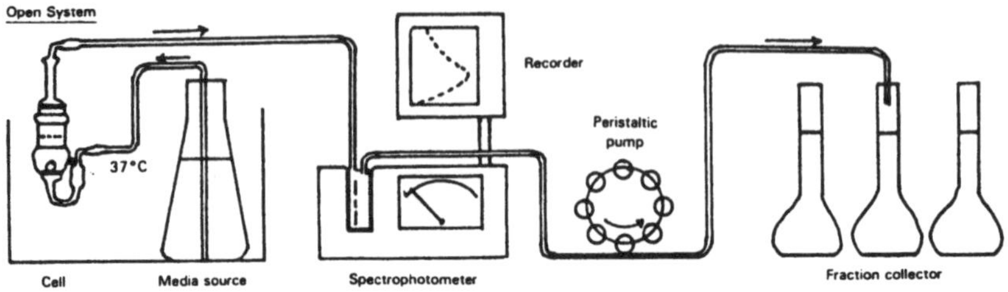

Open system in which pure solvent from the media source contacts the dosage form in the cell. After the absorbance is determined in the spectrophotometer, the samples may be collected for further analytical work. Note that the recorder shows the differential or mg/ml at any instant of solution.

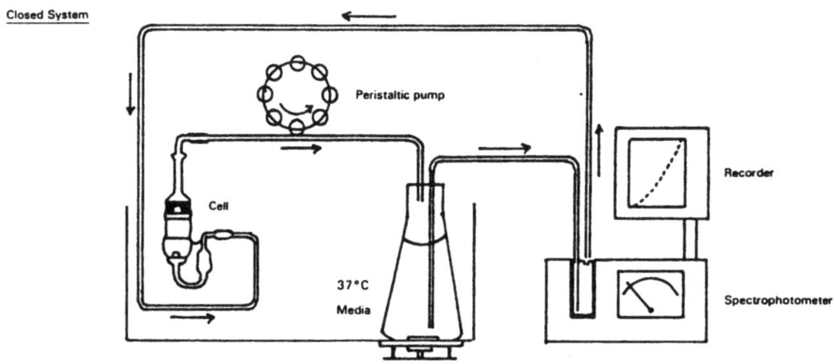

Closed system in which a finite volume of solvent is used. It is returned to the solvent source. Note that the dissolution profile records the cumulative mg/ml drug in solvent against time.

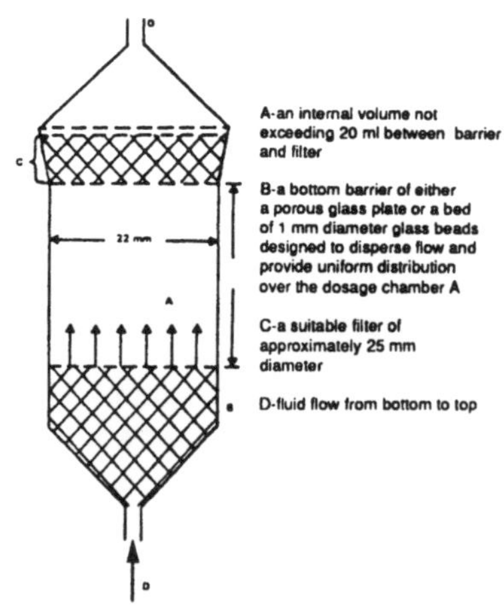

Fig. 3.18 Schematic illustration of open and closed flow through dissolution testing systems. Inset: Schematic diagram of a flow-through cell.

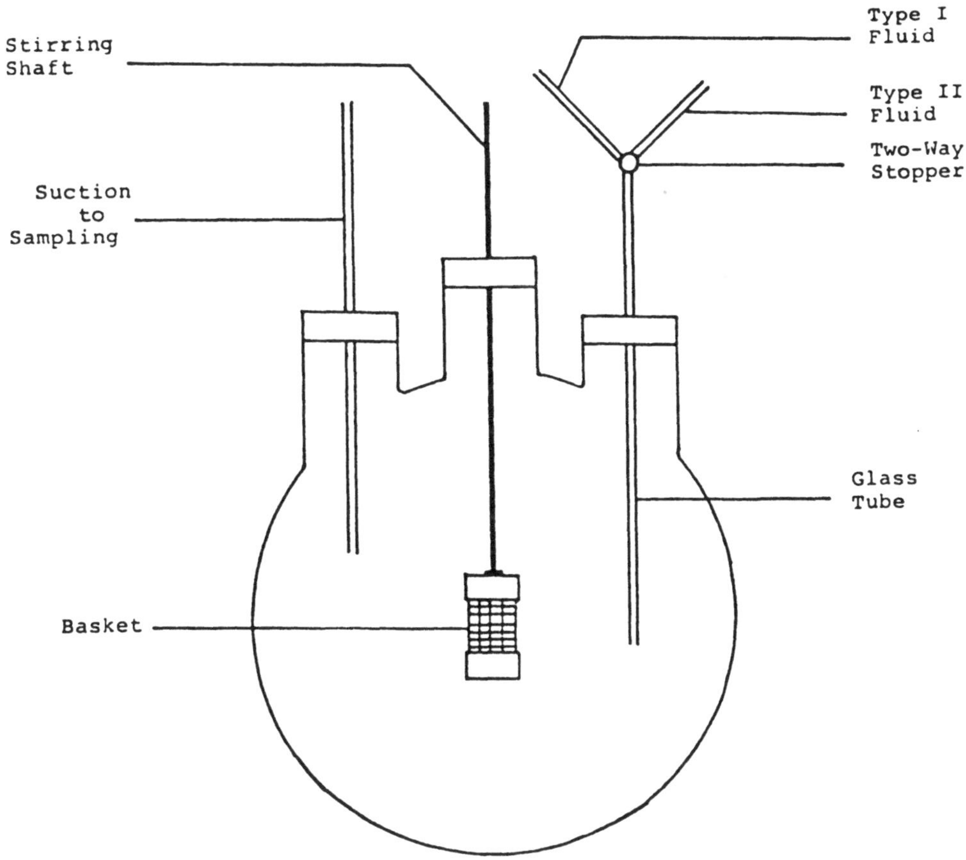

Fig. 3.19 Schematic illustration of a flow-through dissolution testing system by Pernarowski et al.

Dissolution characteristics may be determined by using exactly 1 L of fluid or by operating the apparatus as a continuous-flow system. If operated continuously, the volume of fluid in the dissolution container is slightly greater than 1 L. Dissolution characteristics are based on the amount of fluid pumped through the dissolution container.

This assembly can easily be automated, but at the same time, may be used as a simple flask–stirrer assembly with an auxiliary system for media transfer. The operating characteristics can be altered easily. However, when conditions are fixed, similar dissolution profiles are obtained when drug or tablets from a uniform lot are subjected to the procedure. Moreover, the basket stirrer assembly positions the tablet in the same way from run to run, assisting in producing results characteristic of the product rather than of the apparatus.

Langenbucher Column-Type Flow-Through Method (1969)

The design of this dissolution testing device closely matches the description of a typical flow-through apparatus. An illustrative sketch, together with a few other methods essentially operating on the same principle but with minor modifications, are shown in Fig. 3.20a–c. The dosage form to be investigated (tablet, capsule, granules, etc.) is placed in a vertically mounted dissolution cell on a screen that permits fresh dissolution medium to enter from the bottom. The screen is so constructed as to guarantee an equally distributed laminar flow over the entire cross section of the cell. At a height *h* above the screen, the cell is closed by a second screen, which filters the liquid and prevents the removal of undissolved particles. The dissolution medium—water or simulated gastric or intestinal fluid—is pumped through the cell by means of

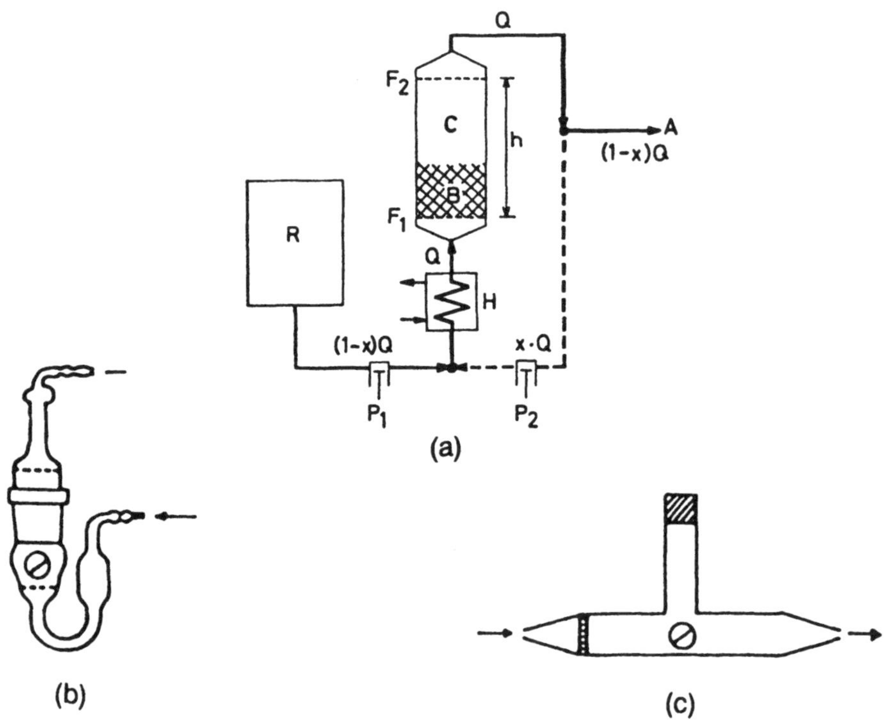

Fig. 3.20 Schematic illustration of a flow-through dissolution testing system by Langenbucher. (a) B, particle bed; C, cell; F_1, F_2, screens; H, heat exchanger; h, height of the cell; P_1, P_2, volumetric pumps; R, liquid reservoir; x, circulation factor; Q, xQ, $(1 - x)Q$, volumetric flow rates. (b) and (c) Designs of flow-through cells.

a peristaltic or metering pump from a reservoir after having passed the heat exchanger for temperature control. The eluate leaving the cell is analyzed for drug content, either continuously or at fixed intervals.

One particular feature must be pointed out; different drug amounts are dissolved under identical conditions whenever the parameter's liquid velocity equals the amount of drug per unit cell area. The physical meaning of such an observation is that the dissolution of *N* units of a dosage form (e.g., tablets) studied simultaneously in a cell with a known cross section and volumetric flow rate is the same as the average of *N* runs of single tablets in a cell with known cross section and volumetric flow rate (107).

The cell and the outlet tubes represent a holdup volume for the dissolved drug which corresponds to the lag time between the dissolution of the drug and removal of the solute from the system, whereas in biological absorption, the absorbing membranes may represent a drug-specific resistance to the removal of the material from the site of dissolution. If desired, this resistance can be simulated by recirculating a fraction of the liquid flow through the cell by means of a second metering pump. This simulates the membrane resistance in a quantitative manner. Thus any drug-specific permeability of the membranes can be simulated in a very convenient manner.

Additionally, it must be noted that the fixed-volume method appears to be a borderline case of this generalized model. With a unit circulation factor and a large holdup volume, the dissolution kinetics of this model should correspond completely to those obtained in a stirred beaker.

Continuous-Flow Apparatus by Baun and Walker (1969)

Baun and Walker (56) designed an apparatus which they termed a constant-circulation apparatus. The primary principle was that of the Wiley apparatus as reported by Meyers (114) with several modifications. Figure 3.21 illustrates the principal components of the system. The apparatus consists of a glass dissolution cell in which the dosage form to be tested is placed, a reservoir for the dissolution medium, a continuous-duty oscillating pump, and a suitable water bath in which the dissolution cell and reservoir are partially immersed. The rate of liquid flow through the cell is controlled by setting the variable transformer to a previously determined value. The lower screen of the dissolution cell is a 100-mesh stainless-steel screen, 1.8 cm in diameter.

The dissolution medium is poured into the reservoir and equilibrated at 37°C. The pump is initially primed for higher flow rates, facilitating residual air expulsion. A flow rate of 70 ±2 mL/min is found to be satisfactory. The tablet is dropped into the dissolution cell and the upper screen is inserted on commencement of the dissolution test.

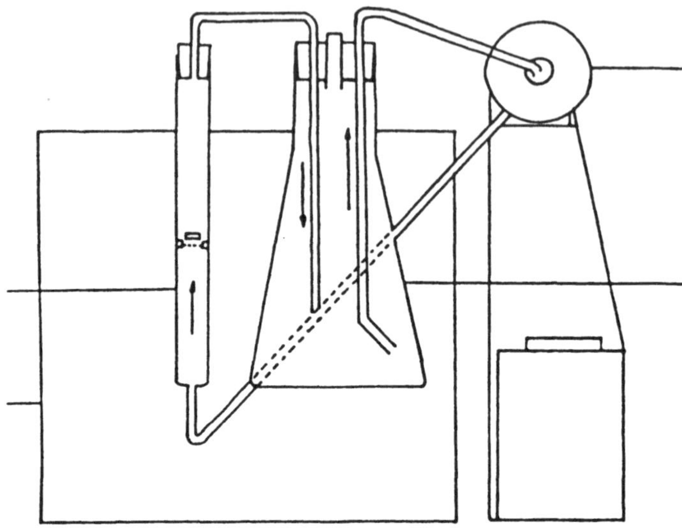

Fig. 3.21 Schematic illustration of a flow-through dissolution testing system by Baun and Walker.

This constant-circulation apparatus lends itself to modification with regard to dissolution chamber and size of chamber if deemed necessary for different-size dosage forms. The use of a reservoir of any size makes it possible to achieve solutions of any degree of saturation, facilitating evaluation of pharmaceutical formulations, particularly in the correlation with in vivo results and the "perfect sink" conditions presented in the literature. Agitation would be provided by a suitable stirring mechanism. For the most part, tablets remain below the screen, but depending on density, trapped air, and so on, may rise and roll against the screen, thus influencing dissolution.

The test fluid may be introduced through the top screen, but no data have been presented with reverse flow, which would be useful with certain lower-density dosage forms. The introduction of an opposing stream of dissolution medium from the top of the chamber with a suitable chamber design might provide a suspended system. Needless to say, the specifications could vary but should be standardized in the light of reproducibility and laminar and turbulent flow.

Continuous-Flow Apparatus by Tingstad and Riegelman (1970)

The apparatus consists of a cylindrical glass dissolution cell, 6.1 cm long and 1.9 cm in diameter, constructed from two small-volume glass filter funnels (59). A schematic diagram of the assembly is illustrated in Fig. 3.22. The dis-

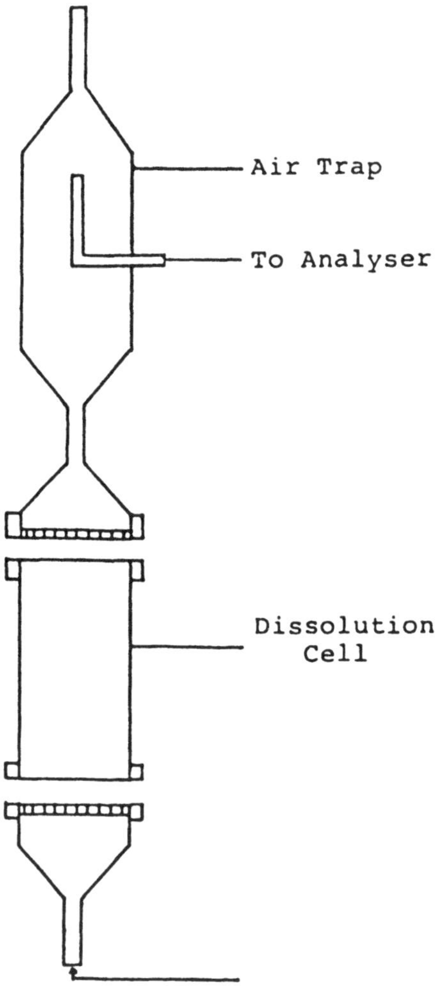

Fig. 3.22 Schematic illustration of a flow-through dissolution testing system by Tingstad and Riegelman.

solution cell facilitates the use of filter membranes of sufficient retentive characteristics, which prevent solid particles from reaching the analyzer. The solvent flow to the system is controlled by external valves, with the excess capacity of the pump being recirculated to the reservoir. The air trap prevents air bubbles from distorting the analytical reading.

The assembly is submerged in a constant-temperature bath, including a flowmeter, lower filter, dissolution cell, and lower part of an upper filter piece/air trap. On equilibration, the pump is turned on and the flow is regulated to the desired flow rate. The air outlet, open when the pump is turned on, is closed to the analyzer as soon as the liquid level in the air trap is above the outlet tube.

It should be emphasized that the apparatus described is a prototype, and numerous improvements are both possible and probable as more experience is gained. The cross-sectional flow or solvent flow is a variable that must be taken into account. The volume of the dissolution cell should be minimized to optimize homogeneity of the system. In addition, the size and shape of the air trap should be altered to optimize shape and minimum size, as any mixing and pooling of solution beyond the dissolution cell tends to distort the analytical tracing. The system should lend itself easily to automation.

There is little doubt that based on theoretical considerations, this method is superior to present methods for both fundamental and practical studies. It possibly has the inherent flexibility that may allow it to meet, with appropriate modification, most or all of the requirements listed for the ideal dissolution-rate method.

Flow-Through Modified Column Apparatus (1972)

A schematic illustration of the entire apparatus is given in Fig. 3.23. The dissolution cell is available in two sizes. The solvent reservoir consists of a 4-L flask submerged in a constant-temperature water bath (62). The bath temperature is closely monitored and adjusted to 37 $\pm 1\,^{\circ}C$ for any given flow rate. It is not necessary to place the cell itself in a bath, making the system more convenient and useful for routine studies. For closer temperature control, however, a second bath for the cell is recommended.

A filter holder, employing a 14M-size nylon filter, is attached to the flexible tubing in the reservoir. This keeps the dissolution chamber free from extraneous particulate matter. The pump is a variable-speed peristaltic tubing pump with solid-state speed control with a pump head capable of delivering 7 to 150 mL/min. This type of pumping system allows the use of 0.1 *N* HCl without causing pump deterioration or solvent contamination. Additionally, it permits the use of different flow rates for different experiments while holding a given flow rate constant during each experiment. Furthermore, it eliminates the need for a flowmeter in the system and allows for more convenient flow control than does a centrifugal pump, where bypass valves must be used.

The tubing from the pump is connected directly to the bottom of the dissolution cell, which is a commercially available ultrafilteration cell. The system takes standard 13- and 25-mm filters. The Teflon-faced stainless-steel support screen, with a sealing gasket, rests on the bottom half of the filter holder and

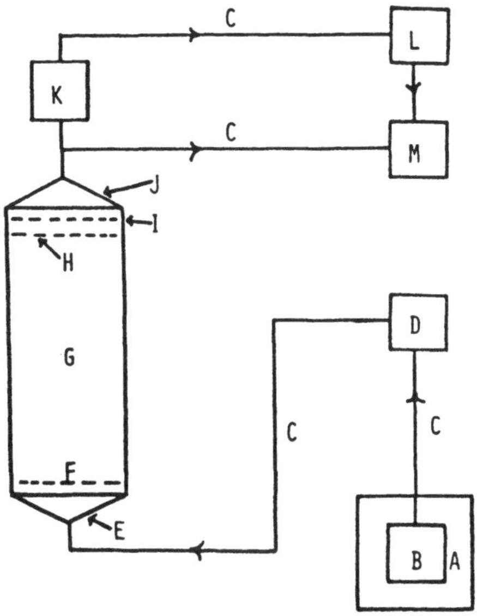

Fig. 3.23 Schematic illustration of a flow-through dissolution testing system with a modified column system by Tingstad et al. A, Solvent reservoir; B, filter holder; C, flexible tubing; D, pump; E and J, parts of filter holder; G, polycarbonate cylinder; F, support screen; H, filter; I, gasket; K, standard t-tube; L, flow cell; M, receptacle.

no filter is used here. The filter in the solvent reservoir keeps this screen clean. The direction of the flow is such that particles in the sample do not fall through the screen, and the absence of any filter at this site helps ensure uniform flow into the chamber. Another support screen and gasket, with a 14M nylon filter, are placed at the top of the cylinder. The lower screen and the upper filter thus form the boundaries of the system in which undissolved sample material is free to move. The low volume of the chamber reduces homogeneity problems to a minimum, even at low flow rates. Because of its lower volume, the 13-mm cell is preferred; however, it tends to clog more rapidly due to the small cross-sectional area of the filter (62).

The top of the cell is connected to flexible tubing. This facilitates disassembling the cell and also changing the effluent tubing system for different types of experiments. If continuous monitoring is not needed, this tubing system can be disconnected and a short delivery tube leading directly to the receptacle can be used.

Multichamber Continuous-Flow Apparatus by Cakiryildiz et al. (1975)

The dissolution system consists of a six-channel peristaltic pump, a thermostated water bath with a magnetic stirring plate for six beakers, an additional smaller water bath, an analyzer equipped with an automated cell changer and recorder, and five identical independent dissolution units with a sixth for recirculation of a reference solution (75). From the reservoir, the dissolution medium goes (via the pump) to the flow-through quartz cell, to the bottom of the dissolution cell, and from its top, returns to the reservoir (see Fig. 3.24 for a sketch of this device).

The dosage form under investigation is placed on top of a bed of glass beads (0.2 mm, 20 g) in the dissolution cell and the cell is closed. One liter of simulated gastric fluid USP (without pepsin) is used for drug powders. Less liquid is employed for capsules and tablets, so that maximum concentration of drug in solution does not exceed 10 to 15% of its saturation solubility. A flow rate of 8.0 ±0.2 mL/min is used for drug powder and the same of 16 ±0.5 mL/min is employed for capsule dissolution studies. These rates minimize pressure buildup at the membrane filter. A flow rate of 33 ±1.0 mL/min is maintained for tablet dissolution studies.

The apparatus, as described, lends itself to mechanical abrasion (scratching) by glass beads. A more serious drawback is the low recovery observed in powder studies due to retention of undissolved drug in scratches on the inner wall of the cell. However, the apparatus is versatile enough to determine dissolution patterns of drug powders and of tablet and capsule formulations with any change of the experimental setup. In addition to being capable of showing formulation differences, the apparatus is sensitive enough to reveal process changes (75).

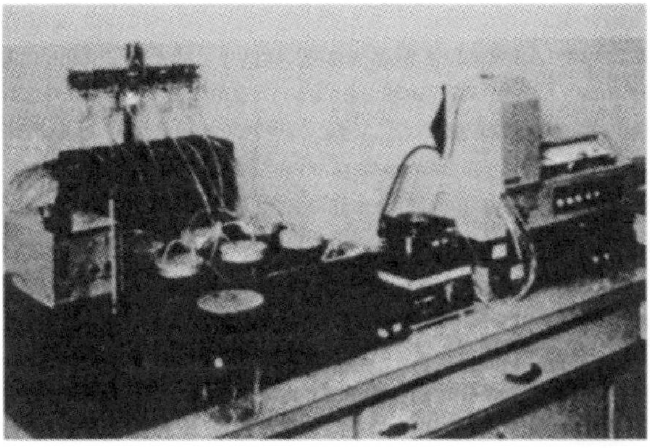

Fig. 3.24 Schematic illustration of a flow-through dissolution testing system by Cakiryildiz et al.

Continuous-Flow Apparatus by Takenaka et al. (1980)

This apparatus is a modification of a basket–stirrer–beaker assembly adapting to flow-through mechanics. The in vitro release of the drug from a dosage form (e.g., tablet) is measured by employing an in vitro simulator device consisting of a flow-type dissolution container in which the pH of the medium was changed continuously from 1.3 to 7.0 to simulate the pH change of tablets exposed to the GI tract (115). The schematic diagram of the assembly is shown in Fig. 3.25.

The dissolution test is carried out by placing a tablet in a USP basket. The basket is set at 1 ±0.2 cm from the bottom of the container. The basket was rotated at 94 rpm. Three hundred milliliters of simulated gastric fluid (pH 1.3) are introduced into the dissolution container, followed by the addition of simulated intestinal fluid (pH 7.5) at a rate of 1.27 ±0.2 mL/min. Simultaneously, the agitated dissolution medium is removed at the same rate to the collecting reservoir using a peristaltic pump. According to this techniques, the volume of the dissolution medium in the container is held at 300 mL, while the pH of the medium is gradually changed. The pH change in the dissolution medium is closely monitored by a pH electrode.

Aliquots of 2.0 mL of the dissolution medium in the apparatus and the reservoir are sampled at prescribed intervals using a syringe and then filtered, if necessary, through a Whatman number 42 filter paper. Aliquots of distilled water (same volume and temperature) are added immediately to the dissolution container to keep the volume of the dissolution medium constant during the test.

After 2.5 to 3.5 h, when the pH became less acidic (i.e., 6.8 to 6.9), the peristaltic pump was stopped. This ensures that the simulated conditions of the

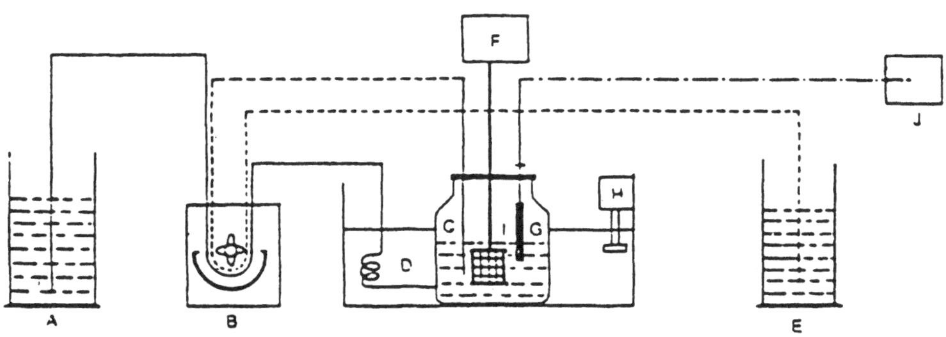

Fig. 3.25 Schematic illustration of a flow-through dissolution testing system by Takenaka et al. A, Simulated intestinal fluid reservoir; B, peristaltic pump; C, dissolution container; D, water bath; E, collecting reservoir; F, motor; G, pH electrodes; H, thermoregulator; I, USP dissolution basket; J, pH meter.

dissolution medium corresponded to the intestinal medium. Thereafter the pH is held constant at 6.8 to 6.9.

This apparatus is very easy to work with and can easily be monitored and controlled for reducing variability (116). Additionally, it is amenable for automation. This apparatus can prove to be very helpful for evaluating release of experimental formulations of prolonged-release dosage forms.

SPECIAL METHODS

Numerous types of apparatus for dissolution testing, in addition to the ones described and/or mentioned above, have been described in the literature during the past three decades. Some of them are indeed highly sophisticated and at an early stage of development may have represented interesting approaches to dissolution methodology but are now not more than museum pieces. Methods like the rocking cylinder (48), rotating bottles (117,118), Desaga Resomat apparatus (119), and Sartorius dissolution model (120–122), just to mention a few, are now considered as unsuitable for common use. However, a few of these can prove to be very useful for experiments that warrant special circumstances. Such apparatus needs recognition in view of its possible use by investigators with special interests in mind. In the following sections we address the descriptive relative merits of these few.

Tape Method (1965)

In this method described by Goldberg et al. (123), a weighed quantity of particles is dusted onto a pressure-sensitive tape mounted on a frame. The entire assembly is inserted into a beaker. The dissolution of the drug into the stirred dissolution medium is monitored by the removal of samples at known time intervals. The dissolution data were reproducible and were found to fit the extended Hixon–Crowell method (124) quite well. The method has also been used to study the dissolution properties of several drugs, alone and when present as solid dispersions and eutectic mixtures (125–127).

Pressure-Controlled Apparatus (1979)

A special modification of the USP basket method led to the development of apparatus employing pressurized air for the purpose of agitation. The design of this apparatus, illustrated in Fig. 3.26, consists of two tubes, one tube being 28.4 cm × 3.4 cm ID and the other 29.4 cm × 2.8 cm ID, connected in turn by two tubes, each of 4.7 cm × 1.0 cm ID (128). Air at pressures of 40, 43, 46, 50, and 55 mmHg is used to provide agitation to the dissolution medium. The basket is positioned 15.7 cm away from the bottom of the larger-diameter tube. Air bubbles are avoided by the use of a venting tube at the top of this

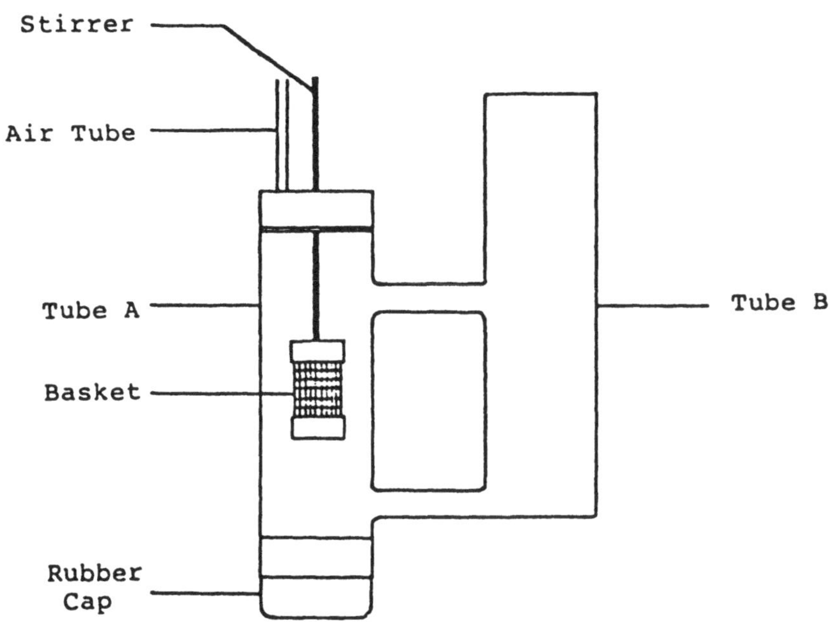

Fig. 3.26 Schematic diagram of pressure-controlled dissolution testing system by Nasir et al.

tube. The cylindrical basket, made of stainless-steel 40-mesh wire cloth, is 3.66 cm high and 2.5 cm in diameter. The basket consists of a solid metal top with a small vent. The basket, loaded with the dosage form to be tested, is suspended in the larger-diameter tube.

At the bottom of the tube with the larger diameter is a porcelain stone projecting through the circular hole in the center. The stone is encircled by a 40-mesh stainless-steel screen inside a rubber stopper supported by a stainless-steel sleeve. An opening at the bottom of the porcelain stone is connected by 5.5-mm polythene tubing to an air pump through a mercury manometer.

The temperature of the dissolution medium is maintained at 37°C and the dosage form within the basket is suspended in the medium. Airflow is controlled by a pump attached with a mercury manometer. The circulation of the dissolution medium is maintained by air pressure. The aliquots are withdrawn from the smaller-diameter tubes.

This method uses air pressure for agitation, in contrast to the official method, where the medium is deaerated to avoid air bubbles. This dissolution apparatus is reported to have yielded results comparable with the Levy method at an air pressure of 46 mmHg. No excessive settling of particles and no clogging of screen is observed in addition to complete dissolution of the dosage form under investigation. Poor agreement was observed at all pressures in the dissolution rates of drugs tested in USP dissolution apparatus compared to the new apparatus. The possibility exists, however, that tablets with significantly different properties may produce contrary results.

Perturbed Angular Correlation Method by Beihn and Digenis (1981)

A novel noninvasive technique was developed to measure dissolution of the water-soluble component of a solid dosage form using indium-111 and perturbed angular correlation (129). In principle, this method measures the conversion of one distinct state of nuclei to another, illustrating a phase change from solid indium chloride to liquid indium chloride. The method involves time-delayed coincidence counting of two cascading γ-rays that exhibit angular correlation. This angular correlation can be perturbed if the intermediate excited state of the nucleus is reoriented due to an interaction with its environment. When such an interaction occurs, as in a phase change (solid to liquid), the perturbation changes can be shown by anisotropy. A highly perturbed condition in the solid state results in low values (0.02 to 0.04), while increasing values of anisotropy indicate dissolution. They reach a maximum of 0.14 to 0.15 when the total perturbed physical state, the liquid state, exists. The method illustrates a noninvasive technique for measuring dissolution rates both in vitro and in vivo.

A schematic representation of entire assembly is given in Fig. 3.27. The apparatus consists of a 10-cm × 10-cm single-layer cotton gauze sheet with a mesh size sufficiently small to prevent the dosage form (tablet) or larger particles from falling through. The gauze containing the solid dosage form is suspended 6 cm from the bottom and in the center of a 1000-mL glass beaker containing 700 mL of HCl–water. An assembly comprising a hemostat clamped to the gauze and a ringstand is employed to hold the dosage form in place. The aqueous dissolution medium is stirred with a magnetic stirrer at approximately 100 rpm at 25 to 26°C.

Immediately after the dosage form is immersed and positioned, serial coincident counting on the scalers is initiated, which continues until completion of the experiment. Throughout the experiment, 0.5-mL samples are removed employing a 1-mL tuberculin syringe equipped with a 0.22-μm filter to prevent particles from being collected. These samples are removed at appropriate times and are transferred to sample vials and counted in a well counter.

The data obtained with the perturbed angular correlation method show that this technique, coupled with external scintigraphy, may permit the in vitro and in vivo study of the disintegration behavior of the dosage form. Additionally,

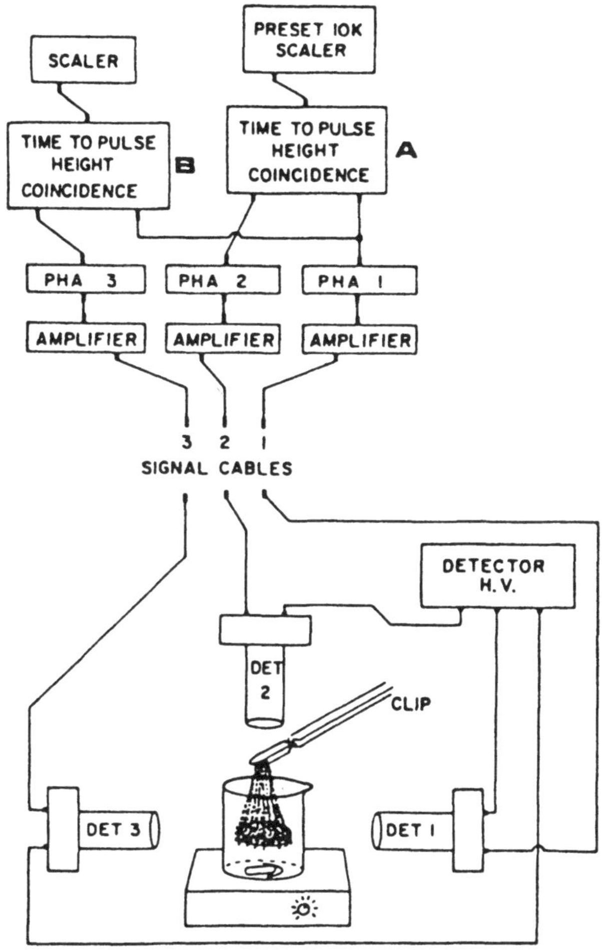

Fig. 3.27 Schematic diagram of the assembly illustrating the positioning of a flat plane around the tablet for an in vitro dissolution experiment using the perturbed angular correlation method.

this technique follows the dissolution pattern of the radionuclide and does not provide information on dissolution of any particular component of the solid dosage form. The technique might prove useful in comparative studies in which various solid dosage formulations could be compared for their disintegration properties.

COMPENDIAL METHODS: PERMISSIBLE VARIATIONS, SPECIFICATIONS, AND DRAWBACKS

It is desirable that the commonly accepted dissolution technique makes use of an apparatus that can be handled as simply as possible (i.e., that it requires a minimum of adjustments of this component's technical information). Additionally, when setting up apparatus for dissolution testing, routine quality control, new drug development, or complying with regulatory requirements, the analyst must consult the latest issue of the compendia, including revisions. The modifications introduced in the dissolution testing methods during recent years are so numerous that even revisions 2 or 3 years old may be outdated.

Currently, as of 1986–1987, only USP/NF, Canadian, and BP (*British Pharmacopoeia*) dissolution test standards are available. Japanese pharmacopoeial dissolution standards are very similar to those of USP/NF. The USP/NF paddle apparatus (method 2) and flow-through apparatus are scheduled to be adopted by European pharmacopoeias. The basic official methods are outlined in each of the compendia. However, the specifications as to dissolution medium composition, basket mesh, stirring rate, and so on, may vary for individual drug monographs. In the following sections we address basic USP/NF dissolution testing methods and point out the permissible variations and their limitations.

USP/NF Method 1 (Rotating Basket Method)

The USP/NF rotating basket method of dissolution testing essentially consists of an 1-in.-diameter × 1 3/8-in.-high stainless-steel 40-mesh wire basket rotated at a constant speed ranging between 25 and 150 rpm. It is immersed in 900 mL of dissolution medium in a flask of 1000 mL capacity. The medium in the flask is maintained at a constant temperature of 37 ±0.5°C by means of a suitable water bath.

The rotating basket method in the USP XX/NF XV and BP are almost similar. Table 3.2 lists the most significant differences observed in the dimensions and positioning of the apparatus, including other general features as well. The stainless steel (type 316) employed for the fabrication of the basket is not totally resistant to corrosive media (e.g., dilute acid). Consequently, plating of gold up to 1×10^{-4} in. thickness is permitted by both USP/NF and BP for use in acid media. Certain analytical procedures such as fluorometric determinations are sensitive to the presence of nickel and chromium, components of type 316 stainless steel. In such cases the basket as well as the bottom part of the basket's drive shaft and its retaining spring warrants gold plating.

Method 1 requires a 40-mesh screen for the basket unless otherwise indicated in a specific monograph. However, studies employing 10-, 20-, 30-, and

Table 3.2 Comparison of Specifications Recommended for Official Dissolution Testing Methods

	Compendium		
	Rotating basket (method 1)		Rotating paddle (method 2)
Parameter	USP XXI/NF XV	BP	USP XXI/NF XVI
General			
Water bath temperature (°C)	36.5–37.5	37	36.5–37.5
Dissolution medium	As specified in monograph, or 900 mL	As specified in monograph, or 1000 mL	As specified in monograph, or 900 mL
	Dissolved gasses must not interfere with the test	Deaeration required	Dissolved gases must not interfere with the test
Required samples	6 + 6 + 12 sequenced until specification is met	5 + 5 sequenced for 100% of 5	6 + 6 + 12 sequenced until specification is met
Shaft speed (rpm)	As specified in monograph, 20–150 4%	As specified in monograph 20–150 5%	As specified in the monograph 20–150 4% lower speed preferred
Shaft diameter (mm)	6–10.5	Approx. 6	9.5–10.5, lower part polyfluorocarbon coated if desired
Centering	2 mm at all points	2 mm at all points	2 mm at all points
Eccentricity	No significant wobble	No perceptible wobble	No significant wobble
Sampling point	Halfway from top of basket to top of fluid; no closer than 1 cm to side of flask	Halfway between basket and side at middle of basket	Halfway between top of blade and top of fluid; no closer than 1 cm to side of flask
Flask	Cylindrical with spherical bottom 16–17.5 cm high, 10–10.5 cm ID plastic or glass	Cylindrical, flat-bottomed, glass	Cylindrical with spherical bottom 16–17.5 cm high, 10–10.5 cm ID, plastic or glass
Basket position (cm)	2.5 ± 0.2	2.0 ± 0.2	2.5 ± 0.2
Sinkers			Stainless steel or glass helix

40-mesh screens have been reported (130). Usually, it is observed that 40-mesh screen tends to clog and the apparent rate of dissolution is lowered. Baskets with a wide variety of mesh openings are available, and it is anticipated that as long as the deaggregated particle size is consistent, a variation in mesh size may assist in solving some difficult dissolution problems.

It must be noted that USP XX/NF XV rotating basket (method 1) is also employed as an unofficial test for dissolution testing of suppositories and microencapsulated particles. Dissolution testing of dosage forms is discussed in Chapter 7.

USP/NF Method 2 (Rotating Paddle Method)

For all practical purposes the compendial specifications outlined for this method are identical to method 1 except that the paddle is substituted for the rotating basket. These specifications are listed in Table 3.2. It must be noted that investigators might be tempted to view the paddle as a crude agitating device similar to other stirring devices common to the laboratory. On the contrary, the paddle is a precisely defined, close-tolerance instrument and must be selected carefully. Additionally, it should be regularly inspected and handled with the same care as for any delicate instrument.

To get consistent results from flask to flask, certain dimensions and tolerances for the paddle should be critically assessed. The contour of the paddle blade must not include any sharp edges at the tips, which will not produce turbulent flow patterns. No significant wobble should be produced during operation. Coating the paddles with polyfluorocarbon to prevent corrosion and entry of unwanted ions into the medium is suggested by USP/NF. Due to the variations inherent in the coating process, which may result in coat stripping and flaking, it is recommended that the paddles be closely inspected routinely. Also, because of the precise geometry required for repeatability of this method, the stirring paddle has been specified to be stainless steel rather than glass, with a detachable blade.

USP/NF permits variation in the paddle method involving the use of a helix of nonreactive material as a "sinker" for floating dosage units. Anchoring accomplished by such a device has been severely criticized, particularly by European scientists (131). Several unique solutions have been suggested by many investigators; however, the problem has not yet been solved satisfactorily or clearly.

Shortcomings of Official and Recommended Methods

The rotating basket device (method 1) was adopted by the USP XVIII/NF XIII in 1970 and is now, in modified form, one of the official methods for the dissolution test of solid pharmaceutical formulation (39). This device suffers from several drawbacks (132–145). An inadequacy of mixing at slow speed, clogging of mesh openings by drug or excipient particles, deterioration of the basket after exposure to hydrochloric acid, abrasion of tablets in multilaminated baskets, entrapment of air bubbles at the top of the basket assembly, hindered visual inspection of the disintegration process, and inconvenience for cleaning the setup after testing are but a few that have been recorded over the years. It is sometimes difficult to adjust the basket or to keep it in proper position during the entire experiment. One of the major problems encountered while employing the basket method is "coning" of the dissolution test material. This occurs when a dosage form breaks up and the fragments fall to the bottom of the dissolution vessel and form a cone of material; hence sampling is not accomplished from a well-stirred medium. These and many other facts not mentioned above cast doubt on the utility of the rotating basket methodology as a whole. The search for principal alternatives seems to be the other way to circumvent these difficulties.

The rotating paddle method (method 2), based principally on Levy's classical beaker method (18) and Poole's stirred flask apparatus, was modified a number of times before it was finally recommended officially (146–148). Formulations with dense excipients tend to mound at the bottom of the dissolution vessel at moderate revolutions of the paddle. On the other hand, floating dosage forms must be submerged by some means. "Sinkers" are recommended, but no agreement has yet been achieved on a suitable design, and reproducibility remains poor (146–150). Furthermore, such dosage forms need to be shielded from paddle agitation to avoid mechanical destruction. Coated or sustained dosage forms often produce erratic dissolution profiles which are caused by the paddles knocking lumps out of the dosage form and/or fracturing the coating. To minimize interlaboratory variations, these and other shortcomings warrant extremely strict regulations for the construction of the apparatus.

The stirrer itself, along with its fixation to the shaft, the vertical distance of the blade from the bottom of the vessel, has to be controlled separately by means of a needle gauge attached to the end of the shaft to prevent wobbling of the shaft. The rotational speed of the stirrer is subject to rather stringent standardization. The sampling point needs to be well defined to circumvent possible problems of nonhomogeneity of the bulk medium. Even the sampling probe can influence the test results (151).

Considerable disagreement still exists about the size and shape of the dissolution vessel (three-necked round-bottomed flask, cylindrical vessel with round or flat bottom). It discloses a serious shortcoming of this method as a whole, which is inherent in a system agitated with a mechanical stirrer, and thus cannot be overcome by minor technical improvements alone.

The basket-rack assembly, which is now the third official method of the USP XX/NF XV for dissolution testing, suffers from similar insufficiencies as the foregoing two methods (39). This device, originally designed for tablet disintegration testing, dates from 1946 (152).

The recent philosophy in approaching dissolution testing has deprived the disintegration test of its previous importance. Certainly, the latter will be replaced totally by real dissolution procedures in the near future.

FABRICATION OF NEW DISSOLUTION TESTING DEVICES

It has now been recognized that dosage forms with different in vitro dissolution rates *should* correlate with the observed in vivo availability when dissolution is rate limiting in vivo. If they do not, either the in vitro dissolution method used is incorrect or the in vitro differences obtained are simply not significant in vivo.

It seems unrealistic to devise different devices, models, or systems for different drugs and formulations, especially since there is essentially one basic model in vivo. In this chapter we have shown that there are a multitude of devices used in dissolution testing. Many of these suffer from deficiencies, such as too intense agitation, absence of sink conditions, and the inability to program progressive changes in the dissolution environment. Consequently, they fail to stimulate in vivo conditions.

Interest has focused on designing "the" in vitro dissolution testing device that can positively characterize the role of the dissolution process in bioavailability. Such an apparatus should meet the following criteria:

1. The fabrication, dimensions, and positioning of each component must be specified precisely.
2. Simplicity of design, convenience of operation, and flexibility in use under a variety of test conditions must be the overriding considerations.
3. The apparatus should be sensitive enough to reveal process changes and be capable of showing formulation differences. However, it should yield reproducible results upon repeated testing under identical conditions.
4. The apparatus should permit controlled variable intensity of mild, uniform, nonturbulent liquid agitation.
5. The apparatus should provide and maintain nearly perfect sink conditions during in vitro dissolution rate determinations (i.e., the drug concentration in the dissolution medium should not exceed 10 to 20% of its solubility).
6. The apparatus must provide a convenient means for introducing the dosage form under investigation (tablet, capsule, etc.) into the dissolution

medium, in addition to holding it at a fixed position completely immersed in the medium.

7. To retain its microenvironment, the test sample must be subjected to minimal mechanical impacts, abrasion, and wear during the entire test period.
8. The dissolution medium container must be closed to prevent loss of medium due to evaporation, thermoregulated at fixed temperature, and preferably transparent to permit visual observation.
9. The apparatus must lend itself to easy withdrawal of representative fluid samples of the bulk medium for analysis, either by manual or automated methods, without interrupting medium agitation. An automated system should permit continuous filtration efficiently without encountering operational and/or analytical difficulties.
10. The apparatus must be applicable for the evaluation of disintegrating, nondisintegrating, dense or "floating" tablets and capsules, finely powdered drugs, and all other types of solid drug forms.
11. The apparatus should be rugged enough so that critical parameters result in good interlaboratory agreement.

The recent sharp increase in the amount of dissolution testing carried out by the pharmaceutical industry reflects growing recognition of the technique's value. Dissolution tests are critical and difficult to carry out properly. If one is to obtain correct results, care and attention must be given to those aspects that have been identified as crucial.

Present methods suffer from the disadvantage of stirring or rocking as a device for ensuring homogeneity and moving solvent/solute molecules. Due to this empirical nature, they cannot be related to fundamental dissolution rate equations except by including them in a catch-all constant, which is a very superficial solution to the problem. As a result, it is crucial that the various test systems be standardized as much as possible: one stirring rate, one type of container, one type of solvent, and so on. But this greatly reduces investigative flexibility, which is a primary requisite for a good standard method. Furthermore, with such rigid constraints, the procedures will be less quantitative and less meaningful.

CONCLUDING REMARKS

For obvious reasons, it would be ideal if one relatively simple and inexpensive apparatus and method could be used to determine the dissolution rates of most drugs and drug products. However, standing in the way of a one-method concept is the fact that a great variety of factors influence the results obtained from dissolution-rate tests.

The real question to be addressed is how far the results of in vitro studies permit inferences to be made regarding bioavailability (153). In most cases it can reasonably be concluded that such inferences should be limited to the actual quantities measured. However, such restricted testing methods also have advantages, in particular less scatter and simpler study conditions. It is important to employ test conditions similar, at least in principle, to those found in vivo.

Controversy still exists as to the usefulness and validity of the in vitro dissolution method as far as correlation with in vivo results is concerned. The development of an in vitro method that can serve to predict the in vivo performance of a specific drug would be the first step toward developing and designing of dissolution systems. Unquestionably, poor in vitro–in vivo correlations may in some instances reflect the variability of the in vitro dissolution procedure employed, as well as inter- and intrasubject variation in vivo. No universal dissolution test method has yet been devised that in every instance gives the same rank order for in vitro dissolution and in vivo availability for different formulations or batches.

The current proliferation of dissolution testing methods presents no real advances in terms of devising a realistic model. Our efforts must be geared along two related channels:

1. Generation of more quantitative data on in vivo conditions that prevail
2. Employing this information to refine those in vitro dissolution testing devices that appear to offer most promise in achieving in vitro–in vivo correlations

There is presently an acknowledged scarcity of data showing correlation between in vitro–in vivo performance of drugs and drug products. However, the great current interest and activity in this area indicate that more and more data are forthcoming. With the increased accumulation of knowledge in this area, difficulties, problems, and deficiencies in the in vitro methods will be exposed, necessitating refinement in equipment and procedures. The more flexible the standard method is, the more easily it will lend itself to modifications warranted by new findings.

REFERENCES

1. W. Hanson, *Handbook of Dissolution Testing*, Pharmaceutical Technology Publications Springfield, Oreg. (1982) p. 6.
2. D. Cox, C. Douglas, W. Furman, R. Krichhoefer, J. Myrick, and C. Wells, *Pharm. Technol.*, *2*(4), 40 (1978).
3. W. Hanson, *Pharm. Technol.*, *1*(5), 30 (1977).
4. K. Thakker, N. Naik, V. Gray, and S. Sun, *Pharm. Forum*, *6*, 177 (1980).

5. A Sarapu, A. Lewis, and M. Grostic, *Pharm. Forum, 6*, 172 (1980).
6. K. A. Lees, *J. Pharm. Pharmacol., 15*, 143T (1963).
7. A. B. Morrison and J. A. Campbell, *J. Pharm. Sci., 54*, 1 (1965).
8. J. A. Hersey, *Manuf. Chem. Aerosol News*, p. 32 (Feb. 1969).
9. U. V. Banakar and L. H. Block, *Pharm. Technol., 7*, 107 (1983).
10. L. Klein, *Bull. Biol. Pharm.*, 273 (1932).
11. G. H. Elliott, *Pharm. J., 131*, 514 (1933).
12. E. Nelson, *J. Pharm. Sci., 47*, 297 (1958).
13. G. Levy, *J. Pharm. Sci., 52*, 1039 (1963).
14. W. S. Wruble, *Am. J. Pharm., 102*, 368 (1930).
15. J. C. Souder and W. C. Ellenbogen, *Drug Stand., 26*, 77 (1958).
16. W. I. Higuchi and E. N. Heistand, *J. Pharm. Sci., 52*, 67 (1963).
17. W. I. Higuchi, E. L. Rowe, and E. N. Heistand, *J. Pharm. Sci., 52*, 162 (1963).
18. G. Levy and B. A. Hayes, *N. Engl. J. Med., 262*, 1053 (1960).
19. E. L. Parrott, D. E. Wurster, and T. Higuchi, *J. Pharm. Sci., 44*, 269 (1955).
20. E. Nelson, *J. Pharm. Sci., 46*, 607 (1957).
21. E. Nelson, *J. Pharm. Sci., 47*, 300 (1958).
22. A. G. Mitchell and D. J. Saville, *J. Pharm. Pharmacol., 19*, 729 (1967).
23. E. Sheffer and T. Higuchi, *J. Pharm. Sci., 52*, 781 (1963).
24. J. F. Broadbent, A. G. Mitchell, and W. J. O'Reilly, *J. Pharm., 47*, S46, S92 (1966).
25. I. C. Edmundson and K. A. Lees, *J. Pharm. Pharmacol, 17*, 193 (1965).
26. G. Levy and B. A. Sahli, *J. Pharm. Sci., 51*, 58 (1962).
27. J. W. Wood, J. E. Syarto, and H. Letterman, *J. Pharm. Sci., 54*, 1068 (1965).
28. W. E. Hamlin, E. Nelson, B. E. Ballard, and J. G. Wagner, *J. Pharm. Sci., 51*, 432 (1962).
29. G. Levy and W. Tanski, Jr., *J. Pharm. Sci., 53*, 679 (1964).
30. G. Levy and R. H. Gumtow, *J. Pharm. Sci., 52*, 1139 (1963).
31. E. J. Middleton, J. M. Davis, and A. B. Morrison, *J. Pharm. Sci., 53*, 1378 (1964).
32. B. Caleswick, B. Katchen, and J. Black, *J. Pharm. Sci., 54*, 1277 (1964).
33. D. Cook, H. S. Chang, and C. A. Mainville, *Can. J. Pharm. Sci., 1*, 69 (1966).
34. V. Walters, *J. Pharm. Pharmacol., 20*, 2285 (1968).
35. L. C. Schroeter and J. G. Wagner, *J. Pharm. Sci., 51*, 957 (1962).
36. A. Richter, B. Myhre, and S. C. Khauna, *J. Pharm. Pharmacol. Suppl., 21*, 4095 (1969).
37. D. C. Cox, C. C. Douglas, W. B. Furman, R. D. Kirchhoefer, J. W. Myrick, and C. E. Wells, *Pharm. Technol., 2*, 41 (1978).
38. D. Cook, H. S. Chang, and C. A. Mainville, *Can. J. Pharm. Sci., 1*, 69 (1966).
39. *United States Pharmacopeia*, XX rev., *National Formulary*, XV rev., United States Pharmacopeial Convention, Rockville, Md. (1980).
40. P. T. Shah and W. E. Moore, *J. Pharm. Sci., 59*, 1034 (1970).
41. R. E. Shepherd, J. C. Price, and L. A. Luzzi, *J. Pharm. Sci., 61*, 1152 (1972).
42. T. E. Needham, R. E. Shephard, and L. A. Luzzi, *J. Pharm. Sci., 62*, 470 (1973).

43. G. Haringer, B. J. Poulsen, and R. N. Havemeyer, *J. Pharm. Sci.*, *62*, 130 (1973).
44. A. C. Shah, C. B. Peot, and J. F. Ochs, *J. Pharm. Sci.*, *62*, 671 (1973).
45. A. C. Shah and J. F. Ochs, *J. Pharm. Sci.*, *63*, 110 (1974).
46. G. Levy, *J. Mond. Pharm.*, *3*, 237 (1967).
47. M. Gibaldi and S. Feldman, *J. Pharm. Sci.*, *56*, 1238 (1967).
48. H. MacDonald, F. Pisano, J. Burger, A. Dornbush, and E. Pelcak, *Drug Inf. Bull.*, *3*, 76 (1969).
49. J. Poole, *Drug Inf. Bull.*, p. 8 (Jan./June 1969).
50. M. Gibaldi and H. Weintraub, *J. Pharm. Sci.*, *59*, 725 (1970).
51. A. Ferrari and A. Khoury, *Ann. N.Y. Acad. Sci.*, *153*, 660 (1968).
52. H. Koch, *Oesterr. Apoth. Ztg.*, *31* 1, 245, 353, 924 (1977).
53. H. Koch, *Oesterr. Apoth. Ztg.*, *32* , 177 (1978).
54. H. Koch, *Oesterr. Apoth. Ztg.*, *33* , 119, 681 (1979).
55. P. Niebergall, E. Sugita, and R. Schnarre, *J. Pharm. Sci.*, *60*, 1575 (1971).
56. D. C. Baun and G. C. Walker, *J. Pharm. Sci.*, *58*, 611 (1969).
57. E. G. Rippie and J. R. Robinson, *J. Pharm. Sci.*, *58*, 428 (1969).
58. K. Marshall and D. B. Brooke, *J. Pharm. Pharmacol.*, *21*, 790 (1969).
59. J. E. Tingstad and S. Riegelman, *J. Pharm. Sci.*, *59*, 692 (1970).
60. H. Andersgaard, P. Finholt, P. Gjermundsen, and T. Hyland, *Acta Pharm. Suec.*, *8*, 403 (1971).
61. H. W. Dibbern and E. Wizbitzki, *Pharm. Ztg.*, *116*, 1848 (1971).
62. J. Tingstad, E. Gropper, L. Lachman, and E. Shami, *J. Pharm. Sci.*, *61*, 1985 (1972).
63. D. C. Monkhouse and J. L. Lach, *J. Pharm. Sci.*, *61*, 1430 (1972).
64. S. I. Borst and W. Wald, *Can. J. Pharm. Sci.*, *7*, 18 (1972).
65. P. Seth, *Pharm. Acta Helv.*, *47*, 457 (1972).
66. R. L. Nedich and D. O. Kildsig, *J. Pharm. Sci.*, *61*, 214 (1972).
67. H. Kala, M. Dittgen, G. Zessin, and H. Moldenhauer, *Pharmazie*, *28*, 408 (1973).
68. U. Boggs and A. Darr, *Pharmazie*, *28*, 112 (1973).
69. P. Pothisiri and J. T. Carstensen, *J. Pharm. Sci.*, *62*, 1468 (1973).
70. J. Tingstad, E. Gropper, L. Lachman, and E. Shami, *J. Pharm. Sci.*, *62*, 293 (1973).
71. H. G. Kwee and G. A. Ulex, *Pharm. Ind.*, *36*, 576 (1974).
72. J. Cobby, M. Meyerson, and G. Walker, *J. Pharm. Sci.*, *63*, 732 (1974).
73. P. Schwarge and H. Hittinger, *Pharm. Ind.*, *36*, 732 (1974).
74. R. V. Bathe, O. Haflinger, F. Langenbucher, and D. Schonleber, *Pharm. Acta Helv.*, *50*, 3 (1975).
75. C. Cakiryildiz, P. J. Mehta, W. Rahmen, and D. Schoenleber, *J. Pharm. Sci.*, *64*, 1692 (1975).
76. M. J. Grooves, M. H. Alkan, and M. A. Deer, *J. Pharm. Pharmacol.*, *27*, 400 (1975).
77. A. C. Shah and K. G. Nelson, *J. Pharm. Sci.*, *64*, 1518 (1975).
78. J. V. Fee, D. J. W. Grant, and J. M. Newton, *J. Pharm. Sci.*, *65*, 48 (1976).

79. F. Langenbucher and H. Rettig, *Drug Dev. Ind. Pharm.*, *3*, 241 (1977).
80. C. Merle, C. Mangin, and A. M. Guyot-Hermann, *Bull. Soc., Pharm. Lille*, *1977*, 87 (1977).
81. *Pharm. Ind.*, *43*, 334 (1981).
82. D. E. Wurster and G. P. Polli, *J. Pharm. Sci.*, *50*, 403 (1961).
83. D. E. Wurster and G. P. Polli, *J. Pharm. Sci.*, *53*, 311 (1964).
84. E. L. Parrott, D. E. Wurster, and T. Higuchi, *J. Pharm. Sci.*, *44*, 269 (1955).
85. D. E. Wurster and G. P. Polli, *Farm. Buc.*, *12*, 261 (1964).
86. M. Gibaldi and S. Feldman, *J. Pharm. Sci.*, *56*, 1238 (1967).
87. E. Marlowe and R. F. Shangraw, *J. Pharm. Sci.*, *56*, 498 (1967).
88. R. B. Barzilay and J. A. Hersey, *J. Pharm. Pharmacol*, *20*, 2325 (1968).
89. V. E. Krogerus, E. R. Kristoffersson, and P. Kahela, *Farm. Notisbl.*, *76*, 122 (1967).
90. H. Weintraub and M. Gibaldi, *J. Pharm. Sci.*, *59*, 1972 (1970).
91. W. Rothe and J. Schellhorn, *Pharm. Ind.*, *41*, 485 (1979).
92. K. Munzel, *Arch. Pharm.*, *293*, 766 (1960).
93. M. Pernarowski, W. Woo, and R. D. Searl, *J. Pharm. Sci.*, *57*, 1419 (1968).
94. H. Moller, *Pharm. Ind.*, *45*, 617 (1983).
95. E. L. Parrott, *J. Pharm. Sci.*, *64*, 878 (1975).
96. I. W. Kellaway and C. Marriott, *J. Pharm. Sci.*, *64*, 1162 (1975).
97. S. L. Lin, J. Menig, and C. J. Swartz, *J. Pharm. Sci.*, *59*, 989 (1970).
98. K. A. Khan and C. T. Rhodes, *Can. J. Pharm. Sci.*, *8*, 29 (1973).
99. R. J. Whithey and A. J. Bowker, *J. Pharm. Pharmacol.*, *24*, 345 (1972).
100. C. F. Lerk and M. Lagas, *Pharm. Weekbl.*, *112*, 925 (1977).
101. T. W. Underwood and D. E. Cadwallader, *J. Pharm. Sci.*, *61*, 239 (1972).
102. R. J. Whithey, *J. Pharm. Pharmacol.*, *23*, 573 (1971).
103. H. Moller, *Pharm. Ztg.*, *127*, 2045 (1982).
104. H. Moller, *Pharm. Ztg.*, *127*, 1453 (1982).
105. F. Langenbucher, *J. Pharm. Sci.*, *58*, 1265 (1969).
106. T. M. Rust, summary of a paper given to Sotax AG, CH-4008, Basel (1985–86); Deutsche Arzneimittel Codex, West Germany (1984).
107. P. Schwarze and H. Hittinger, *Pharm. Ind.*, *36*, 732 (1974).
108. G. K. Bolhuis, C. F. Lerk, and K. Zuurman, *Pharm. Weekbl.*, *108*, 49 (1973).
109. H. Lapidus and N. G. Lordi, *J. Pharm. Sci.*, *55*, 840 (1966).
110. C. F. Lerk and K. Zuurman, *J. Pharm. Pharmacol.*, *22*, 319 (1970).
111. D. L. Simmons, A. A. Legore, P. Picotte, K. S. Lee, and N. N. Joshi, *J. Pharmacokinet. Biopharm.*, *3*, 39 (1975).
112. D. Ganderton, J. W. Hadgraft, W. T. Rispin, and G. A. Thompson, *Pharm. Acta Helv.*, *42*, 152 (1967).
113. K. Toth, Z. Feher, E. Lindner, G. Nagy, and E. Pungor, *Magy. Kem. Lapja*, *34*, 77 (1979).
114. E. L. Meyers, *Drug Cosmet. Ind.*, *87*, 622 (1960).
115. H. Takenaka, Y. Kawashima, and S. Y. Lin, *J. Pharm. Sci.*, *69*, 1388 (1980).
116. U. V. Banakar, Ph.D. dissertation, Duquesne University, Pittsburgh, Pa. (1985).
117. I. Bohrer, J. Prochazka, and P. Schmidt, *Dtsch. Apoth. Ztg.*, *119*, 1406 (1979).

118. D. Chiaramonti, C. Giani, and F. Innocenti, *Farm. Ed. Prat.*, *25*, 257 (1970).
119. H. W. Dibbern, *Arzniem.-Forsch./Drug Res.*, *16*, 177, 1304 (1966).
120. H. Stricker, *Arzniem.-Forsch./Drug Res.*, *20*, 391 (1970).
121. H. Stricker, *Pharm. Ind.*, *31*, 794 (1969).
122. H. Stricker, *Pharm. Ind.*, *33*, 157, 446 (1971).
123. A. H. Goldberg, M. Gibaldi, J. L. Kanig, and J. Shanker, *J. Pharm. Sci.*, *54*, 1722 (1965).
124. A. W. Hixson and J. H. Crowell, *Ind. Eng. Chem.*, *23*, 923 (1931).
125. A. H. Goldberg, M. Gibaldi, and J. L. Kanig, *J. Pharm. Sci.*, *55*, 482 (1966).
126. A. H. Goldberg, M. Gibaldi, and J. L. Kanig, *J. Pharm. Sci.*, *55*, 487 (1966).
127. A. H. Goldberg, M. Gibaldi, J. L. Kanig, and M. Mayersohn, *J. Pharm. Sci.*, *55*, 581 (1966).
128. S. S. Nasir, L. O. Wilken, Jr., and S. M. Nasir, *J. Pharm. Sci.*, *68*, 177 (1979).
129. R. M. Beitin and G. A. Digenis, *J. Pharm. Sci.*, *70*, 1325 (1980).
130. D. M. Patel et al., *Pharm. Forum*, p. 376 (July/Aug. 1980).
131. D. Brossard, Ph.D. dissertation, Université René Descartes de Paris (May 1981).
132. W. F. Beyer and D. L. Smith, *J. Pharm. Sci.*, *60*, 496 (1971).
133. J. T. Carstensen, T. Y. Lai, and V. K. Prasad, *J. Pharm. Sci.*, *66*, 607 (1977).
134. K. Embil and G. Torosian, *J. Pharm. Sci.*, *68*, 1336 (1979).
135. E. A. Hardwidge, A. C. Sarapu, and W. C. Laughlin, *J. Pharm. Sci.*, *67*, 1732 (1978).
136. G. Harringer, J. B. Poulsen, and R. N. Havemeyer, *J. Pharm. Sci.*, *62*, 130 (1973).
137. S. A. Howard, J. W. Mauger, A. Kwangsopha, and D. A. Pasquerelli, *J. Pharm. Sci.*, *68*, 1542 (1979).
138. K. A. Khan and C. T. Rhodes, *Can. J. Pharm. Sci.*, *8*, 29 (1973).
139. S. Lin, J. Menig, and S. J. Swartz, *J. Pharm. Sci.*, *59*, 989 (1970).
140. G. L. Mattock, I. J. McGilveray, and R. D. Hossie, *J. Pharm. Sci.*, *61*, 460 (1972).
141. J. R. Rosolia, J. R. O'Connell, J. R. Bavitz, and J. F. Restaino, *J. Pharm. Sci.*, *61*, 1638 (1972).
142. J. S. Tempio and H. C. Caldwell, *J. Pharm. Sci.*, *69(3)*, IV (1971).
143. H. Moller, *Pharm. Ind.*, *45*, 617 (1983).
144. R. J. Whithey and A. J. Bonker, *J. Pharm. Pharmacol.*, *24*, 345 (1972).
145. W. Rothe and J. Schellhorn, *Pharm. Ind.*, *39*, 801 (1977).
146. W. Rothe and J. Schellhorn, *Pharm. Ind.*, *40*, 645 (1978).
147. W. Rothe and J. Schellhorn, *Pharm. Ind.*, *41*, 785 (1979).
148. H. Moller, *Pharm. Ztg.*, *127*, 2045 (1982).
149. H. Moller, *Pharm. Ind.*, *48*, 514 (1986).
150. C. E. Wells, *J. Pharm. Sci.*, *70*, 232 (1980).
151. S. Gershberg and F. D. Stoll, *J. Am. Pharm. Assoc. Sci. Ed.*, *35*, 284 (1946).
152. H. W. Dibbern, *Pharm. Ind.*, *46*, 387 (1984).

ADDITIONAL READING

Langenbucher, F., D. Benz, and W. Kurth, *Pharm. Ind.*, *51*, 1276 (1989).

FOUR

Automation in Dissolution Testing

William A. Hanson
Hanson Research Corporation
Chatsworth, California

Albertha M. Paul
Zymark Corporation
Hopkinton, Massachusetts

THE CONCEPT OF AUTOMATION

System Concept

A dissolution test consists of more than one procedure. The entire test is a series of procedures any one of which may be manual or automatic. An important concept in planning automation is to survey the test as a whole system and decide which of the discrete operations should be automated (1). Illustrations on automation in dissolution testing are to be found in Figs. 4.1–4.12.

Selection of Procedure to Automate

When we use the word *automate*, we should specify which procedure(s) are to be automated. For example, a person may state, "I want to automate my dissolution testing" when he means that he wants only to do automatic sample collecting. When specifying an automated dissolution system, one should clearly indicate the level of automation desired.

Cost-Effectiveness

Automation is not a panacea (2). Its cost-effectiveness is analyzed by comparing the advantages with the disadvantages. In this analysis one should consider the probability of adding degrees of automation to various additional procedures in the future as demand develops.

Robotics

The term *robotics* is often used in discussions of automation. It has come to imply the use of a robotic hand or arm but is not limited to this. In a more general sense, mechanical devices that do human tasks may be a part of any automated system. The robot arm is superbly adaptable to some dissolution problems and its application is included in all sections of this chapter.

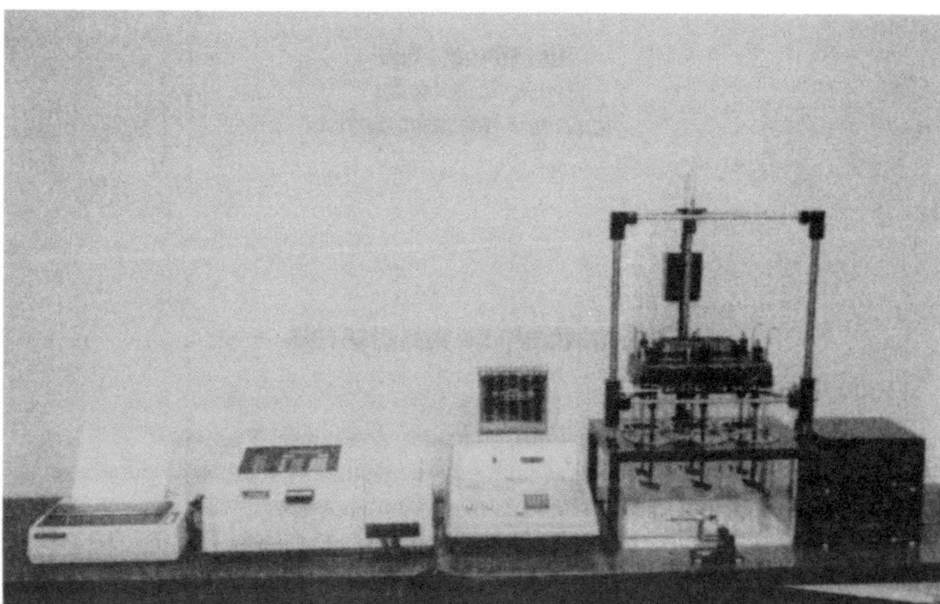

Fig. 4.1 Menu-driven automated dissolution system using a programmable spectrophotometer with seven flow cells. Sampling acquisition, UV detection, and data reduction are complete. (Courtesy of Beckman Instruments.)

GENERAL PRINCIPLES OF AUTOMATION

Advantages

The user can benefit from several advantages once the dissolution test, which is routinely conducted, is automated.

Accuracy

Although opinions vary, it is the author's experience that automated methods tend to provide more repeatable results than comparable manual procedures. This advantage, however, can only be realized when the automated hardware is carefully designed. Precise time, for example, is more likely with automatic methods since the time point is determined by an electronic clock and the time duration of the procedure is similarly controlled.

Timing

Electronic timing, however, can introduce errors. For example, although the exact time of reading absorbance in a flow cell always repeats with electronic timing, the hardware may fail to allow a few seconds for the contents of the flow cell to stabilize. (This stabilization always occurs with manual procedures.) Absorbance differences of 1 or 2% are commonly observed between readings of dynamic versus static flow cell contents.

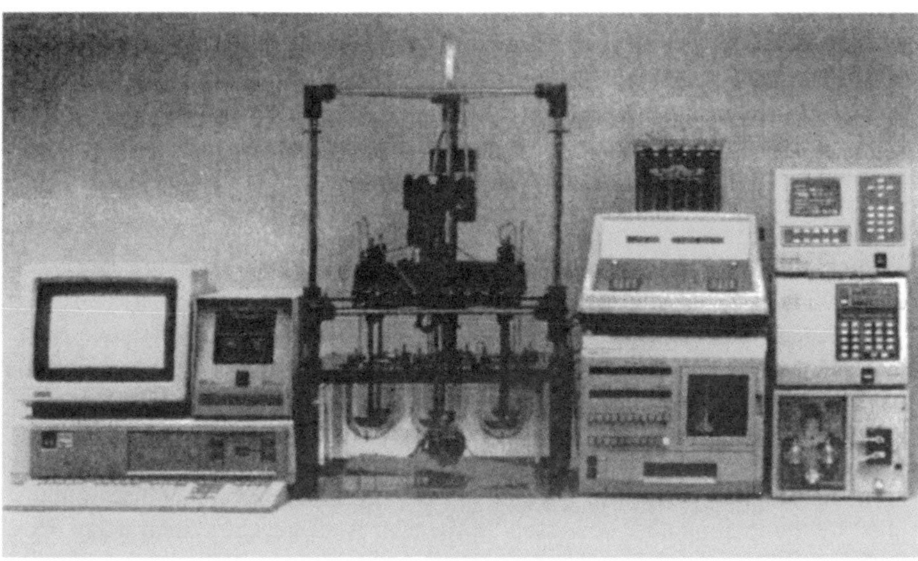

Fig. 4.2 HPLC automated dissolution system. Computer menu driven, it withdraws samples, injects into column, and reduces data. (Courtesy of Waters Division Millipore.)

Time Saving

Investigator's time is normally used more effectively when a procedure is automated. An automatic sampling procedure, for example, allows a technician to utilize his or her time for other chores. This may allow an additional dissolution run during a normal work span when the runs are short. It may eliminate the necessity of overtime or second shifts for extended release tests that run over 8 h.

Versatility

It may be surprising to some that versatility can be a benefit of automation. When test protocols change, the setup changes may be much easier in some automated systems than the manual counterpart. Some samplers, for example, can be changed from ultraviolet (UV) to high-performance liquid chromatographic (HPLC) detection by turning a few valves and replacing a carousel. Complete directions for timing and operating a given protocol may be saved on disk or stored in memory with some systems.

Validation

An automated procedure is easily validated by performing the same operation manually and then automatically. The results are compared statistically.

Limitations

Personnel

Although a more efficient use of personnel is almost always a benefit of any degree of automation, the addition of high-cost staff support for automated equipment should be considered. Programmers, maintenance technicians, and higher-educational-level operators may be required.

Synchronizing

Various time problems inherent in a given test may impose severe requirements on the type of automation.

Sequential time demands. Automated sample withdrawal may be classified into simultaneous and sequential sample acquisition. Generally, the finite time used to withdraw/deposit a sample and be ready for the next sampling is the minimum time duration between sampling periods for a simultaneous system. This can practically be held to 2 min in commercial equipment. The duration between sampling periods in a sequential system, however, is this time multiplied by the total number of vessels in the test. A sequential system using six flasks would have a minimum sample interval of 6×2 min (12 min).

Archiving. Archiving of samples in the system may be necessary. For example, samples may be withdrawn simultaneously into a collector, and sequentially from the collector into the detector. The sequence of detection

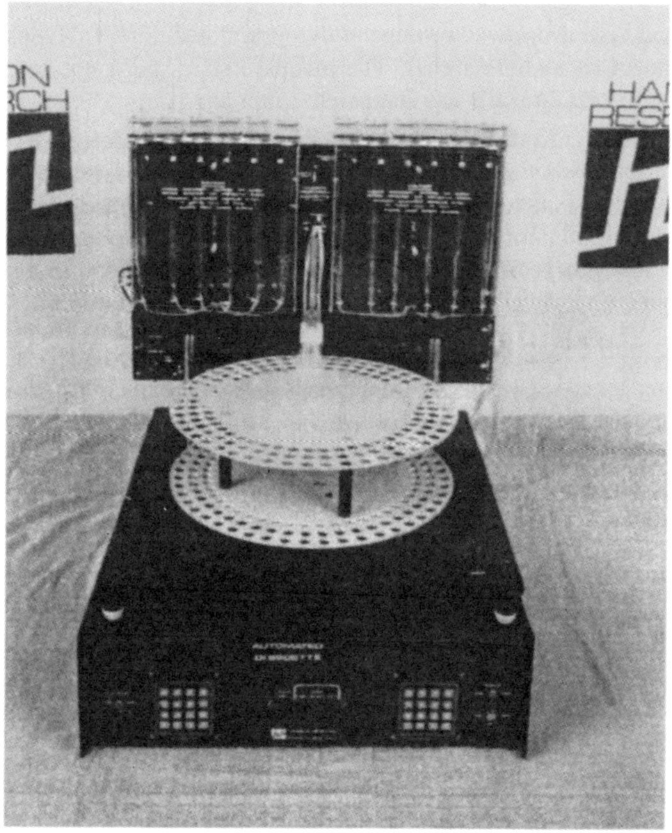

Fig. 4.3 Menu-driven automated sampler capable of replacing sample volume removed. Used for UV, HPLC, and other detection methods. (Courtesy of Hanson Research Corporation.)

analysis becomes independent in time from the sequence of withdrawing samples. This is particularly important when chromatographic column time may not conveniently match sample interval time. A recent commercial system completely automates the sampling–detection–data processing cycle by loading an HPLC automated injector carousel at convenient sampling-time intervals, and withdrawing samples for column analysis in the time window between sample deposit periods. The entire system is computer driven (3).

Staggering starts. Sequential sampling requires staggered start of vessels. Robotic automation such as the Zymark systems (discussed later in this chapter) has no problem with staggered starts. Other automated systems supply controlled "pill droppers" or depend on manual addition of the dosage form on command of an audible signal. The manual "start" does not become burdensome until 12 or 24 starts are staggered 2 min apart.

Evaporation. Archiving of samples leads to problems of evaporation or deterioration with time or temperature. Evaporation is generally controlled with septums mounted on the receiving vials in the collector. However, none of the evaporation control methods currently available commercially are completely satisfactory. Special apparatus holding the collector in a temperature-controlled bath has been used to avoid temperature deterioration.

Cleanup and Setup Requirements

These are generally longer for automated systems than for a manual system. This is not necessarily a disadvantage in completely automated systems that repeat (robotic systems). The problem is being gradually reduced as manufacturers supply stored program controls and provide self-cleaning programs for their systems.

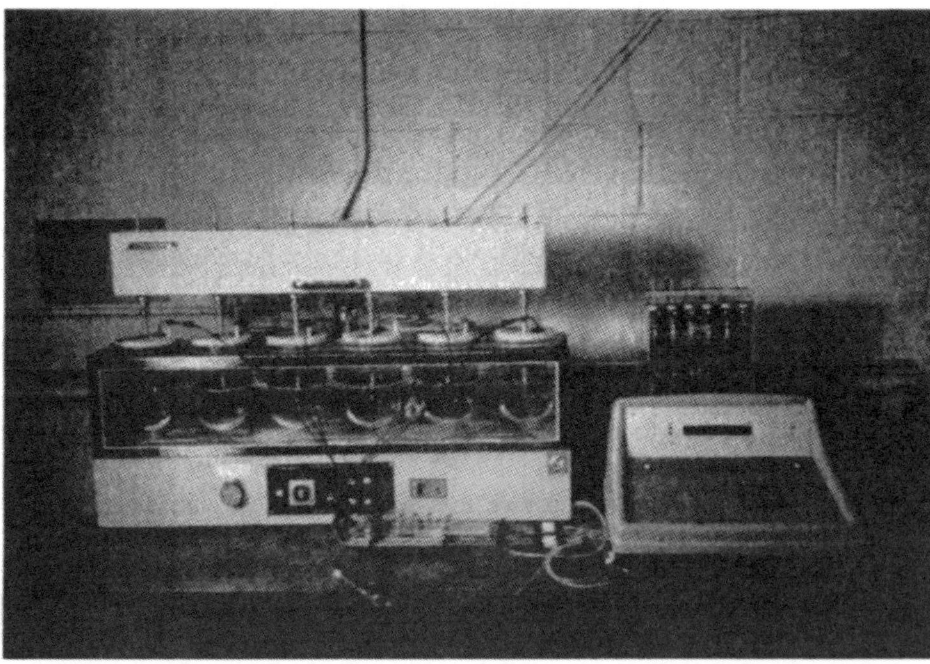

Fig. 4.4 Automated sampler probes attached to Toyama dissolution station. Probes such as this adapt to all commercial dissolution stations. (Courtesy of Hanson Research Corporation.)

Versatility

Versatility was described in the preceding section as a possible advantage for automated systems. Some systems, however, are supplied by detector manufacturers and restricted to their type of detection. Most UV automated procedures and dissolution software, for example, cannot be adapted to HPLC or other wet chemistry detection methods.

Lack of Versatility

Lack of such versatility may not be a handicap when the system is dedicated, but can be a serious limitation for the laboratory attempting to automate for multiple protocols. Such versatility is a big advantage in product development, analytical development, stability, and similar activities.

Failures

Equipment failures may be catastrophic in an automated system. This is particularly true in quality control installations where dissolution testing is a release requirement and thus a part of the production line. Those considering an automated installation should therefore carefully consider redundancy (e.g., two separate six-flask dissolution stands with two motors/controls instead of one 12-drive unit). Adequate spare components should be kept handy to minimize downtime. Finally, if possible, automated equipment should be so designed that in case of an emergency, manual methods can be used to maintain some degree of performance.

SELECTING AN AUTOMATED SYSTEM

Unit Operations

The first step in specifying an automated system is to consider each unit operation carefully. Each unit operation should be evaluated as a candidate for automation using the criteria of advantages and disadvantages previously outlined.

Classifying Unit Operations

These unit operations are superbly defined in detail in the outstanding review of automation presented by Compton and Hinsvark (1). A simplified outline more adaptable when considering automated equipment might list the following.

Setup

Practically, automation of setup should be considered when a series of back-to-back tests are planned using the exact same protocol. The initial setup is

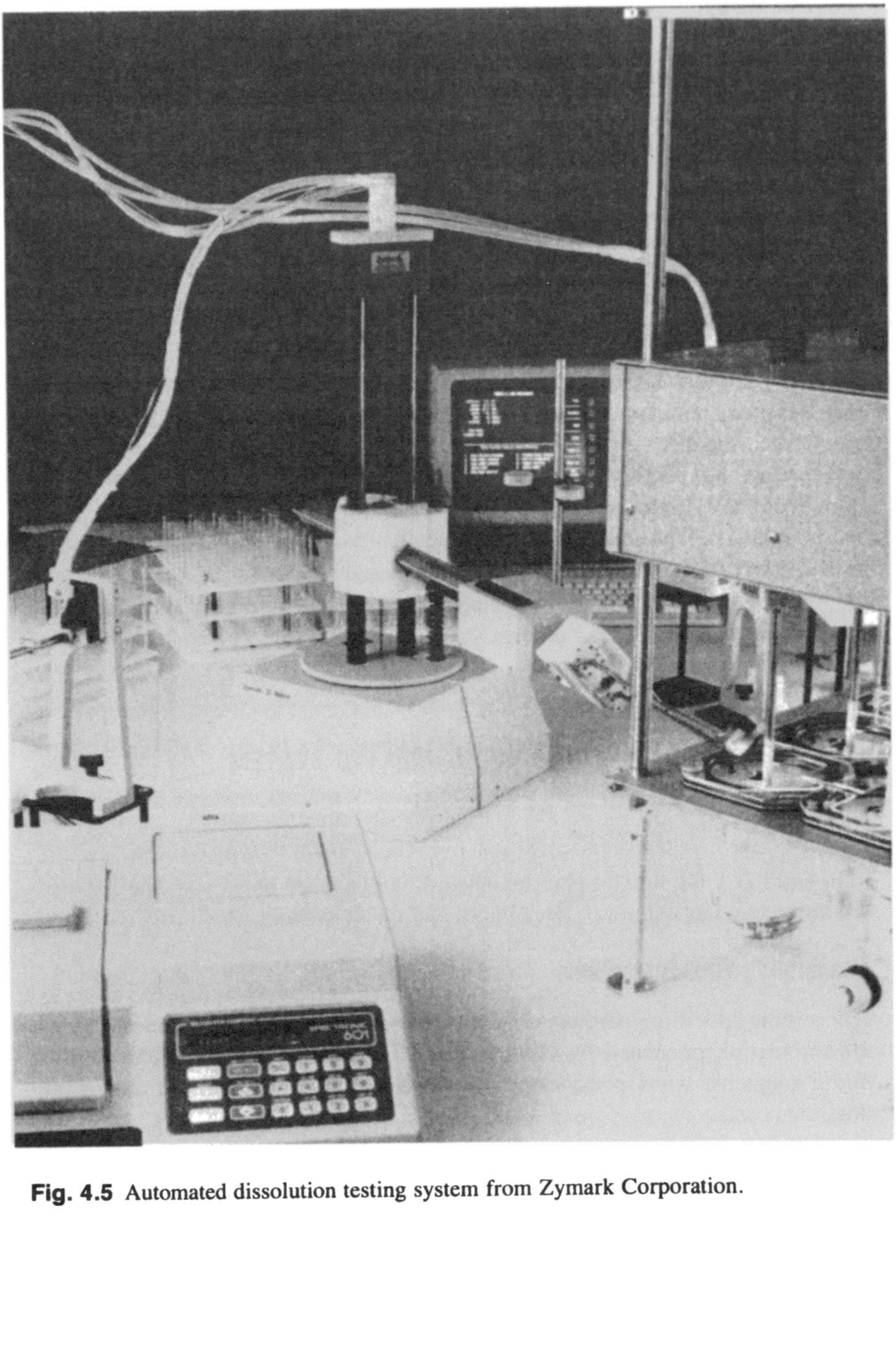

Fig. 4.5 Automated dissolution testing system from Zymark Corporation.

manual, but reestablishing conditions of clean, preheated media and lines ready for the subsequent test involves time and effort that must be included in the list of unit operations considered for automation.

Dissolution

Specific manipulations involving manual or automated procedures include verifying temperature and volume, rpm of stirrer, time zero, introduction of the dosage form, and starting rotation of the stirring mechanism.

Sampling–Analysis–Data Reduction

1. Acquisition of aliquot for analysis. Techniques for in situ UV absorption determination using fiber optics eliminate this step.
2. Determination of ingredient released in unit time by a selected method. Methods vary but may require sample preparation. Calculations, statistical manipulations, graphic displays, and data storage may all be included in this operation.

Systems Analysis

If one considers a completely automated system from setup through data reduction, it is still necessary to select and specify details for each of these operations. The design of such a system is almost a project in itself, requiring a careful systems analysis. Such services are available commercially, but the user will still be asked to specify certain constraints. Therefore, this discussion will be organized to consider specifications for each of the foregoing operations separately.

Automating Setups

Before a dissolution session is started, the stirring device, flasks, and lines must be cleaned, fresh media must be added, and the temperatures must be validated. Validation of other parameters may be required. Examples include tablet weights, stirring speeds, establishing blank and standards, and test background absorbance (4). Setup *must* be automated if more than one complete test is desired without human attendance. It need not be automated if only one test is planned without human intervention.

As of this writing, the automated washing of vessels and stirrers and replacement with fresh media may represent not only the most expensive unit of automation, but may dictate the approach to automating other units. For example, if a robot station is selected as the method of washing and preparing vessels, the robot station may then be the economical method of choice for sampling, dropping dosage forms, pH change, and so on.

Broadly speaking, complete automation of setup is economically justified when the same protocol is run back to back either in a relatively short time duration or at intervals occurring at inconvenient times, such as the middle of the night. But in time-release tests covering long periods of time, the percentage of technician hours devoted to setup may be a small percentage of the total and not worth the investment. Technician hours are not the only factor to consider, however. An extensive discussion and formal procedure of evaluation is available from Zymark (5).

Completely automated setup systems enabling back-to-back unattended dissolution procedures have been offered by the Zymark Corporation using a robot arm with robot stations (4). Perkin-Elmer has also entered this field. Robotic systems not using a robot arm are offered by Erweka and Pharmatest from West Germany and by Sotax from Switzerland. One must make one's own evaluation of the relative merits of these systems. Each has its strong and weak points. A partial automation of the setup procedure providing addition of fresh preheated, deaerated, measured media to six vessels in less than 4 min has been available for several years (6).

Automating the Dissolution Procedure

For this discussion we cover only the use of apparatus 1 and 2 compendia requirements for various dosage forms (7). This unit operation classification includes the starting of the test, introduction of the dosage form, maintenance and monitoring of the required temperature, speed, and pH (e.g., the process of dissolving the dosage form under rigorously defined conditions).

General description. In the manual operation the dosage form is placed in the basket (apparatus 1) or dropped into the flask (apparatus 2) at time zero. The speed and temperature have been adjusted and are visually monitored through sensors throughout the test. Depending on the method, the stirring device may be lowered (simultaneously or sequentially) into premeasured position at time zero.

Commercial availability. All of these operations except placing the tablet into the basket (apparatus 1) can easily be automated. Stirring speed and temperature are controlled by feedback sensors whose output may also be transferred to data recording to provide monitoring printouts at desired times. Various automated devices for introducing the dosage form are offered by all manufacturers of automated systems. As of this date only the robot arm has been successful in changing the dosage form in the basket. It also seems more adaptable to monitoring of pH.

Change of pH: simple addition or replacement. Some product protocols require a change in pH during the test. The most common method is to start the test with a reduced media volume (such as 700 mL) for the acid phase and addition of up to 200 mL of alkali buffer for the alkaline phase. Other requirements (such as simulating the rotating bottle method) require more sophisticated step changes. The most drastic requirement is complete removal and

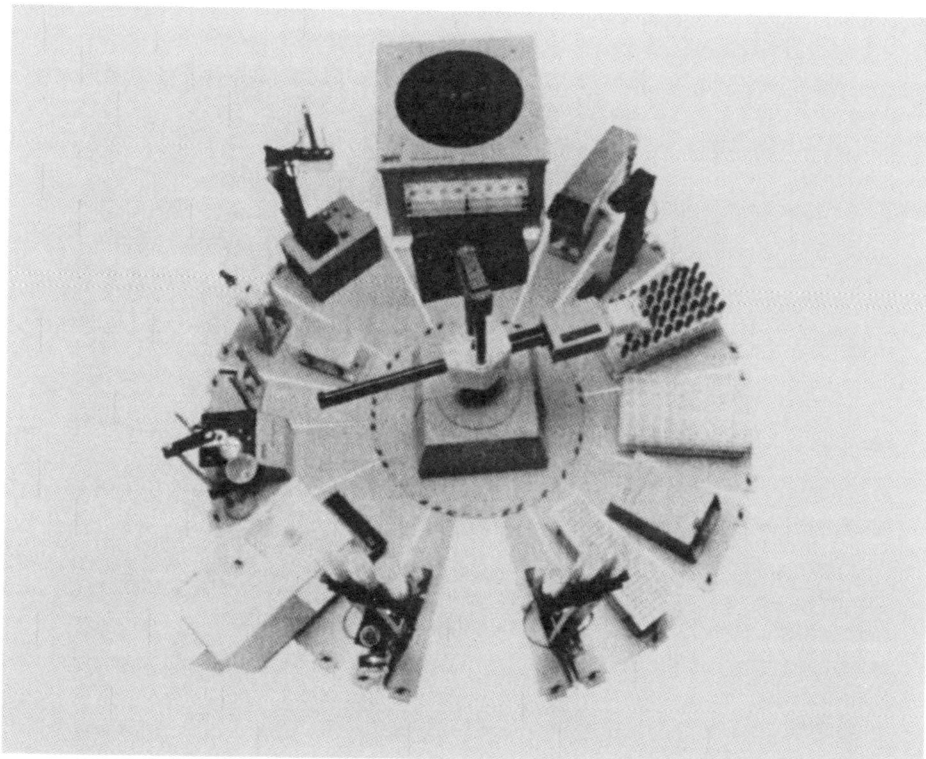

Fig. 4.6 Laboratory robotic system configuration for HPLC sample preparation. (Courtesy of Zymark Corporation.)

replacement of the media at a given point. Any of these requirements may be automated with commercially available equipment.

Simple addition of an alkali buffer can be achieved by using a timer and pump to feed a premeasured amount into each flask. The calculation of unit concentration change is introduced into data reduction. Incremental additions require more sophisticated equipment to ensure volumetric accuracy (6). If a robotic system is installed, the robot station can be programmed to add the buffer at appropriate times (4). This approach uses less than final flask volume to start, such as 700 mL increased by buffer addition to 900 mL.

For low-solubility drugs where sink conditions are violated with less than 900 mL, Hanson Research has commercial pH adjustment apparatus that withdraws media and replaces the exact volume with buffer. Volumes possible are up to 50 mL per change. The Zymark robotic dissolution system can be programmed to accomplish pH change through this type of transfer, offering an

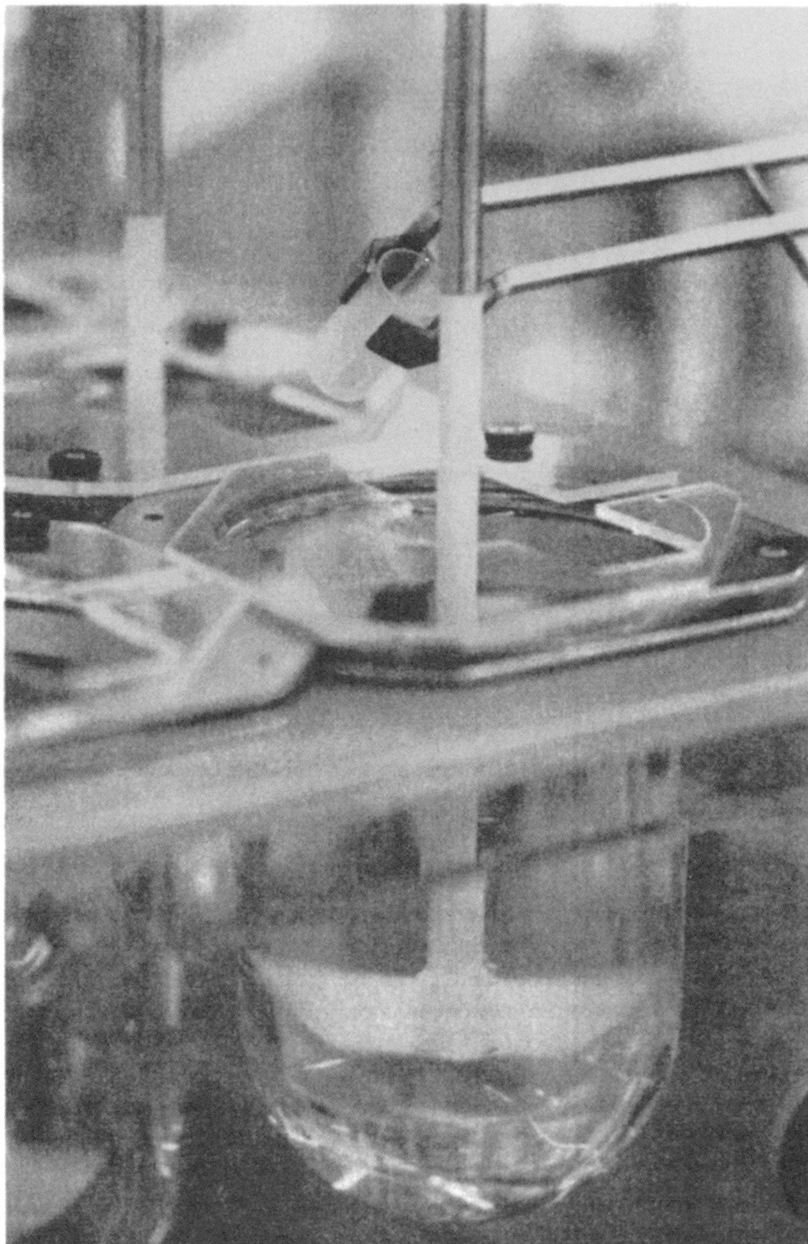

Fig. 4.7 Adding a sample (dosage form to be tested) to the dissolution testing vessel using the general-purpose hand and special sample pouring fingers on the Zymark system.

automatic selection of four buffer sources (4). It can also successfully remove all the medium and replace it with new.

Automating Sampling Procedures

Of all the operations, sampling procedure is generally the most time consuming and labor intensive (1). We borrow the Zymark criteria for strategic evaluation of automation (5) to expand the considerations for automating sampling beyond more efficient use of personnel. Application flexibility, safety, faster turnabout, employee motivation, data audit trail, and accuracy may each be a reason for automating sampling. Where limited resources are available, sampling may be confidently selected as the first unit operation to be automated (1).

Questions to consider. The following questions are considered before choosing a sampling system.

1. Is this equipment to be dedicated to one product or method of detection? (If not, you may wish to compromise some features to gain versatility.)
2. How many samples per set (6, 12, or more) now and in the future, and how many sampling intervals, are needed? (This will determine the number of collector vials you need if the samples are archived at any point; for example, six samples each taken 10 times will require a minimum of $6 \times 10 = 60$ sample vials.)
3. What is the minimum time used by proposed system to complete one cycle of sampling? (This may limit your choice of system; for example, if a cycle of sampling takes longer than your minimum sampling interval, the system cannot function.)
4. Do you wish to vary sampling-time intervals, such as some 10 min followed by 1-h intervals? (Some sophisticated commercial systems require equal sample intervals.)
5. Will the total volume of aliquots withdrawn over the total test significantly alter flask medium volume? (A media replacement sampler will avoid this situation, which may cause problems with "sink" on low-solubility drugs or require special data manipulation to compensate.)
6. Does the sampling system use materials such as flexible tubing and plastics that may adsorb the ingredient you are testing? For example, nitroglycerin and some steroids and prostaglandin derivatives (8) adsorb significantly on plastic surfaces other than polyfluorocarbon. Future problems may be avoided by selecting samplers with only polyfluorocarbon, 316 stainless, and glass wetted surfaces.
7. Does the sampler synchronize with your detector? (HPLC or detectors with some sample preparation requirements may need to archive samples between sample withdrawal and sample detection.)

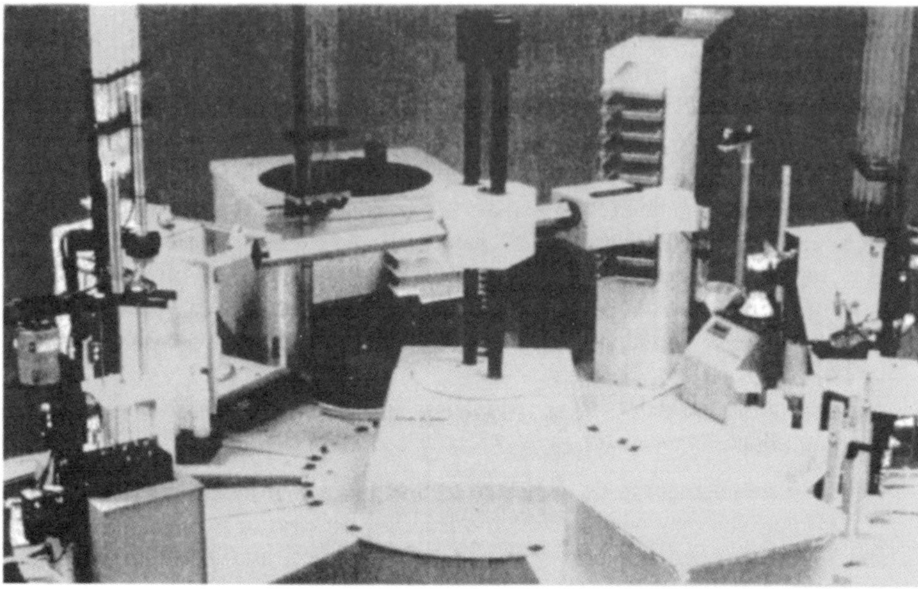

Fig. 4.8 Laboratory robotic system configuration for drugs in biological fluids by Zymark Corporation.

8. What kind of filtration will you need? (Provision for backflush may be necessary for accuracy and to avoid clogging.)
9. Will the system work on fluids with a high surfactant content value? (This should be questioned and specified on a new application.)
10. What protocol details must you meet that cannot be changed to match the demands of the automated sampler? (A thorough listing may avoid problems when the system is installed.)

Classification: continuous and intermittent flow. These systems move a stream out of the dissolution vessel and return it through a separate line. They are classified as continuous even though the flow is turned on and off intermittently. These systems should provide for automatic flow reversal to backflush the filters.

1. *Intermittent-Flow Archiving*. Archiving of samples achieves one objective that may not always be considered; in case of failure in one sampling cycle, archived samples are available for subsequent reanalysis. We say that this will not happen, but those of us familiar with the real world like the security of being able to recheck one or more sample cycles to avoid aborting the

entire test and repeating, a procedure demanding many hours. Archiving samples will provide this security.

These continuous-flow or intermittent-flow systems are also commonly available where detection involves a flow cell (e.g., where UV absorbance is the detection method selected). They rarely provide for archiving of samples. They have been applied to HPLC by inserting an injection valve in place of the flow cell, but this is generally not successful because column time rarely synchronizes with sample interval time.

2. *Advantages and Disadvantages*. Simplicity and neatness is one of the major advantages observed while using intermittent-flow archiving. Beckman has pioneered in UV systems using multiple flow cells, drawing simultaneous samples but measuring absorbance in six (or seven) parallel sample lines sequentially. Their Hanson Dissoscan dissolution package for the DU-60 series spectrophotometers enables all polyfluorocarbon tubing to avoid sorption and can easily be expanded to handle 12 sample sources. LKB offers similar apparatus but cannot expand to 12 or use polyfluorocarbon tubing throughout. Hewlett-Packard offers a dissolution kit for its diode array spectrophotometer, which provides multiple-component analysis. Their system uses one flow cell but several sample lines, diverting sequentially through a valve to the flow cell.

Simultaneous sampling through individual sample lines avoids flask-to-flask carryover problems. The continuous sampling system returns the sample to the vessel, and no media replacement is necessary to maintain sink conditions.

Most commercial continuous systems require positioning of sample probes in the vessel at all times. Unless the probe diameters are restricted to very small diameters, flow pattern disturbances may alter dissolution results (9). Beckman avoids this problem with their Dissoscan by using a discrete sampler that removes the sample probe when samples are not being withdrawn. Peristaltic pumps are generally used in these systems. They suffer from the inherent requirement for the use of flexible tubing, which may adsorb active ingredients (8).

These applications depend on "washing" the stream path by using some time to pump solution before determining absorbance. This adds minutes to each sampling interval, extending the time needed to the point where 5-min sample intervals may not be possible.

The commercial systems available (Beckman, Hewlett-Packard, LKB, and others) include dissolution-data processing formats that are adequate but may not meet individual protocol requirements. They cannot easily be modified by the user. Many formats include a preset sampling interval and do not provide for programming different times into separate sample intervals. LKB attempts

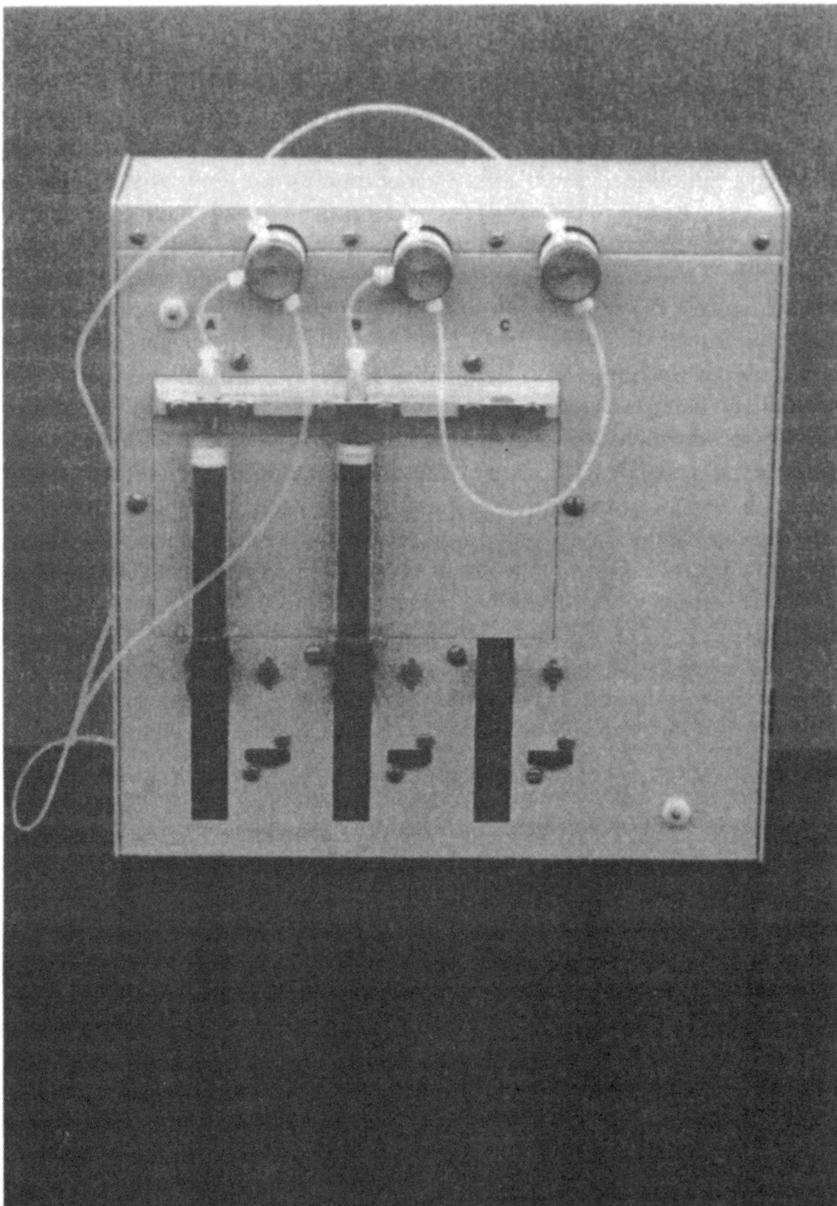

Fig. 4.9 Master laboratory station used to withdraw samples from the dissolution testing vessels on the Zymark system.

to avoid this problem by printing data at any interval selected, but such data are extrapolated and might not be acceptable in a particular protocol requirement.

Some questions that need to be addressed include the following:

1. Can this system later be adapted to total automation?
2. What variety of sample volume and total number of samples are available?
3. What provision is made to avoid evaporation errors during archiving?
4. Are commercial sipper systems available to remove the samples from the collector if included?

Classification of sampling systems: discrete. Discrete systems withdraw an aliquot from each dissolution vessel. This is deposited in a collector, archived, and/or manually or automatically sipped into a detector train such as UV, HPLC, atomic absorption (AA), gas chromatography (GC), or other. Discrete systems usually include an archiving step but not always. The Beckman dissolution package, for example, is offered with the Hanson Dissoscan, which simultaneously removes discrete aliquots for UV analysis and returns them to the source without archiving. The Hanson Gt operates sequentially in the same manner.

Advantages include shorter time periods of actual media aliquot removal and thus less potential disturbance of the flow dynamics in the dissolution flask. These may easily return a portion of the aliquot through the same line, providing for filter backflush or using robotic techniques (5). Filters may be changed between each sampling interval.

Many discrete systems do not replace the aliquot volume because in most cases the sample is a small enough percentage of the total that sink conditions are not appreciably compromised and the change can be compensated for in data reduction. In situations where this is not convenient, suitable media replacement is made available by several manufacturers.

Discrete systems are by their nature more sophisticated than continuous-flow or intermittent procedures. They may be more expensive to begin with and require more maintenance. Since discrete systems are intermittent, the process control logic and fluid hardware is easily adapted to simple media changes, such as pH modification. The Hanson Dissoette incorporates such accessory functions. Robotic systems are almost always discrete and also offer pH change capabilities.

Hidden problems in sampling. Some hidden problems of automated sampling can be cited.

1. *Sample Probes*. Many commercial automated samplers do not provide sample probe systems and users are left to their own ingenuity to make this

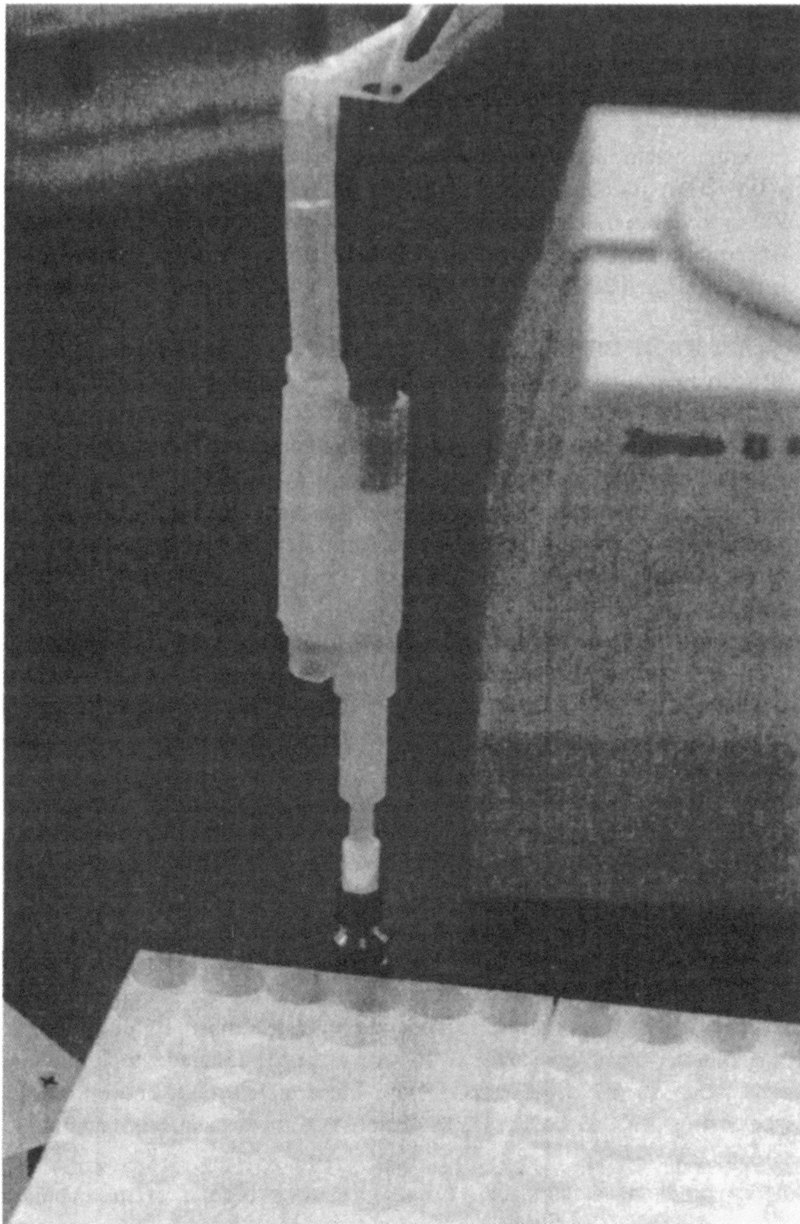

Fig. 4.10 Confirming the attachment of the filter on the sipper/fill hand using the filter confirm station on the Zymark system.

hookup. This requirement has always been supplied by Hanson (Autoprobe) VanKel (automated sample probes) and as of this writing is becoming more common with all manufacturers (Pharmatest, Erweka, Distek, Sotax, Toyama, etc.). Hanson and VanKel probe systems may be withdrawn to avoid flow disturbance. A universal automated probe system that can also include media replacement lines (The Snake) is now available to fit all dissolution test stands, no matter who the manufacturer.

2. *Filters*. Continuous unidirectional flow not only clogs filters but can produce errors due to accumulated particulates that provide a local dissolution "hot spot" where the solute–solvent interface shear is drastically increased. Filtration at pore sizes less than 1 μm drastically slows flow rates with pressure differentials of less than 10 psi. This limits positive-displacement pumping that draws through such a filter. The tendency is to use glass matt filters, due to sorption problems on many materials and the wetting characteristics of fluorocarbon materials.

3. *Sorption*. Fluorocarbon, glass, and stainless (316 only) are the only materials that do not significantly sorb some drugs, particularly nitroglycerin and some steroids (8).

4. *Surfactants*. Surfactants in dosage forms can lead to disastrous bubble problems in flow systems.

5. *Evaporation*. Archiving systems are subject to evaporative losses that are not consistent. Various solutions to this are available, such as septums and plugs for vials. Automated equipment, however, must be capable of puncturing these septums.

Automating Analysis Procedures

In the context of dissolution, unit operations may be divided into two separate procedures, sample preparation and detection. In HPLC, for example, the sample is first prepared in the column and then detected, often by UV. In the spectrophotometric determination of absorbance by UV, the sample must often be first diluted. Both sample preparation and detection may be automated.

UV absorbance. UV absorbance is the most popular method of detection used in dissolution. It is simple, inexpensive, and direct, generally requiring no sample preparation other than filtration. Dilution or concentration can be effectively mimicked by varying the optical path length of the cuvette.

UV spectrophotometric analysis is automated in all cases by substituting a flow cell for the manual cuvette. The flow cell is filled with sample using either continuous or discrete samplers. Samplers that allow the contents of the cell to stabilize (e.g., stop the flow) before reading absorbance are to be preferred. Extremely short optical paths (<0.5 mm) may cause difficulty with air bubbles.

A broad range of spectrophotometers is available with varying degrees of sophistication and capabilities. For many dissolution applications an inexpensive single-cell single-wavelength instrument coupled with a sampler feeding the flow cell and a printer output triggered by the sampler is adequate. Modern instruments can also include microprocessor-aided setup wavelength selection, automatic baseline control, and other helpful features. These are termed *programmable instruments*.

Dissolution programs are offered by many spectrophotometer manufacturers. Beckman has pioneered in this field and currently offers a complete dissolution program, including graphics, that handle up to 12 dissolution vessels with its DU-60 series. LKB provides an attractive package handling six vessels, with control and data processing supported by an IBM-PC computer. Hewlett-Packard supplies a dissolution package for its diode-array spectrophotometer capable of multicomponent analysis of samples from three separate six-vessel baths. These dissolution programs suffer from the requirement of equal sampling intervals, although LKB offers a printout that extrapolates selected sampling points.

In situ UV analysis using fiber optics has been experimented with using equipment from Guided Wave, Rancho Cordova, Calif. This technique has many problems to resolve before being practically applied to dissolution, but it has the potential advantage of eliminating the sampler.

HPLC. In the past decade, HPLC has advanced in popularity as the analytical procedure selected for dissolution. By its very definition, it includes sample preparation. As the drug delivery preference tends more and more to controlled-release preparations, the problems of monitoring polymer excipients and degradation products during dissolution accelerate the trend toward HPLC. It also has the inherent advantage of multicomponent identification.

HPLC is an analytical method that is also simple and inherently automated. Complete unattended automation of the sampling, analysis, and data reduction phases in dissolution awaited solution to the problem of time mismatch in attempts to synchronize sample intervals with column times. This is now available from Waters Division of Millipore Corp., Milford, Massachusetts (3). This system combines a computer-directed sequence in which the samples are archived directly in their autosampler during a time "window" during which column injection is stopped.

Most HPLC equipment manufacturers offer their own version of an autoinjector. Vials may be filled by sampling equipment and later inserted into the autoinjector for off-line analysis where dissolution operations and analytical operations are in separate departments. This solution is particularly attractive for the laboratory, which may prefer UV absorption for one procedure and HPLC for another. The same automated sampler may be used for both.

GC. As more emphasis is placed on transdermal delivery systems, the low concentrations involved suggest GC as a preferred analytical procedure. Com-

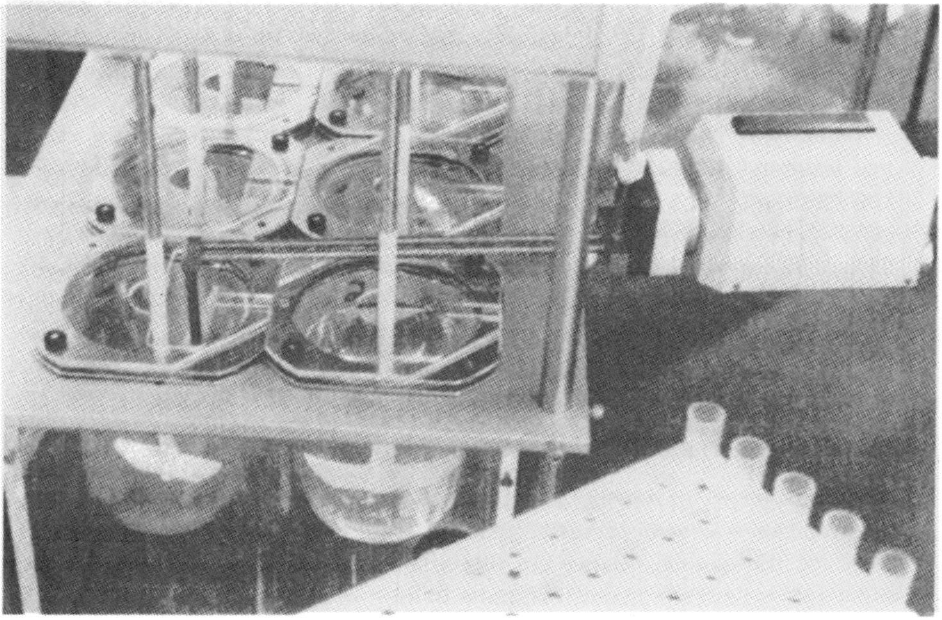

Fig. 4.11 Washing the dissolution testing vessels using the wash/aspirate hand on the Zymark system.

mercial instrumentation has not yet provided for GC on-line automation in dissolution testing.

Other analytical methods. Other analytical methods have been applied to automated dissolution systems by adapting commercial samplers to specially designed detectors. These include fluorescence, pH, and specific ion detectors. The ingenuity of the analyst and instrument designer are needed for these special applications.

Automating Data Reduction

Several commercial dissolution software packages are available for analytical instruments described in this chapter. These are generally free-standing data processing programs with various formats. They almost always include mean, standard deviation, and high–low values for each sample group and offer both raw data and computations such as percent dissolved. Graphic presentations are included. Some provide overlay capabilities for comparison of different runs. Others may be individually programmed to print "pass" or "fail" conclusions.

Source codes are not normally available for these programs. The user is thus precluded from making minor variations. This is not necessarily due to fear of copyright violation. Rather, software suppliers fear loss of control over the performance of their products.

Sometimes the data processing is performed manually. In such cases a normal printout is satisfactory. Users may write their own simple programs for keyboard entry on a personal computer or avail themselves of many packages commercially available (e.g., Data-Pak, Hanson Research, Northridge, California). Integration of data output with departmental computer systems is not a serious problem if the detector can supply a standard RS-232 communications link and the system controller can provide a proper time signal.

AUTOMATING TRANSDERMAL DISSOLUTION TESTING

Importance of Transdermal Dissolution

In this chapter we have concentrated on automating the compendial dissolution test procedures using apparatus 1 and 2 (7). Alternative drug delivery systems involving transdermal patches are receiving a great deal of attention and we might anticipate that a major revolution in drug delivery is imminent. Dissolution characteristics of these devices are being studied widely. As it was 20 years ago with oral dosage forms, a myriad of dissolution procedures have been suggested. One would suspect, however, that one or both of two methods will prevail (10).

One method in wide use consists of apparatus 2 (the paddle method) employing a screen holder on the bottom of the flask to which the transdermal device is attached. This method has the advantage of not requiring excessive investment in new equipment and being supported by a substantial data base on system variables (11).

Reciprocal transdermal dissolution testing was originally developed by Alza Corporation of Palo Alto, California. This method employs an up-and-down reciprocating motion similar to the USP disintegration test (7). The transdermal patch is attached to a wire that moves up and down in a test tube for a period of time, then transferred to a successive series as the test continues. In practice, several tubes are arranged in rows and columns in a water bath. Commercial equipment (RTD) is available from the Alza Corporation, Hanson Research in Northridge, California, and a limited-capacity unit (the Biodis) that can be adapted is available from VanKel. The Hanson apparatus offers an accessory that automatically delivers samples to HPLC vials.

Percutaneous Absorption Methods

Transdermal research using the Franz or Valia-Chien side-by-side cells presents very special problems. Complete unattended automation is not

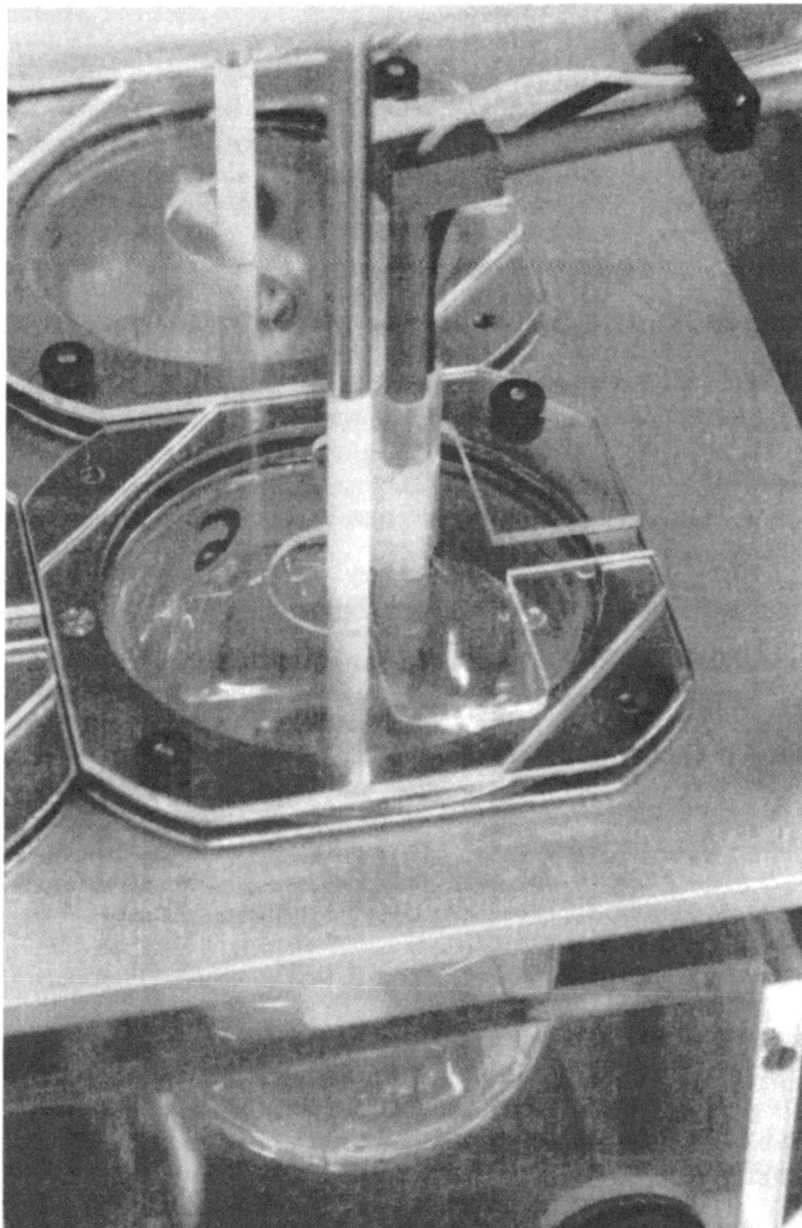

Fig. 4.12 Filling the dissolution testing vessels using the sipper/fill hand on the Zymark system.

currently available, although the robot might offer some attractive possibilities (5). Automated sampling is difficult because of (a) the necessity of preventing bubble introduction against the membrane, (b) extremely minute sample volumes, and (c) maintaining acceptable dissolution volume stability as samples are removed. Commercial samplers are currently under study by several laboratories (e.g., the Microette system; information available from Crown Glass, Somerville, New Jersey, or Hanson Research, Chatsworth, California).

Problems in Transdermal Dissolution

Transdermal devices present some special problems in dissolution testing not always present with oral dosage forms. Active ingredient concentrations at exceedingly low levels require more sophisticated detection procedures such as HPLC and GC. Detection of excipient materials and degradation products inherent with longer dosage periods suggest the need for multicomponent information. Larger sample lots than the 6 or 12 generally used in oral dosage dissolution are generally used and combined with extended sampling periods running into days or weeks.

Advantages of Reciprocal Transdermal Methods

The reciprocating dissolution test procedure adapts to these requirements better than apparatus 2 in the following ways. Much smaller dissolution volumes (5 to 20 mL) are easily used. Thus higher concentrations of released drug are available. The equipment lends itself to massive sample volumes and extended test runs. Twenty-four samples with 12 individual sampling intervals that run unattended are handled with equipment currently available. Since each test run is separated and retained after sampling, the entire test is archived. If stability is not a problem, this provides a measure of cost-effectiveness security (e.g., a 2-week run is not necessarily lost if one or two tests abort).

SUMMARY

Automation should be considered as a step-by-step adaptation, not as all or nothing. The procedures selected for automation should, however, be considered for their impact on later addition of automated steps. If not, one may be locked into obsolete expensive hardware incapable of change.

Automation of the sampling process is generally considered first because it is most time consuming. A wide variety of sampling hardware is available. Each system has its advantages and disadvantages. These should be considered in the light of future requirements as well as current needs. The key consideration in planning automation is to compare versatility with completeness. These two features tend to be mutually exclusive.

REFERENCES

1. B. J. Compton and O. N. Hinsvark, *Pharm. Technol.*, pp. 28–32 (Aug. 1986).
2. W. A. Hanson, *Handbook of Dissolution Testing*, Pharmaceutical Technology Publications, Springfield, Oreg. (1982).
3. *Automated Dissolution HPLC System*, Waters Division, Millipore Corporation, Milford, Mass. (1988).
4. A. M. Paul, K. S. Good, K. A. Tucker, and J. R. Strimaitis, *Automated Dissolution Testing with the Zymate II Laboratory Robotic System*, Zymark Corporation, Hopkinton, Mass. (1988).
5. *Laboratory Robotics Handbook*, Zymark Corporation, Hopkinton, Mass. (1988).
6. *Media-Mate*, Hanson Research, Northridge, CA.
7. *United States Pharmacopeia*, XXI rev., *National Formulary*, XVI rev., United States Pharamacopeial Convention, Rockville, Md. (1985).
8. G. W. Halstead and D. L. Theis, *J. Pharm. Sci.*, *74*, 1086 (1985).
9. T. S. Savage and C. E. Wells, *J. Pharm. Sci.*, *71*, 670 (1982).
10. PMA Committee, *Pharm. Forum*, *12*, 1798 (1986).
11. V. P. Shah, N. W. Tymes, W. Ment, and J. P. Skelly, *Pharm. Forum*, *14*, 3458 (1988).

ADDITIONAL READING

Figazzotto, A. C. and J.G. White, *Drug Dev. Ind. Pharm.*, *14*, 1799 (1988).
McCarthy, J.P., *Pharm. Techn.*, *12*, 72 (1988).

FIVE

Factors That Influence Dissolution Testing

INTRODUCTION

It has long been recognized that the availability of a drug for gastrointestinal absorption from solid dosage forms is often reflected by in vitro dissolution rates. It is also recognized that the rate-determining step in the absorption of drugs is generally the dissolution rate of drugs in the gastrointestinal fluids rather than the rapidity of their diffusion across the gut wall. These observations have stimulated research in dissolution-rate studies. Consequently, with the passing of years, dissolution testing has emerged to the single most important test that is employed not only as a quality control tool, but also in the development of dosage form(s), solid dosage forms in particular.

The dissolution-rate data can be meaningful only if the results of successive tests on the same dosage form are consistent within reason. The dissolution test should yield reproducible results even when it is performed in different laboratories or with different personnel. To achieve high reproducibility, all variables that influence the test should be clearly understood and possibly controlled.

Dissolution rate is influenced by many factors. The variety of factors that can affect the dissolution rate in vitro is considerable, and a large part of the literature is concerned with identifying and evaluating the extent to which these factors are involved. Hanson (1) has listed more than a dozen common random input variables that influence the dissolution rate of a drug from a dosage form (refer Table 5.1). Wagner (2), on the other hand, suggests that the factors affecting dissolution rate of drugs from capsules and tablets in vitro and in vivo are similar to those that affect disintegration time of tablets and capsules (see Table 5.2).

The various factors affecting the dissolution rate of a drug from a dosage form fall in six main classes:

1. Factors related to the physicochemical properties of the drug
2. Factors related to drug product formulation
3. Factors related to dosage form
4. Factors related to dissolution testing device
5. Factors related to dissolution test parameters
6. Miscellaneous factors

It must be stated at the outset that this classification is oversimplified for the purpose of understanding their influence on the dissolution process. Additionally, in most cases more than one factor is concomitantly in operation. Consequently, it is rather difficult to get a true appreciation while evaluating the influence of any one of these factors on the overall dissolution-rate process. In this chapter we elucidate the various factors that influence the dissolution process by presenting data illustrating the degree of effect. It is hoped that this approach will result in gaining a better and fuller appreciation for the relative magnanimity of the role that these factors play in dissolution testing of dosage forms.

FACTORS RELATING TO THE PHYSICOCHEMICAL PROPERTIES OF THE DRUG

The physicochemical properties of the drug substance can assume a primary role in controlling its dissolution from the dosage form. It is well known that the aqueous solubility of the drug is one of the major factors that determines its dissolution rate. Some studies have actually concluded that the drug solubility data can be used as a rough predictor of the possibility of any future problems with bioavailability, a factor that should be taken into consideration in the formulation design. Some of the more prominent physicochemical properties of the drug that influence the dissolution rate are discussed below.

Solid-Phase Characteristics

The solid-phase characteristics of drugs, such as amorphicity and crystallinity, have been shown to have a significant effect on the dissolution rate. Numerous

Table 5.1 Random Input Variables Influencing Dissolution Testing

Variable	Maximum Allowable	Excess Commonly Seen	Effect of Excess	Methods of Control
1. Eccentricity	±2mm (compendium) ±3/4 mm (optimal)	2–5 mm	+4–8%	Straighten shafts; use wide shaft guide points
2. Vibration	0.1 mil displacement at vessel	0.2–0.9 mil	+5–10%	Eliminate source
3. Alignment	1.5° to perpendicular	2–7°	+2–25%	Adjust alignment in field
4. Centering	±2 mm (compendium)	±2–6 mm	±2–13%	Center individual flasks
5. Agitation rate	±4%	±10%	Linear	Use better, smoother control, or use synchronous drive
6. Dissolved gas	Deaerated	Bubbles form	±50%	Deaerate media by various methods
7. Media pH	0.00 accuracy	±0.05	±10%	Check buffers or deaerate; calibrate the pH meter
8. Media contamination	ppm	Ions, surfactants	Substantial	Carefully control media
9. Evaporation	None	2–5%	Linear	Use flask covers
10. Temperature	±0.05 (compendium) ±0.01 (optimal)	1–2°	Linear	Monitor individual flasks; allow adequate equilibrium
11. Flow pattern	No interference	Turbulence from probes	Substantial	Remove probes
12. Sampling position	Compendium	±0.5 cm	Little	Use care
13. Filters	No sorbing	Considerable blockage	Significant	Use bidirectional filter flow; check sorbing
14. Detection	Use standard	Interference	Considerable	Use standard
15. Sorbtion	None	Considerable	Significant	Check materials

Source: Ref. 1.

Table 5.2 Factors Influencing Dissolution Rate of Drugs from Tablets and Capsules

I. Environmental factors during dissolution
   1. Intensity of agitation, rate and type of flow of fluids, and geometrical factors
   2. Concentration gradient (i.e. the difference in concentration between the solubility of the drug in the dissolution medium and the average concentration in the bulk fluid)
   3. Composition of the dissolution medium; pH, ionic strength, viscosity, surface tension, etc., are all important and are determined by the composition of the medium
   4. Temperature of dissolution medium

II. Factors related to the physicochemical properties of the drug
   A. Factors affecting solubility
      1. Polymorphism
      2. Amorphous state and solvation
      3. Free acid, free base, or salt form
      4. Complexation, solid solutions, and eutectics
      5. Particle size
      6. Surfactants
   B. Factors affecting surface area available for dissolution
      1. Particle size
      2. Manufacturing variables

III. Factors related to the composition and method of manufacture
   A. Tablets
      1. Amount and type of diluent or filler and other adjuvants, such as neutral salts
      2. Type of tablet manufacture employed
      3. Granule size and size distribution
      4. Amount and type of disintegrant and method of incorporating it
      5. Amount and type of surfactant (if any) and method of incorporating it
      6. Compressional force and speed of compression.
   B. Capsules
      1. Amount and type of diluent or filler and other adjuvants, such as neutral salts
      2. Method used to reduce bulk (e.g., granulating or slugging)
      3. Granule or powder size and size distribution
      4. Amount and type of lubricant and method of incorporating it
      5. Amount and type of surfactant (if any) and method of incorporating it
      6. "Pressure" applied during filling
      7. Composition and properties of the capsule shell

IV. Environmental factors involved with dosage forms
   1. Humidity during manufacture
   2. Storage conditions for dosage forms
   3. Age of dosage forms

Source: Ref. 2.

studies have demonstrated that the amorphous form of a drug usually exhibits greater solubility and higher dissolution rate as compared to that exhibited by the crystalline form. The drugs that abide by this observation are novobiocin, griseofulvin, phenobarbital, cortisone acetate, and chloramphenicol. However, Piccolo and Sakr (3) showed that the dissolution rate of amorphous erythromycin estolate is markedly lower than the crystalline form of erythromycin estolate, as exemplified in Fig. 5.1.

Polymorphism

The polymorphic forms of drugs have shown to influence changes in the solubilizing characteristics and thus the dissolution rate of the drug substance in question. Numerous reports have shown that polymorphism and the states of hydration, solvation, and/or complexation markedly influence the dissolution characteristics of the drug.

The dissolution profiles of chlorpropamide (CPM) polymorphs were investigated employing the USP XIX/NF XIV rotating basket method (4). Four metastable forms exhibited faster dissolution rate than those of the stable form. Ueda et al. (5) further extended the investigation for the dissolution behavior of CPM polymorphs employing a stationary disk method and a dispersed amount method. They reported that the metastable form II polymorph of CPM showed a dissolution phenomenon involving simultaneous phase change from metastable form to stable form during dissolution. The dissolution curves of CPM polymorphs are illustrated in Fig. 5.2, which demonstrates the influence

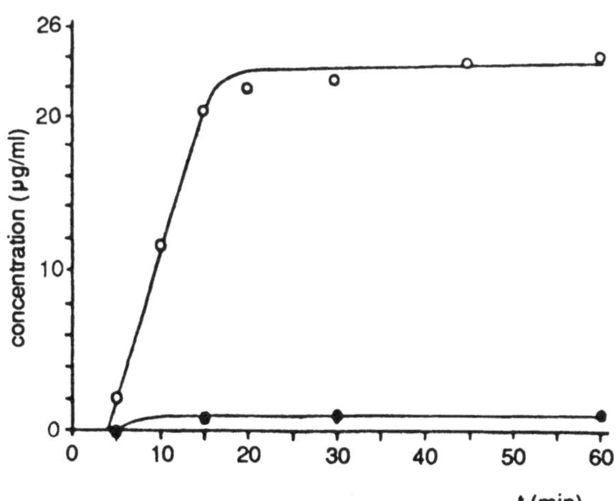

Fig. 5.1 Dissolution performance of erythromycin estolate. ○, Crystalline form; ●, amorphous form. (From Ref. 3.)

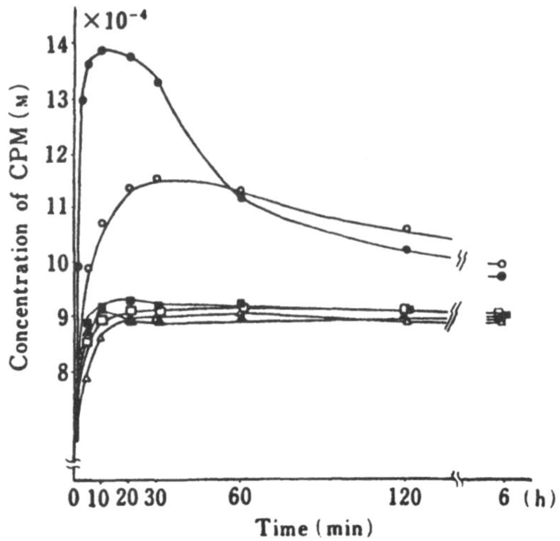

Fig. 5.2 Dissolution profiles of chlorpropamide polymorphs in 50 mL of KCl–HCl buffer (pH 2.0, 30°C). □, Form A; ■, form B; ○, form C; ●, form II; △, form III; ▲, form V. (From Ref. 5.)

of polymorphism on the dissolution rate of a drug. Other drugs that exhibit influence on the dissolution behavior include tolbutamide (6), phenylbutazone (7), erythromycin (8), ampicillin (9,10), chloramphenicol (11), anhydrous griseofulvin and its chloroform solvate form (12), and others.

Coprecipitation and/or Complexation

Numerous reports have shown that coprecipitation with polyvinylpyrrolidine (PVP) can markedly influence the dissolution of drugs (13–16). In most instances, coprecipitation as well as complexation is employed for enhancing the dissolution characteristics of the drug substance. The mechanism for this enhanced dissolution has been the subject of debate. Several authors have proposed that the increased drug dissolution rate results from the formation of an energetic amorphous drug phase (14,17,18). Others have attributed the effect to the drug being molecularly dispersed (19). Yet others claim that complexation with PVP while there is formation of a coacervate is responsible for accelerated dissolution rates (20–22).

Hydroflumethiazide–PVP coprecipitates were investigated for their dissolution rates and were compared to that of pure crystalline drug (15). The coprecipitate supported the existence of high-energy amorphous drug phase in systems containing more than 40% PVP. Additionally, dissolution data suggested that the solubility of this phase was four times that of the crystalline drug.

Corrigan and Holohan (23) prepared hydroflumethiazide–PVP complexes by spray drying the drug with PVP. These systems were amorphous, as confirmed by differential scanning colorimetry at low PVP weight fractions. The apparent solubility of the drug in these complexes increased with increasing PVP content, reaching a plateau value approximately four times that of the pure crystalline drug. Dissolution studies with compressed disks supported the apparent solubility data. The results were attributed to the increased free energy and entropy associated with the spray-dried drug, resulting in different orders of organization. The results for the dissolution profiles of hydroflumethiazide from the various drug–PVP systems are illustrated in Fig. 5.3. Although coprecipitation has been employed primarily to enhance the dissolution rate of sparingly soluble drugs, it has also been used to retard the release rate of drugs as a method of prolonging the drug action (24).

Particle Characteristics

According to Nernst–Brunner theory, the dissolution rate is directly proportional to the surface area of the drug. Since the surface area increases with decreasing particle size, higher dissolution rates may be achieved through the reduction of particle size. This effect has been highlighted by the superior dissolution rate observed after micronization of certain sparingly soluble drugs as opposed to the regularly milled form. However, when employing this technique to enhance dissolution, it is important to recognize the fact that it is the

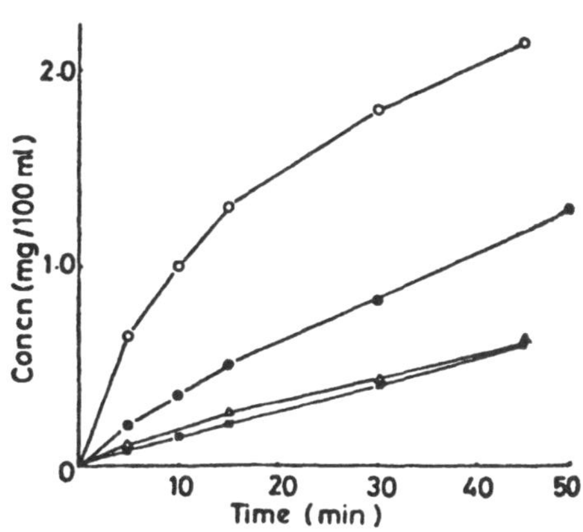

Fig. 5.3 Dissolution profiles of hydroflumethiazide (HDFT) from HDFT–PVP systems. ○, Spray-dried with 20% PVP; ●, spray-dried with 5% PVP; △, mixture containing 20% PVP and spray-dried HDFT; ■, Mixture containing 20% PVP and crystalline HDFT. (From Ref. 23.)

effective surface area that has to be increased. The effective surface area is the surface area available to the dissolution fluid. If the drug is hydrophobic and the dissolution medium has poor wetting properties, reduction of particle size may lead to decreased effective surface area and hence a "slower" rate of dissolution, as shown in Fig. 5.4. By and large, this parameter has been investigated extensively for the purpose of enhancing the dissolution rate of poorly soluble drugs, as illustrated in Fig. 5.5 (25–27).

The mechanism by which the reduction in particle size improves dissolution is usually through enhancement of the drug solubility. It is assumed that the drug solubility is independent of particle size. However, the drug solubility and surface area can be correlated by the *Ostwald–Freundlich equation*:

$$\ln C_s = \frac{2M\gamma}{\rho RT}\frac{1}{r} = \frac{\alpha}{r} \tag{5.1}$$

where C_s is the solubility of the drug, M the molecular weight, ρ the density, γ the interfacial tension or surface free energy of the solid, T the temperature, R the gas constant, and r the radius of the particle.

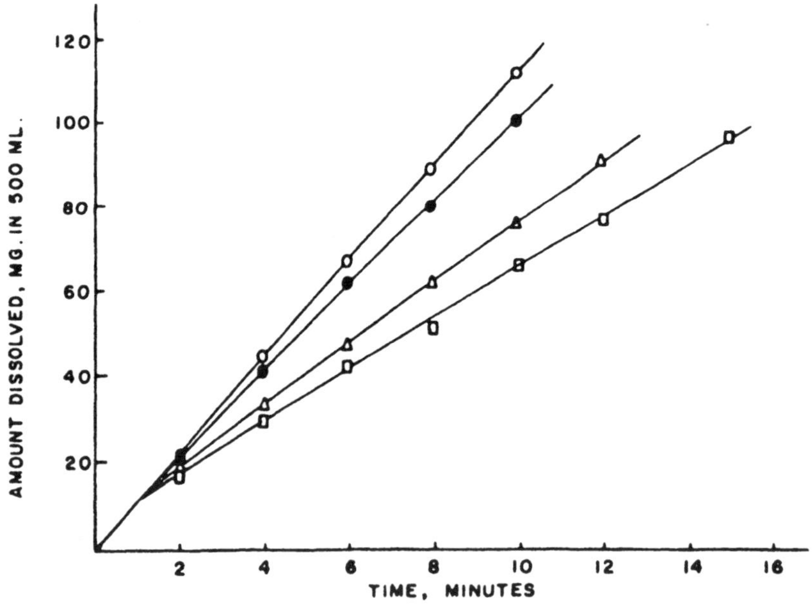

Fig. 5.4 Effect of particle size on the dissolution of phenobarbital. Key for various particle sizes tested: □, 0.07–0.15 mm; △, 0.15–0.25 mm; ●, 0.25–0.42 mm; ○, 0.42–0.71 mm. (From Ref. 25.)

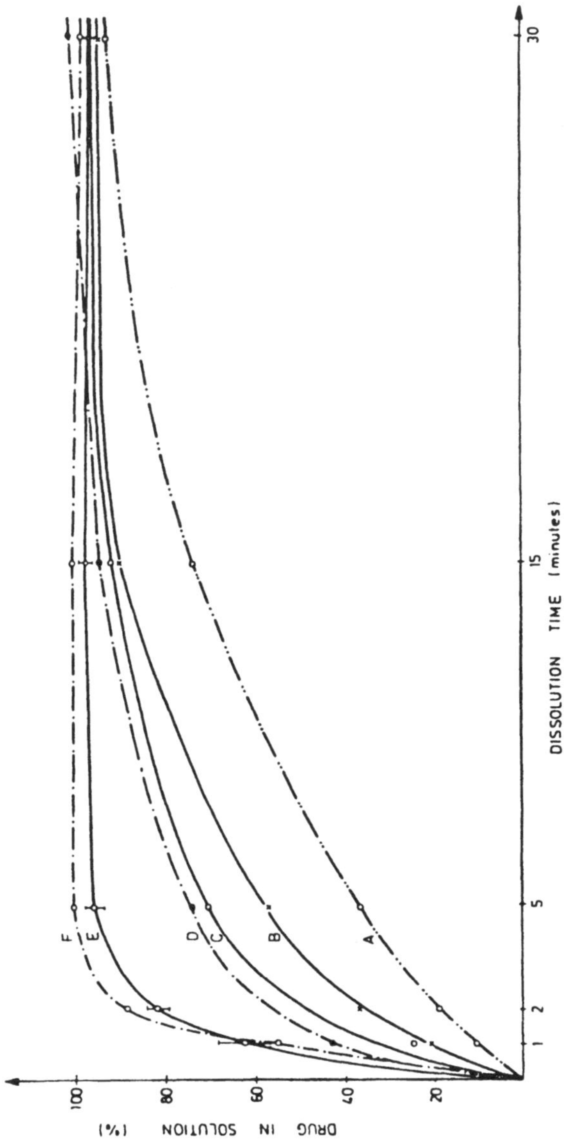

Fig. 5.5 Change in dissolution rate of metronidazole in water as a result of change in particle size. A, 400–500; B, 125–200 μm; C, 2.4 μm; D, 2.4 μm (0.05% aqueous sodium cholate solution); D, 44 μm; E, 1.75 μm F, <1.0μm (From Ref. 26.)

Equation (5.1) implies that the solubility is inversely proportional to particle radius. Consequently, it is more appropriate to view C_s as the solubility of the microparticles and C_s' as the solubility of the macroparticles as given in the following equation:

$$C_s = C_s' e^{\alpha/r} \tag{5.2}$$

This expression is indicative of the fact that unless the particles are reduced to microlevels, it will not affect the solubility appreciably.

Particle characteristics other than particle size that affect the rate of dissolution include particle shape and particle density. These properties indirectly affect the effective surface area by modifying the shear rate of the fresh solvent that comes in contact with the solid (28).

FACTORS RELATED TO DRUG PRODUCT FORMULATION

A variety of factors concerning the formulation of a drug product can directly influence the dissolution rate of the active ingredient contained within it. Once these factors are completely characterized, one can use this information to achieve custom-tailored drug dissolution profiles. This information is then employed in the development of optimally effective dosage forms.

The effects of various formulation factors on the dissolution rate and subsequent bioavailability of the active ingredients from solid dosage forms, such as tablets and capsules, have been well documented by several investigators since the early 1960s. Although the magnitude and significance of these effects must be determined individually for each product, the forthcoming discussion will serve as a guideline for the scientist during the various stages of product development.

Excipients and Additives

Most solid dosage forms incorporate more than one excipient for various purposes together with the active ingredient in the formulation. It has been shown that the dissolution rate of a pure drug can be altered significantly when mixed with various adjuncts. These adjuncts include diluents, binders, lubricants, granulating agents, disintegrants, and so on. In the following discussion we address the influence of excipients on the rate of dissolution of the active ingredient from a dosage form.

Commonly used diluents and disintegrants, such as various grades of lactose and starch, in the preparation of tablets and capsules have been shown to influence the dissolution rate of a drug. Levy et al. (29) studied the effect of starch on the rate of dissolution of salicylic acid tablets manufactured by a dry, double-compression process. An approximate threefold increase in the dissolution rate was observed when the starch content was increased from 5% to 20% in the formulation (Fig. 5.6). This observation was attributed to improved and more complete disintegration. Later it was suggested that the fine starch particles form a layer on the outer surface of the hydrophobic drug particle. This association results in imparting hydrophilic character to the granule and thus increased effective surface area and rate of dissolution.

Several other studies have been reported in the literature employing a variety of diluents and test substances (30,31). While developing a product, it is important to consider the effect of diluent particle properties as well as excipient dilution (drug/excipient ratio) on the dissolution rate. Also, drug–excipient as well as excipient–excipient interactions can influence the rate of dissolution.

Kornblum and Hirschorn (32) evaluated excipient dilution effects on dissolution rate. The data obtained demonstrated the importance of the excipient/

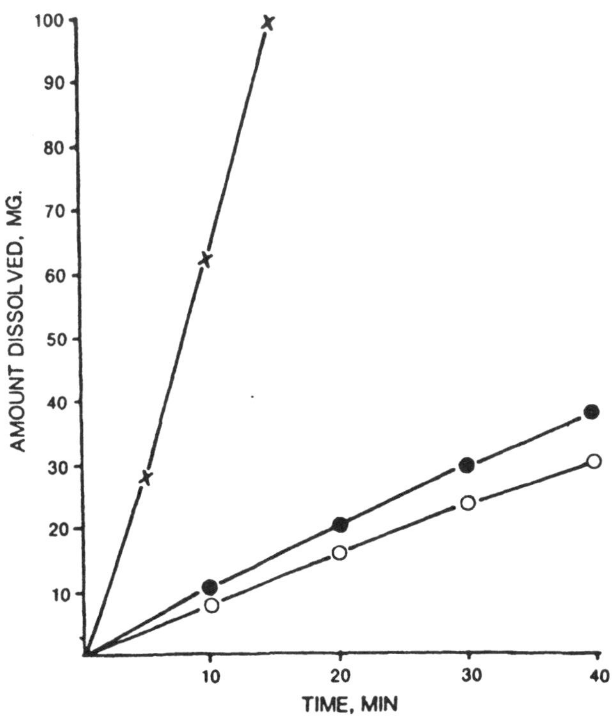

Fig. 5.6 Effect of pharmaceutical additives (starch) on the dissolution of salicylic acid. O, 5%; ●, 10%; x, 20% starch in granules. [From G. Levy et al., J. Pharm. Sci., *52*, 1050 (1963).]

drug ratio to optimal dissolution rate. Further, employing a quinazoline compound as a test substance, they found that dissolution rate increased as the excipient/drug ratio increased from 3:1 to 7:1 to 11:1 (33).

Westerberg et al. (34) evaluated six different carrier materials possessing varying solubility characteristics on dissolution rate of griseofulvin under sink conditions by preparing ordered mixtures. Highly soluble carrier materials gave extremely fast dissolution, due to the fact that the drug was delivered as free, well-dispersed primary particles, after rapid dissolution of the carrier particles. Compared to griseofulvin agglomerates, practically insoluble carriers yielded a limited increase in dissolution rate. This was attributed to the increased influence of diffusional transport and to some extent by a decrease in the surface area participating in dissolution. Compared to griseofulvin agglomerates, the use of hydrophobic carrier decreased the dissolution rate.

Chowhan and Chi (35) prepared capsules by thoroughly mixing magnesium stearate with drug and either cornstarch or pregelatinized starch. These capsules behaved quite differently. The disintegration time and the drug dissolution rate of capsules containing pregelatinized starch were not affected when the powders were thoroughly mixed with magnesium stearate. Under similar conditions, however, capsules containing cornstarch showed an increase in disintegration and a decrease in drug dissolution rate when mixing time with magnesium stearate was increased, as shown in Fig. 5.7. These results suggest that drug–excipient and excipient–excipient interactions are the major factors influencing both disintegration time and drug dissolution rate.

Particle Size

Several investigators have concluded that in most instances, reduction in particle size of drugs contained in tablets or capsules will enhance dissolution and absorption. This can most likely be attributed to the procedures employed in tablet production; that is, mixing the drug with usually hydrophilic diluents and subsequent granulation will result in a more hydrophilic surface, even for originally hydrophobic drug particles. Additionally, the gastrointestinal fluids have good wetting properties, so that reduction in particle size will increase the effective surface area of the drug even if the drug retains its hydrophobic properties after tabletting.

Finholt et al. (25,36) have extensively evaluated the effect of particle size on the dissolution rate of drug from granules and tablets. Figures 5.8 and 5.9 illustrate this phenomenon with phenacetin and phenobarbital as the test compounds. Several other investigators have reported similar results (26,30,37,38).

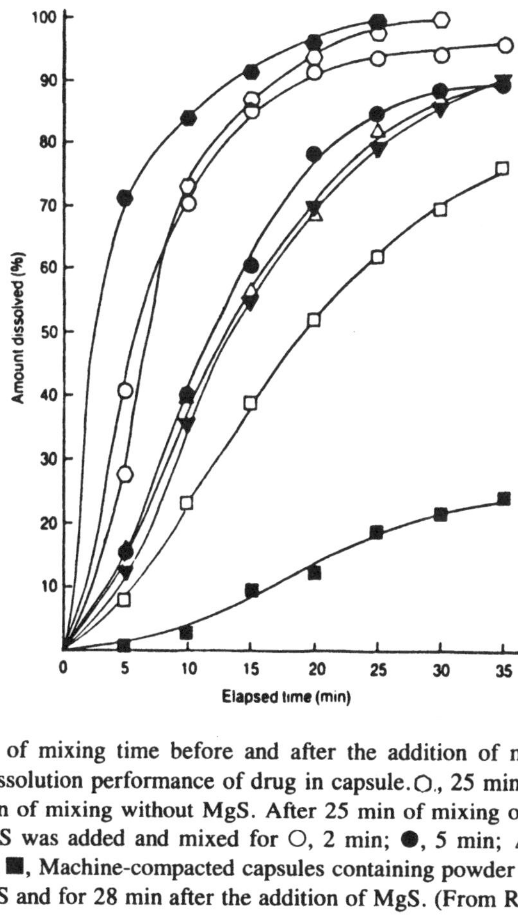

Fig. 5.7 Effect of mixing time before and after the addition of magnesium stearate (MgS) on the dissolution performance of drug in capsule. ○, 25 min of mixing without MgS; ●, 53 min of mixing without MgS. After 25 min of mixing of drug, cornstarch, and lactose, MgS was added and mixed for ○, 2 min; ●, 5 min; △, 10 min; ▼, 20 min; □, 28 min. ■, Machine-compacted capsules containing powder were mixed for 25 min without MgS and for 28 min after the addition of MgS. (From Ref. 35.)

Granulating Agents and Binders

It has been reported by several investigators that binders and/or granulating agents incorporated in tablet formulation and other solid dosage forms can markedly influence the dissolution characteristics of the drug from the dosage form. Solvong and Finholt (39) have shown that phenobarbital tablets granulated with gelatin solution provide a faster dissolution rate in human gastric juice than do those prepared using sodium carboxymethylcellulose or polyethylene glycol 6000 as a binder, as shown in the Fig. 5.10. This observation was attributed to the fact that gelatin imparts hydrophilic characteristics to the

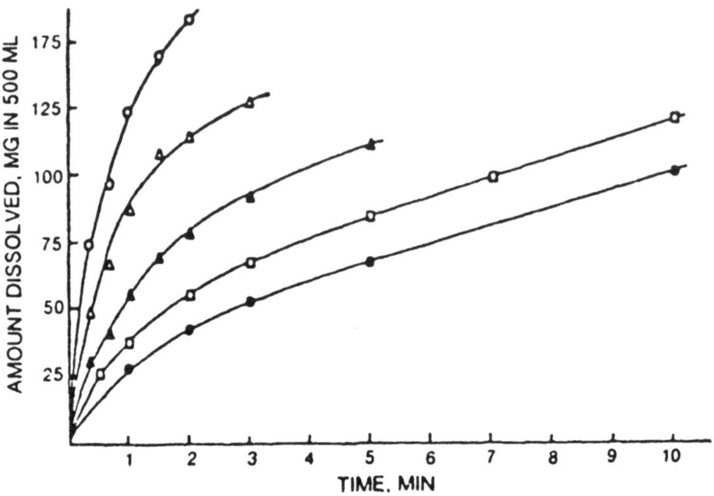

(a)

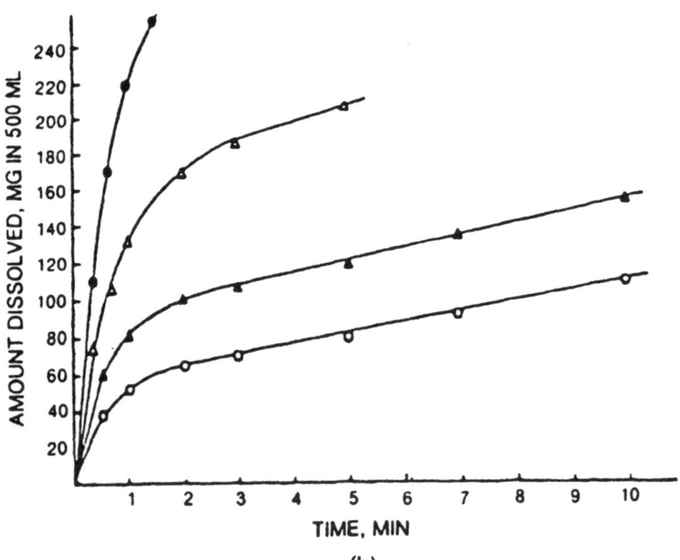

(b)

Fig. 5.8 Influence of particle size on the dissolution of phenacetin (a) and phenobarbital (b) from solid dosage forms. Key for particle sizes employed for investigation: (a) ○, 0.11–0.15 mm; △, 0.15–0.21 mm; ▲, 0.21–0.30 mm; □, 0.30–0.50 mm; ●, 0.50–0.71 mm; (b) ●, 0.07–0.15 mm; △, 0.15–0.25 mm; ▲, 0.25–0.42 mm; ○, 0.42–0.71 mm. (From Ref. 28.)

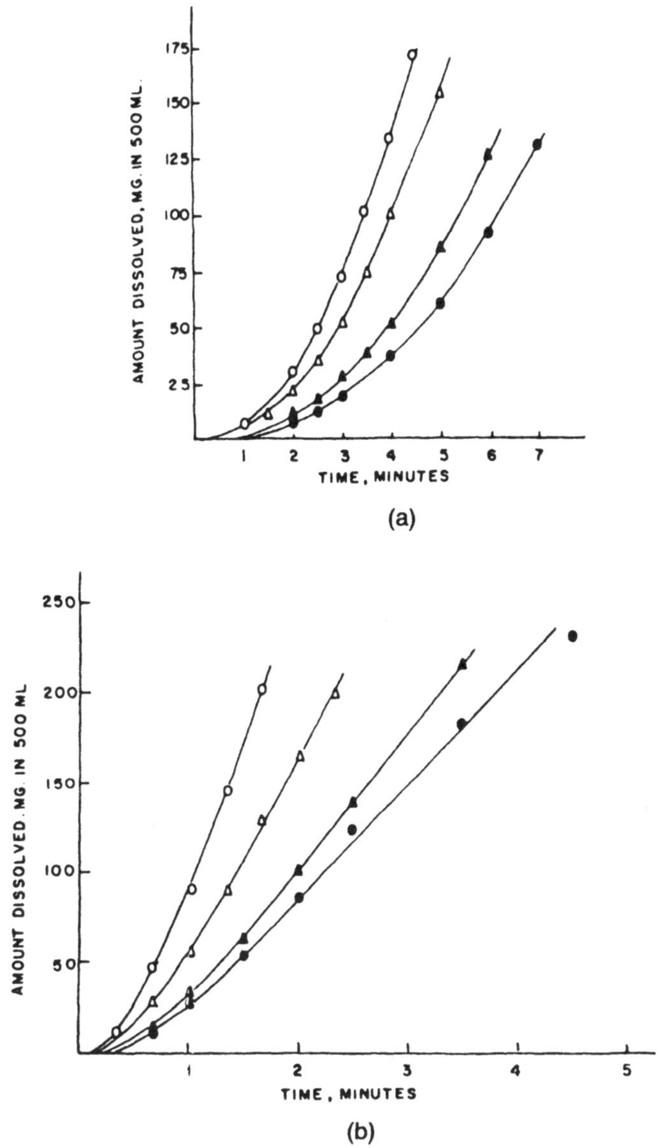

Fig. 5.9 Influence of particle size on the dissolution of phenacetin (a) and phenobarbital (b) from tablets. Key for particle sizes employed for investigation: (a) ○, 0.11–0.15 mm; △, 0.15–0.21 mm; ▲, 0.21–0.30 mm; ●, 0.30–0.50 mm; (b) ○, 0.07–0.15 mm; △, 0.15–0.25 mm; ▲, 0.25–0.42 mm; ●, 0.42–0.71 mm. (From Refs. 25 and 36.)

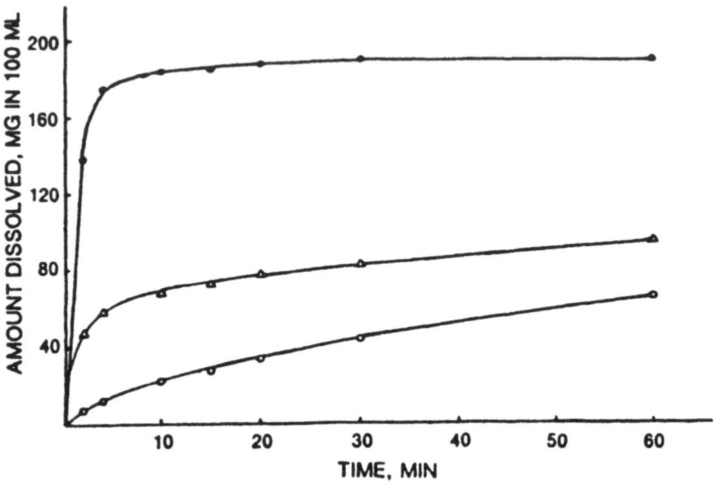

Fig. 5.10 Influence of binders and granulating agents on the dissolution rate of phenobarbital tablets. ●, Gelatin binder; △, CMC; ○, polyethylene glycol 6000. (From Ref. 39.)

hydrophobic drug surface, whereas PEG 6000 forms a complex with poor solubility, and sodium carboxymethylcellulose is converted to its less soluble acid form at the low pH of gastric fluid.

Even gelatin obtained from various processes and origins has been shown to affect the dissolution rate of dosage forms (40). Jacob and Plein (41) compared gelatin with other common binders, such as acacia, ethyl cellulose, and hydroxyethyl cellulose, employing phenobarbital as the test drug. The fastest dissolution rate was observed with 2% gelatin, while a decrease in dissolution rate was observed with 4% gelatin content. Satisfactory tablets were obtained with acacia as binding agent, whereas ethyl cellulose and hydroxyethyl cellulose produced tablets with poor dissolution rates. Similar results were reported by Yen (30). He explained this observation by assuming that upon drying of the granules a film was formed around them. The thickness of the film will depend on the concentration of gelatin. With a water-soluble granulating agent such as Plasdone, a faster dissolution rate was obtained than with gelatin.

Later, Suren (42) compared starch mucilage and Luviskol VA 64 (a vinyl polymer) as binders in the manufacture of amylobarbital tablets. Luviskol gave tablets with a high dissolution rate that was independent of the compression forces employed. However, tablets prepared with starch mucilage gave a slow rate of dissolution that was compression dependent.

Several other studies have been reported in the literature evaluating the effects of various granulating agents and binders on the dissolution rate of tablets (43–46). From these studies it is not possible to comment on which granulating agent is best. As a professional guideline it must be noted that if a fast dissolution rate is desired for a hydrophobic drug, the granulating agent should possess the ability to make the surface of the drug's powdered particles hydrophilic. Gelatin seems to possess this unique property. Additionally, if the granulating agent forms a film around the particle upon drying, it must easily redissolve. If the use of too much binder results in a thick film that is unable to dissolve easily and rapidly, it might result in a decrease in the dissolution rate even if the granulating agent is hydrophilic in nature.

Disintegrating Agents

Several reports have been published in the literature demonstrating the effect of various disintegrating agents on the dissolution rate of tablets (47–49). It must be noted that the type and amount of disintegrating agent employed in the formulation significantly controls the overall rate of dissolution of the dosage form. Jaminet et al. (40) employed several disintegrants in the manufacture of phenobarbital tablets, including Primojel (sodium glycolate of potato starch), Nymcel (polymerized water-soluble brand of sodium carboxymethyl cellulose), and Copagel (low-viscosity grade of sodium carboxymethyl cellulose). The effect on the dissolution rate of tablets by the addition of disintegrant before and after granulation was assessed. When added before granulation, Copagel gave tablets with a remarkably slow dissolution rate. However, when added after granulation, Copagel did not result in lowering the dissolution rate. Primojel was not found to be as effective as expected, particularly on addition after granulation.

Lubricants

Lubricants that are commonly incorporated in the formulation of solid dosage forms fall predominantly in the class of hydrophobic compounds. Consequently, the nature, quality, and quantity of the lubricant added can affect the dissolution rate. Various studies have documented this observation.

The effects of various lubricants on the dissolution rate of salicylic acid tablets were studied by Levy and Gumtow (50). They concluded that magnesium stearate, a hydrophobic lubricant, tends to retard the dissolution rate of salicylic acid tablets, whereas sodium lauryl sulfate enhances dissolution, due to its hydrophilic character combined with surface activity, which increases the microenvironment pH surrounding the weak acid and increases wetting and better solvent penetration into the tablets. Figure 5.11 illustrates the effect of lubricants on the dissolution rate of tablets.

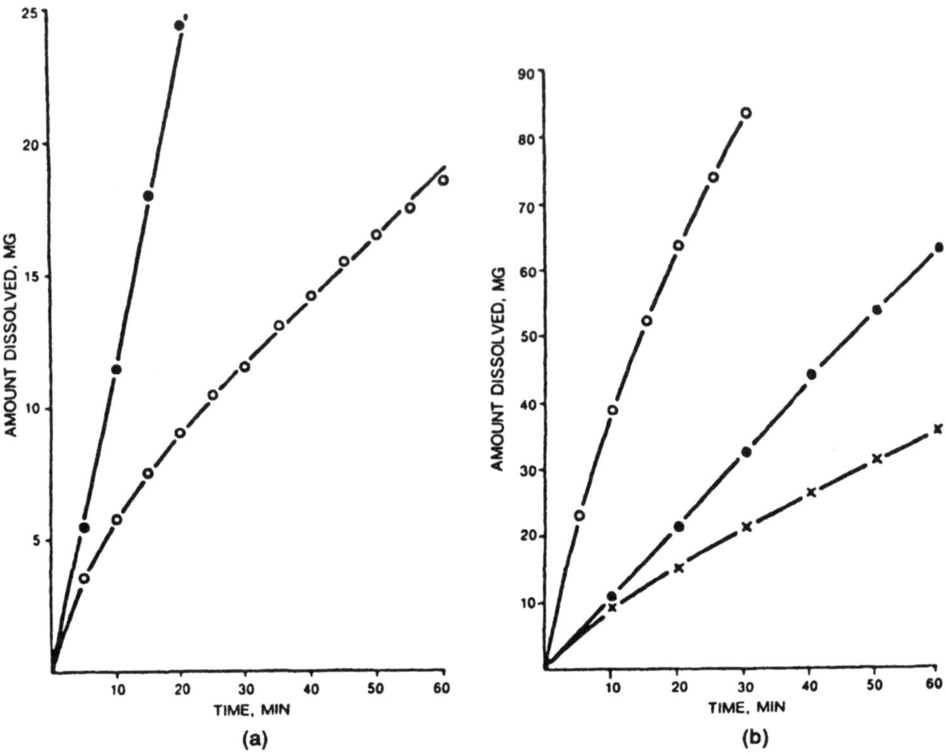

Fig. 5.11 Effect of changes in lubricant (magnesium stearate, MgS) concentration on the dissolution of salicylic acid disks. (a) ○, 3% MgS; ●, no MgS; (b) x, 3% MgS; ●, no MgS; ○, 3% sodium lauryl sulfate. (From Ref. 50.)

Several other studies have been reported which demonstrate the influence of lubricants on the dissolution rate of tablets (31,40,42,51,52). Marlowe and Shangraw (31) employed a water-soluble lubricant composed of a 1:1:2 ratio mixture of DL-leucine, calcium benzoate, and PEG 4000. Using sodium salicylate as the test drug, they compared the influence of this mixture and other conventional lubricants, such as stearates, on the dissolution rate. Surprisingly, the water-soluble lubricant composition did not increase the dissolution rate of sodium salicylate compared with other conventional lubricants.

The effect of lubricants on the dissolution rate of drugs from dosage forms will depend on the properties of the granules, the lubricant itself, and the amount of lubricant used. If the granules are hydrophilic and fast disintegrating, a water-soluble surface-active lubricant will have an insignificant effect on the dissolution. On the other hand, if the granules are hydrophobic, the surface-active lubricant will enhance dissolution.

Some of the superior lubricants, such as stearates and talc, are hydrophobic in nature. They tend to retard the dissolution rate. It is theorized that they decrease the effective drug–solvent interfacial area by changing the surface characteristics of the tablets, which results in a reduction of wettability, prolonging its disintegration time and decreasing the area of the interface between the active ingredient and solvent. However, it must be noted that if the amount of lubricant used is very small ($<1\%$), the retarding effect may be negligible.

Interfacial Tension Between Drug and Dissolution Medium

The properties of the interface between the drug and the dissolution medium can become a deciding factor as far as dissolution rate is concerned. The characteristics can be modified by the addition of agents that act at the interface, thus facilitating effects that can prove to be advantageous.

Finholt and Solvong (38) studied the effect of polysorbate 80 in varying concentrations on the dissolution rate of a relatively hydrophobic test drug phenacetin. Additionally, they attempted to determine a relationship between the surface tension of the dissolution medium and the time necessary for dissolution of 100 mg of phenacetin (T_{100}). The dissolution medium used was 0.1 *N* HCl.

An increase in the polysorbate 80 concentration from 0 to 0.01% resulted in a significant increase in dissolution rate. However, higher concentrations of the surfactants had very little effect. The surface tension was measured at 20°C. The times necessary for dissolution of 100 mg of phenacetin in the different polysorbate–HCl mixtures were determined. The relationship between the polysorbate concentration and T_{100}, and polysorbate concentration and the surface tension of the dissolution medium, resulted in practically superimposable curves, indicative of a linear relationship between the surface tension of the dissolution medium and T_{100} values. These observations are illustrated in Fig. 5.12.

The solubilities of phenacetin in 0.1 *N* HCl containing 0, 0.001, 0.01, and 0.1% of polysorbate 80 were found to be approximately similar, indicative of an insignificant influence of the surfactant on the solubility of phenacetin. Consequently, it can be concluded that the increase in the dissolution rate of phenacetin could be due predominantly to the decrease in interfacial tension between the drug and the dissolution medium

Given the various drug substances that are hydrophobic, it is more crucial to determine the surface tension of the gastric medium. There are very few articles that report the surface tension of gastric media. Finholt and Solvong

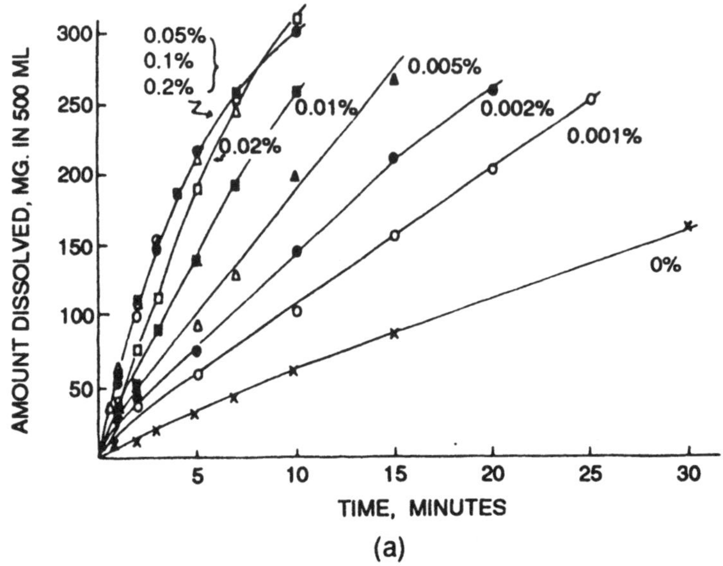

Fig. 5.12 Effect of interfacial tension between drug and dissolution medium on the dissolution rate of phenacetin. (a) Change in concentration of polysorbate in dissolution medium. (b) Relationship between polysorbate concentration of the dissolution medium and time required to solubilize 100 mg of phenacetin; and the relationship between polysorbate concentration of the dissolution medium and surface tension of the same. ○, Time; △, surface tension. (c) Relationship between surface tension, dissolution medium, and time necessary for dissolution of 100 mg of phenacetin. (From Ref. 38.)

(38) determined the surface tension and pH of gastric juice from 27 subjects under fasting and histamine-stimulated secretion conditions. They concluded that the surface tension of human juice is nearly independent of pH and secretion rate, having a value between 35 and 50 dyn/cm.

Other investigations addressing the effect of interfacial tension between the drug and the dissolution medium have been reported (53,54). These investigations attempt to evaluate this phenomenon from in vivo perspective. Suffice it here to say that the surface tension of the dissolution medium *is* an important factor as far as dissolution rate is concerned.

Surfactants

The drugs that are practically insoluble in aqueous medium (<0.01%) are of increasing therapeutic interest, particularly due to the problems associated with their bioavailability when administered orally. It has often been suggested that drugs with low solubilities when incorporated with surfactants can enhance their dissolution rate. Numerous articles addressing the effects of surfactants

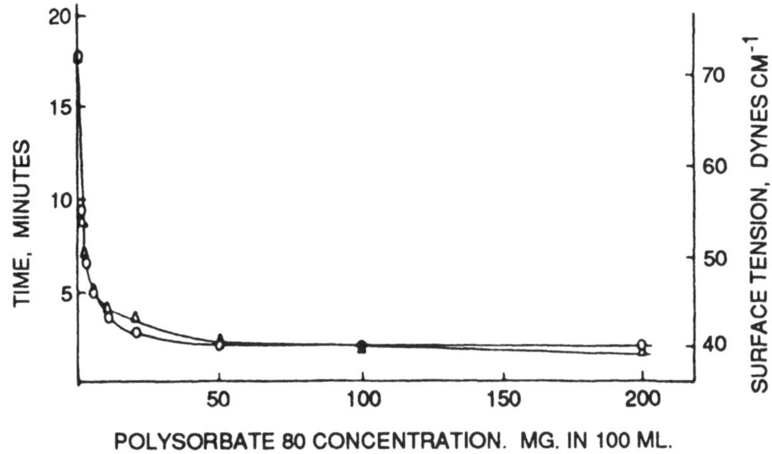

(b)

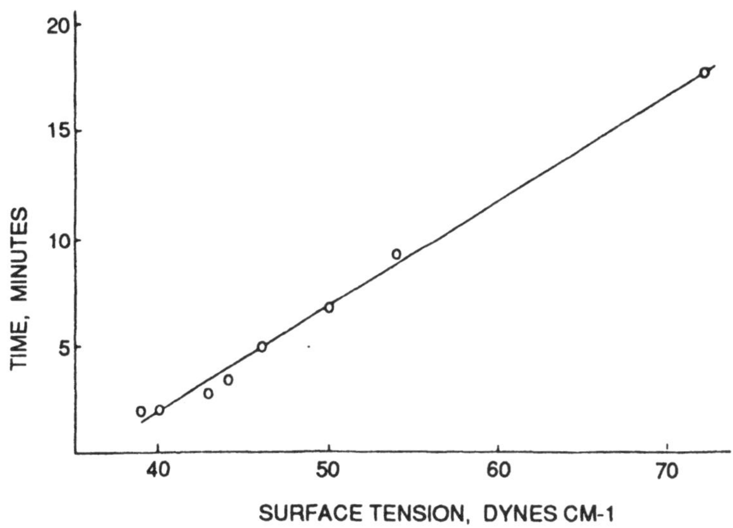

(c)

on the dissolution rate of such drugs have been reported in the literature (39,54–58).

The effects of treatment of cassava starch with sodium lauryl sulfate (SLS) and polysorbate 80 and the method of incorporating the treated and plain starch on the disintegration and dissolution characteristics of sulfadiazine tablets were investigated. Disintegration and dissolution rates were faster with surfactant-treated starch. Polysorbate 80-treated starch exhibited a better dissolution profile than did SLS-treated starch.

The effect of various surfactants on the dissolution rate of three steroids of differing aqueous solubility compressed as tablets was investigated by Fucho et al. (55). At surfactant concentrations below 0.2%, no appreciable effect on either the surface tension of the solution or the solubility of steroids was observed. However, there was some increase in the dissolution rate from tablets in the presence of surfactant. Gibaldi et al. (56) investigated the influence of a nonionic surfactant, polyoxyethylene–lauryl ether (POE-23–lauryl ether), on the dissolution rate of benzoic and salicylic acids. The dissolution rate of benzoic acid was found to increase with increasing concentrations of POE-23–lauryl ether, as shown in Fig. 5.13. They concluded that the dissolution rate of the solid in a micellar solution is not proportional to the solubility of a compound in the dissolution medium.

The increase in drug solubility by surfactant micelles has been demonstrated in vitro for a large number of poorly water soluble compounds, employing synthetic (59) as well as natural surfactants (60–63). Additionally, the method of incorporation of the surfactant in the drug product formulations can markedly influence the dissolution characteristics of the relatively hydrophobic drug. Solvong and Finholt (39) showed that when added with gelatin as the granulating agent and when sprayed on the granules of phenacetin while preparing phenacetin tablets, polysorbate 80 exhibited significantly different dissolution rates, as shown in Fig. 5.14.

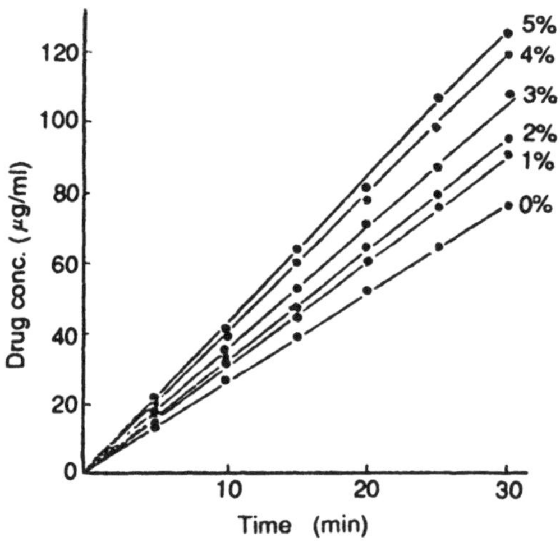

Fig. 5.13 Influence of surfactant (POE-23–lauryl ether) concentration (% w/v) on the dissolution of benzoic acid in water employing rotating disk method at 100 rpm. (From Ref. 56.)

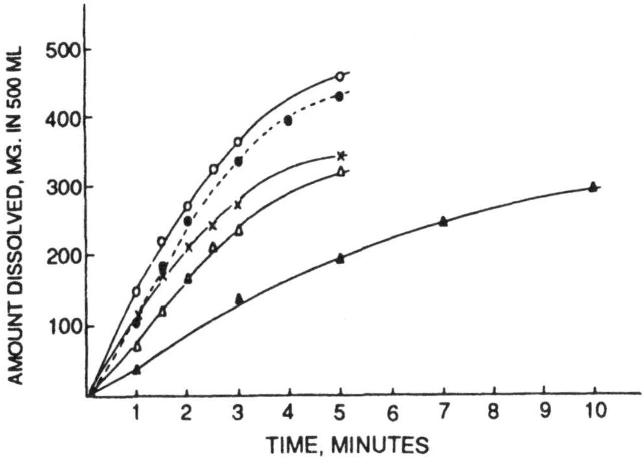

(a)

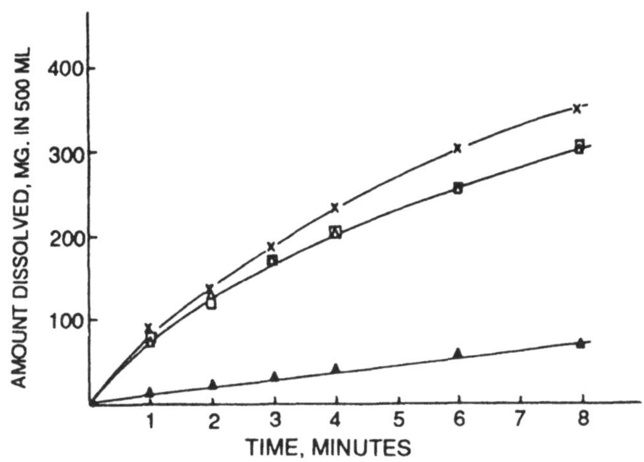

(b)

Fig. 5.14 Effect of surfactant (polysorbate 80, PB80) incorporated in phenacetin (PTN) tablets on dissolution rate. (a) ▲ and ●, PTN tablets from granules I; △, PTN tablets from granules I with 0.1% PB80 dissolved in granulating solution; ○, PTN tablets from granules I with 1% PB80 dissolved in granulating solution; x, PTN tablets from granules I with 0.1% PB80 sprayed on dried granules; ----, dissolution medium: 0.1 *N* HCl, containing 0.2% PB80. (b) ▲, PTN granules II; △, PTN granules II with 0.1% PB80 dissolved in granulating solution; □, PTN granules II with 0.1% PB80 dissolved in granulating solution; x, PTN granules II with 0.1% PB80 sprayed on dried granules. (From Ref. 39.)

FACTORS RELATED TO DOSAGE FORM

Various factors related to solid dosage form have been identified which influence the dissolution behavior of solid dosage forms. Most of the investigations revolve around factors that affect the in vitro dissolution of tablets and capsules. The effects of various formulations and manufacturing process variables on the rate and extent of dissolution and the bioavailability of the active principles from tablets and capsules have been well documented. Although the magnitude and significance of these effects have to be determined individually for each tablet or capsule product, the following discussion can serve as a guideline for the product development scientist during the initial stages of formulation design and development. In the forthcoming sections we focus on the various formulation and processing factors that significantly influence the dissolution characteristics of tablets and capsules.

Manufacturing Procedures

A fairly large number of studies reported in the literature have shown that the process of granulation can markedly influence the dissolution rate of the resultant tablets (31,59,60). Wet granulation, in general, has been shown to improve dissolution rates of poorly soluble drugs by imparting hydrophilic properties to the surface of the granules (28). Additionally, the use of fillers and diluents such as starch, spray-dried lactose, and microcrystalline cellulose tends to increase the hydrophilicity of the active ingredients and thus improve dissolution. Consequently, wet granulation was considered superior to a dry or double-compression procedure. Figure 5.15 shows the effect of different granulation methods on the dissolution rate of tablets.

Finholt (61) conducted an extensive investigation looking into the effects of wet granulation with gelatin and dry granulation of phenobarbital tablets on their dissolution characteristics. Both tablet formulations contained the same amount of drug, filler, and lubricant. A fast dissolution rate was exhibited with both procedures, provided that starch was incorporated in the proper manner when dry granulation method was employed. A much slower dissolution rate was obtained when the drug was dry granulated alone and starch added afterward. In another study, the dissolution rates of phenobarbital sodium from tablets prepared by wet granulation with gelatin and by dry granulation with Avicel were compared. Faster dissolution was obtained with the direct compression method than by wet granulation.

It must be noted that with the advent of newer tabletting machines and materials, it becomes more evident that the careful formulation and proper mixing sequence and time of adding the several ingredients are the main criteria that affect the dissolution characteristics of the tablets, not the method of

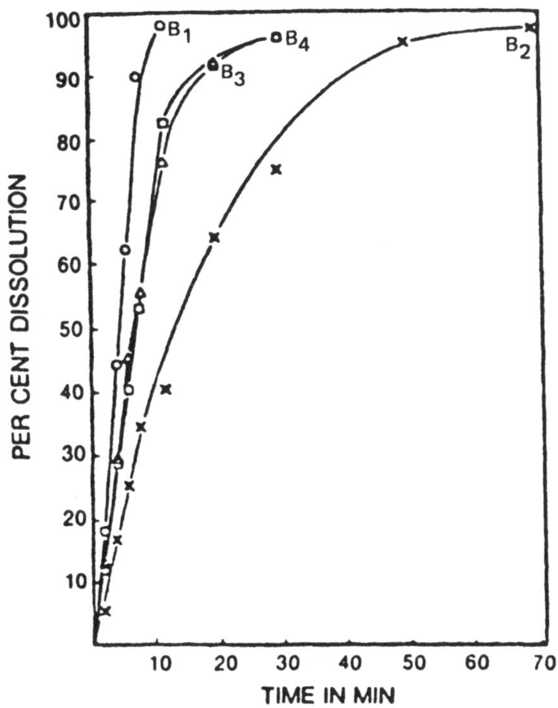

Fig. 5.15 Influence of manufacturing process (method of granulation) on the dissolution rate of tablets. B_1, Direct compression with spray-dried lactose; B_2, wet granulation with ethyl cellulose and lactose; B_3, acacia mucilage and lactose; B_4, starch paste and lactose. (From Ref. 31.)

granulation per se (28). However, there is significant evidence indicating that the manufacturing procedures employed can influence the dissolution rate of tablets.

Granule Size

The size of the granule does not play a role in the dissolution behavior of the dosage form. It is the nature of the granule that can influence the dissolution rate of the dosage form. It has been shown that the granule size probably will have little influence on dissolution rate if the granules are relatively soft and disintegrate easily. However, if they are harder and disintegrate more slowly, the granule size will be of importance and an increase in size will cause a decrease in dissolution rate (30,50,62).

Yen (30) prepared triameterene tablets from granules of different size that were subsequently tested for dissolution rate. He found that the dissolution rate increased with decreasing granule size when terra alba or glycine was the filler. However, when starch was used as the filler, no effect of granule size on dissolution rate was observed. This effect was attributed to the soft nature of granules that contained starch. Levy (50) prepared salicylic acid tablets by double compression. This effect was attributed to the soft nature of granules that contained starch. He found that the dissolution rate of the tablets increased with decreasing granule size. However, this increase in dissolution rate was not strictly proportional to the corresponding increase in the apparent surface area of the granules.

Drug–Excipient Interactions

Studies dealing with the physical interactions between drug particles and excipient particles are essential to the development of fully effective dosage forms (35). These interactions can occur during any unit operation, such as mixing, blending, drying, and/or granulating, resulting in a change in dissolution pattern of the dosage form in question. This topic has been addressed to a certain degree while discussing the effects of additives in a formulation on its dissolution characteristics.

Few studies demonstrating the influence of drug–excipient interactions have been reported (63–67). Two of these investigations have addressed the interaction of tablet disintegrants and magnesium stearate during mixing. The effect of magnesium stearate, a commonly used lubricant, on the disintegration time of tablets containing either potato starch or sodium starch glycolate was found to depend on the swelling properties of the disintegrants. These results were attributed to the formation of a lubricant film during mixing, which resulted in an increase in disintegration time and thus delayed dissolution. The second study evaluated the effect of mixing with magnesium stearate on the dissolution rate of prednisolone from tablets containing either a slightly or strongly swelling disintegrant (66). The dissolution rate of prednisolone was found to depend on the length of time that the ingredients were mixed with magnesium stearate. This was more true for formulations containing potato starch, a slightly swelling disintegrant. A related study indicated that an increase in mixing time of formulations containing 97 to 99% microcrystalline cellulose, another slightly swelling disintegrant, resulted in a decrease in disintegration time, thereby enhancing dissolution rate (68). However, no attempt was made by the authors to explain their results. These published results suggest that prolonged mixing of drug and excipient mixtures with magnesium stearate can have a deleterious effect on tablet disintegration and the rate of dissolution of the drug. In most instances it increases the tablet disintegration time, thereby decreasing the drug dissolution rate.

It is essential that the formulator have a thorough understanding of these interactions so that the most appropriate excipients can be selected to enable the formulation to perform optimally (35). By minimizing if not eliminating these interactions, adverse effects on the performance of the final product can often be avoided. It must also be noted that better process control is also possible with noninteracting drug–excipient combinations.

Compression Force

Research involving the influence of processing variables on dissolution rate is relatively limited in quantity and deals primarily with the effect of force of compression, which is the reflection of the degree of consolidation or compaction. As early as 1953, Higuchi and co-workers in their studies of the physics of tablet compression, demonstrated the influence of the compression force employed in the tabletting process on the apparent density, porosity, hardness, disintegration time, and average particle size of compressed tablets. Bonding of particles and cleavage or crushing of particles are common effects observed on increasing force of compression. In the former case dissolution rates tend to diminish with increasing pressure. However, in the latter case, dissolution rates increased with increase in compressional force. In many instances, both of these factors act competitively, which could result in an ultimate decrease in solvent (dissolution medium) penetrability and hence a decrease in dissolution rate. Depending on which of these two effects dominate, different types of relationships between the compressional force and dissolution rates are observed, as shown in Fig. 5.16 (70–73). Additionally, the high compression may inhibit the wettability of the tablet, due to the formation of a more firm and effective sealing layer by the lubricant under the high pressure and temperature that usually accompanies a strong compression force.

Scores of studies have been reported in the literature demonstrating the influence of force of compression on the dissolution rate of tablets (7,33,73–77). Smith and co-workers (73) studied the relationship between dissolution rate and compression force for tablets of lithium carbonate containing polyvi-

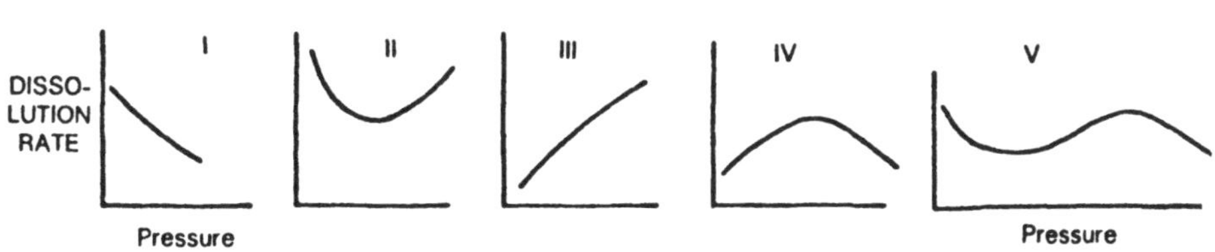

Fig. 5.16 Various types of relations observed between applied compressional force during tableting and dissolution rate of tablets. (From Ref. 28.)

nylpyrrolidone as a binder. A maximum dissolution rate at relatively low consolidation apparently depended on the deformation characteristics of the granules. Tuladhar et al. (7) investigated the relative change in particle size of the drug during the compression process. Assessment was made by comparing the dissolution rates of the drug particles before and after compression. Phenylbutazone was employed as the test compound together with lactose and Avicel as binders. With a low drug concentration (10%) in the tablet, the diluent protected the drug particles from bonding together. Significant differences in the dissolution rate were observed when the force of compression was varied over the range 0 to 150 $MN \cdot m^{-2}$. Ganderton et al. (72) examined the dissolution rate of penindione tablets prepared by wet granulation. At low pressures the tablets were easily penetrated by the dissolution medium, but the tablets did not break up extensively during the dissolution test and the dissolution rate was low. At relatively higher pressures, penetration still occurred quickly, and stress release and loss of small air bubbles caused much more disruption. With further increase in pressure, rebonding of the material occurred and stronger and denser tablets were produced which were less easily penetrated, thus yielding depressed dissolution rates. Figure 5.17 illustrates the effect of compression force on dissolution rate of tablets.

Finally, it must be noted that the effect of an increase in compression force on dissolution rate is dependent on the pressure range evaluated and on the properties of the drug, filler, and binder used. It is really difficult to predict comprehensively the effect on the dissolution rate of an increase in pressure. Other factors involving the methodological character may also play an important role in the overall relationship.

Deaggregation

Deaggregation is often a prerequisite for dissolution. In such instances deaggregation can, in fact, control the rate of dissolution. A close correlation can exist between the rate of deaggregation and plasma levels, as observed for four commercial lots of chloramphenicol capsules (78). The capsule formulation that exhibited most rapid rates of absorption and deaggregation dissolved most rapidly in vitro. The dissolution test was unable to differentiate between the other three formulations.

Two capsule formulations of sodium diphenylhydantoin showed significant deaggregation, dissolution, and thereby absorption rates, as reported by Arnold et al. (79). The formulation that deaggregated rapidly after the capsule shell was dissolved resulted in exposure of a larger surface area. This resulted in rapid dissolution at neutral pH but less rapid dissolution when both preparations were first exposed to 0.1 *N* hydrochloric acid. The aggregation of the other formulation inhibited the conversion of most of its sodium salt to the free

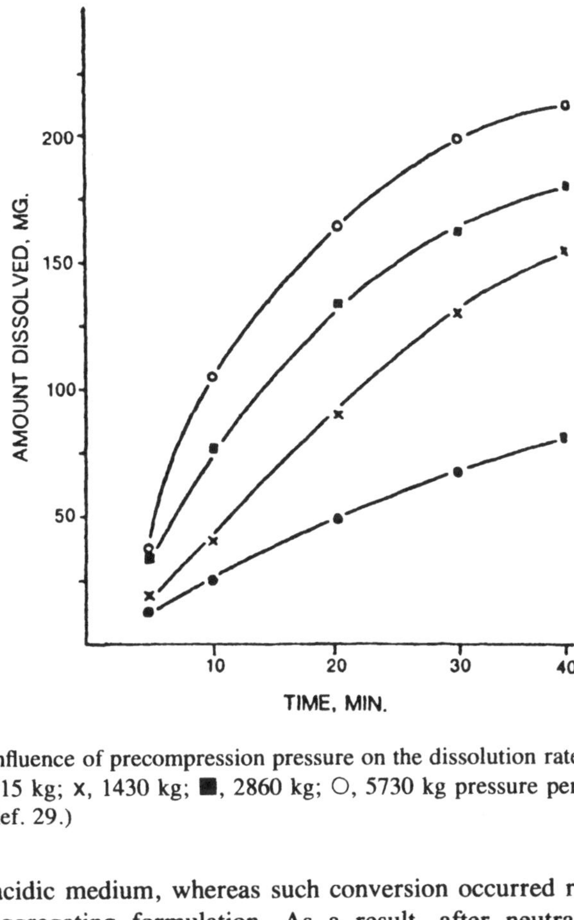

Fig. 5.17 Influence of precompression pressure on the dissolution rate of salicylic acid tablets. ●, 715 kg; x, 1430 kg; ■, 2860 kg; ○, 5730 kg pressure per square centimeter. (From Ref. 29.)

acid in an acidic medium, whereas such conversion occurred readily with the rapidly deaggregating formulation. As a result, after neutralization of the medium, the latter dissolved and absorbed more readily and rapidly than did the former.

Storage of Dosage Form

Storage under less than optimal, if not adverse conditions of temperature and humidity are not uncommon in many parts of the world. The packages used for the dispensing of medication are often less than adequate. These conditions may adversely affect the quality of pharmaceutical preparations (80–83). It might be expected that the effect of aging of tablets, capsules, and other solid dosage forms should always result in a decrease in dissolution rate. However, work done in this area indicates that an increase in dissolution rate may also be found. In many cases, however, there is no effect at all.

Gouda et al. (80) evaluated the effects of storage on the dissolution behavior of nitrofurantoin (NTF) solid dosage forms. The results did not show any change in weight variation and content uniformity upon storage under various storage conditions. NTF capsules containing microcrystals dissolved at a considerably faster rate, as expected. Storage did not markedly alter the dissolution pattern of NTF tablets or microcrystal capsules. However, the dissolution of NTF from macrocrystal capsules was decreased markedly. Macrocrystal capsules stored for 10 weeks in various containers at 40°C and 79% RH all failed to comply with USP XX/NF XV dissolution requirements for tablets. The decrease in NTF dissolution from macrocrystal capsules upon storage compared to microcrystal capsules or tablets was attributed to a physical change involving agglomeration of the particles and may be due to the dissolution conditions adapted.

Alam and Parrot (43) studied the effect of dissolution rate of hydrochlorothiazide (HCTZ) tablets. Tablets granulated with acacia exhibited decrease in dissolution rate during 1 year of aging at room temperature. A similar decrease was observed in tablets stored for 14 days at 50 to 80°C or for 4 weeks at 37°C. For tablets granulated with PVP there was no change in dissolution rate at elevated temperatures, but a slight decrease at room temperature. Tablets granulated with starch gave no change in dissolution rate either at room temperature or at elevated temperatures. Figure 5.18 demonstrates the relationship between the age of phenacetin tablets prepared with gelatin, PEG 6000, and carboxymethyl cellulose and time necessary to get 100 mg of the drug dissolved from the tablets (84).

FACTORS RELATED TO THE DISSOLUTION TESTING DEVICE

Numerous advanced and sophisticated techniques are employed to study the solubility of compounds as well as dissolution of drug products. Most of these techniques make use of some sort of mechanical apparatus. This apparatus is subject to a number of subtle influences that are easily overlooked. Some of the more commonly experienced adverse influences are (a) excessive eccentricity of the agitator device (e.g., the rotating paddle, basket shaft, etc.), (b) vibrations in rotational velocity and acceleration of the rotating element, (c) variations in temperature of the dissolution medium at various positions, and (d) external vibration that may introduce energy into the system by coupling and hence influence flow patterns. Other disturbing factors, such as agitation intensity, are also present which can have deleterious effects on the dissolution process of drugs.

Factors relating to the dissolution testing device discussed below can cause the dissolution results to vary from test to test no matter what testing technique

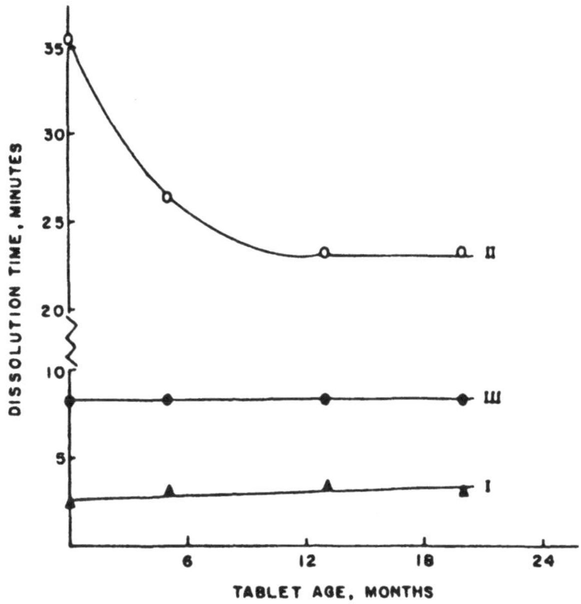

Fig. 5.18 Time required to dissolve 100 mg of phenacetin from tablets I, II, and III as a function of age of the tablets. (From Ref. 84.)

is employed. It must be noted that even with a knowledge of these disturbances, they can be minimized but can never be eliminated entirely. For example, there is currently no testing equipment that is totally free of vibrations. The objective is to hold each disturbance to a practical minimum so that it does not exert a significant influence on the dissolution process. Although certain minimums can be recommended, the reader should be aware that insufficient data are currently available even to predict the multivariant effects of two or more such minimums. They may exert an additive effect or they might cancel out.

Eccentricity of Agitating (Stirring) Element

The current official compendium specifies that the stirring shaft must rotate smoothly without significant wobble. The term *significant* gives the experimenter full right to ensure that such wobble does not significantly affect the dissolution rate. Additionally, USP XX/NF XV states that the axis of rotation of the stirring shaft must not deviate >2 mm from the axis of the stirring vessel. This implies that this specification permits eccentricity up to ±2 mm but that such eccentricity must not significantly affect the dissolution rate. This is certainly an excessive amount.

The effects of eccentricity should not be generalized like those of any random input variable. As one might expect, eccentricity can induce and propagate changes in hydrodynamic conditions and flow patterns that can, in turn, influence the dissolution behavior of the product in question. These effects can vary significantly from method to method as well as from dosage form to dosage form.

Hanson and Hanson (85,86) have studied extensively the effects of these irregularities on salicylic acid and prednisone USP calibrator tablets. The dissolution rate employing the rotating basket, with the eccentricity within the range 2 to 5 mm, increased by approximately 5% over the values obtained when the eccentricity was <2 mm. Similar results were obtained with both calibrators employing the paddle method. The studies suggest that the degree of eccentricity may be more significant with the paddle method than with the basket method and should be limited to 1 mm in order to reduce its influence to an insignificant value. He also indicates that the eccentricity is more prevalent at the junction of the shaft with the paddle blade or the basket. It is extremely difficult to maintain concentricity of a rotating member in this type of equipment. To overcome the problems associated with eccentricity, it is suggested that the shafts be carefully maintained and used in operation. Also, the use of guide bushing is recommended wherever applicable. Two possible ways in which the wobble can be minimized by supporting the rotating shaft are illustrated in Fig. 5.19.

Vibration

The speed of the rotational device selected by official compendium is 100 rpm. Other speeds are specified for certain drugs. Precise speed control is best obtained with a synchronous motor that locks into line frequency (85). Such motors are not only more rugged but are far from reliable. Periodic variations in rpm might result in possible disturbance in rotational acceleration. This phenomenon, present in almost all rotational devices, is commonly referred to as *torsional vibration*. Such vibration indicates a variation in the velocity of rotation for short periods of time. There average velocity was well within ±4% of the specified rate.

Vibration is a common variable introduced into a dissolution system due to various causes. It can effect change in the flow patterns of the dissolution medium. Additionally, it can introduce unwanted energy to the dynamic system. Both effects may result in significant changes in dissolution rate (1).

Numerous articles have appeared in the literature that document the influence of vibration on the dissolution rate (87–89). As early as 1971, Beyer and Smith (87) reported a sixfold increase in the dissolution rate of tolbutamide tablets when the vibration rate at the flask increased from 0.05 mil to 0.8

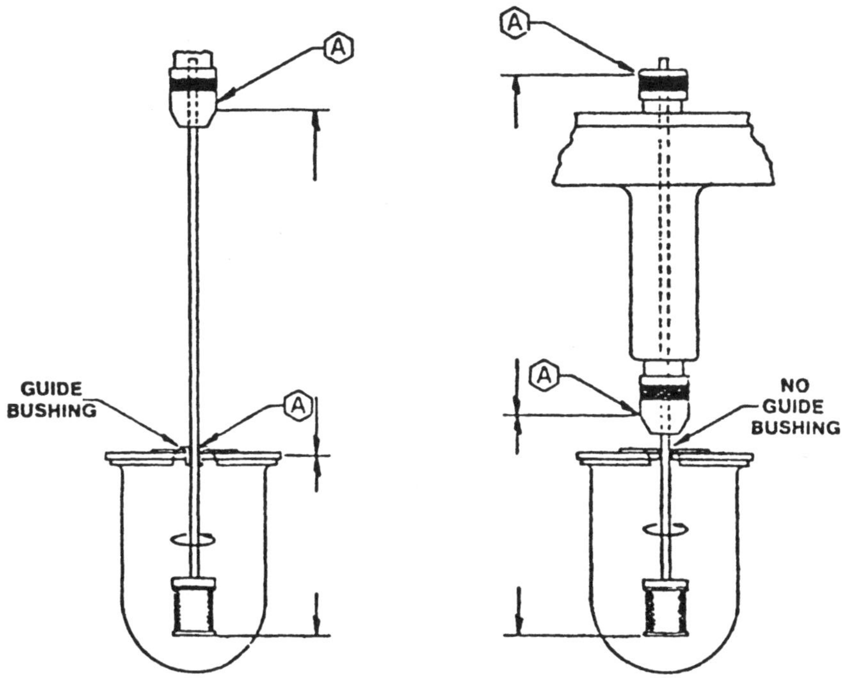

Fig. 5.19 The rotating shaft should be supported at two places (A) to minimize wobble, as shown by the two arrangements depicted. (From Ref. 85.)

mil displacement. Hanson (88) conducted a series of tests to determine the effects of increasing levels of vibration using method 1 and salicylic acid calibrators. In 1979, Cartwright (89) identified the level of vibration near the dissolution flask as a major source of interlaboratory variance in dissolution data.

A substantial portion of the environmental and equipment source of vibration occurs in the frequency range 50 to 60 Hz. Numerous unpublished investigations of vibration spectra have been made on dissolution test equipment. Hanson (1) states that the dissolution rate employing a basket is significantly influenced when horizontal vibration at frequency levels of 50 to 60 Hz exceeds 0.1 mil. With the paddle method, it appears that dissolution rates will be 5 to 10% higher when external vibration at the flask exceeds 0.1 mil, and still greater when it exceeds 0.2 mil in displacement.

Finally, it must be noted that no device is free of vibration. The objective of conducting dissolution testing should be to reduce vibration from external sources to a manageable level that will not introduce significant variation in results from successive dissolution tests on the same product. The USP XX/NF XV requires that no part of the equipment or its environment contribute significant vibration other than that emitted by a smoothly rotating stirring device. Various methods for controlling vibrations have been suggested. The interested reader is referred to the instructional manuals provided by the manufacturer of the dissolution testing device as well as to Ref. 1.

Agitation Intensity

It can be stated with a significant amount of certainty that the degree of agitation, or the stirring conditions, is one of the most important variables to consider in dissolution. Given the background on the various theories of dissolution, it is apparent that agitation conditions can markedly affect diffusion-controlled dissolution, because the thickness of the diffusion layer is inversely proportional to agitation speed. Wurster and Taylor (90) employed the empirical relationship

$$K = a(N)^b \tag{5.3}$$

where N is the agitation rate, K the reaction (dissolution) rate, and a and b are constants. For diffusion-controlled processes, $b = 1$. Dissolution that is interfacial-reaction-rate-controlled will be independent of agitation intensity, and thus $b = 0$.

The agitation intensity within and between the various in vitro dissolution testing devices currently in use can be varied by the dimensions and geometry of the dissolution vessel, the volume of dissolution medium, and the degree of agitation or shaking. Some in vitro dissolution devices that cause to-and-fro motion of the drug particles in the dissolution medium have been criticized by Levy (91) on the grounds that it is virtually impossible to standardize agitation conditions from drug to drug. It is safe to predict that two dosage forms having particles of differing sizes and densities will not experience identical agitation conditions within the same dissolution system, even though the containers are being subjected to the same rate of rotation as of oscillation.

The rotation speed of a stirring device in either method 1 or 2 produces a flow pattern resulting in a changing liquid–solid interface between the dissolution medium and the dosage form. It thus corresponds to the flow rate in the flow-through dissolution apparatus proposed by European scientists (92), for which the flow rate is suggested to fall in the range 10 to 100 mL/min.

The need to ascertain the correct agitation rate and the effect that changes in agitation rate can have on the in vitro dissolution rate have been demonstrated by numerous investigators (93–97). Carstensen et al. (93) studied the relationship between the liquid velocity and the intrinsic dissolution rate according to the Noyes–Whitney equation and Cadwallader's modification. They were able to correlate liquid velocities obtained in various types of dissolution systems with the reported dissolution rates. Levy and Procknal (94) developed the concept of a *rotating disk equivalent* (RDE) in which the intrinsic dissolution-rate data for methylprednisone (polymorph I) determined by a rotating disk method over a wide range of stirring rates was employed as a standard. This approach gave good agreement between the RDE rpm for a particular method when different drugs were used. The effect of agitation intensity on the dissolution rate of aspirin tablets is shown in Fig. 5.20.

The various dissolution testing devices currently in use exhibit a great variation in the hydrodynamics of each system. It is unfortunate that little has been done to quantify these variables in such a way that the agitation intensity of such a system can be related to that of another system. Additionally, there is limited quantitative information on the in vivo hydrodynamics that exist along the length of the gastrointestinal tract. Until such information is available, it will be difficult to develop meaningful in vitro models.

Stirring Element Alignment

It is beyond question true that a misalignment of the rotating shaft's axis to the axis of the dissolution vessel disturbs flow patterns so much so that dissolution-rate data may vary ±25% from test to test. It is unfortunate that

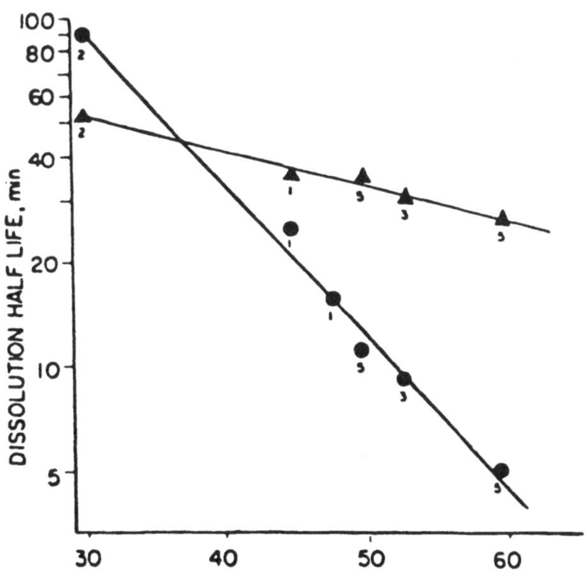

Fig. 5.20 Influence of agitation intensity on the dissolution rate of aspirin tablets. ●, Plain tablets; ▲, tablets with microencapsulated particles. (From Ref. 97.)

more research on this variable has not been published because it appears to be one of the most important external influences in both method 1 and method 2.

The USP XX/NF XV states that the axis of the stirring element must not deviate more than 0.2 mm from the axis of the dissolution vessel, which defines centering of the stirring shaft to within ±2 mm. It also constrains tilt. A series of tests suggest that a tilt in excess of 1.5° may increase dissolution rates using method 2 from 2 to 25% (86). Investigations at DRTL reported decreases in dissolution rates of 30% in prednisone calibrators when method 1 was employed with a forced tilt of 7° (98). Extensive investigations at NCDA concluded that to obtain consistent interlaboratory results, tilt of the rotating shaft in either the basket or paddle method should be avoided (99).

Significant variations in dissolution rates have been reported focusing on the centering of the rotating device employed (98,99). Other studies indicate that significant increases in dissolution rates, up to 13%, may occur when the shaft is offset 2 to 6 mm from the center axis of the flask (85,86). Literature is sparse on methods available to overcome the problems associated with the tilt and centering of the rotating element, which can significantly alter the dissolution test data.

Flow Pattern Disturbances

For dissolution-rate data to be reproducible and reliable, the flow pattern should be consistent from test to test. The geometry and alignment of the stirring device, external vibration, and rotational speed are some of the factors that can influence flow patterns. In 1978, DRTL conducted an extensive examination of these factors and their influence on dissolution testing (100). They concluded that the geometry of the rotating paddle and/or basket, the flask dimensions, and the sampling positions can all introduce various types of flow patterns that can alter the dissolution characteristics of the drug product. Cox et al. (99) further suggested that variations in smoothness of the round-bottomed flask can make significant differences in flow patterns as well.

Investigators in this field have also expressed concern over the return of substantial amounts of dissolution medium to the dissolution container, particularly when the temperature of the fluid is lower than that of the fluid already present in the flask. This can result in changes in the flow patterns. NCDA scientists caution against the permanent intrusion of sampling probes and thermometer troughs into the dissolution flask because of their effects on flow patterns. Automated systems are particularly likely to introduce such disturbances. One automated commercial sampling system minimizes such problems by dipping the sample probe into the medium only while the sample is being removed (20 s) and withdraws it for purging and media replacement.

The influence on flow patterns of the vertical distance of the basket or paddle from the lowest point of the bottom of the round-bottomed flask should also be considered. The official compendium specifies this distance to be 2.5 cm (± 2 mm). Available data and reports (86,100) suggest that this position is not a significant state variable if the distance is held within reasonable limits. It should be noted, however, that there is a need to establish consistent specifications.

Sampling Probes, Position, and Filters

With most automated sampling systems currently in operation, a relatively large filter-tipped probe is immersed in the dissolution medium. Studies imply that a large probe can affect the hydrodynamics of the system and therefore the dissolution rate of some dosage forms, causing results that differ from those obtained by manual sampling (99,101,102). A smaller probe may have less effect on the dissolution rate (103). Savage and Wells (104) studied the effect of sampling probe size and location on the dissolution rate of prednisone tablets. Employing a USP XX/NF XV apparatus 2 with an automated sampling system, dissolution rates were determined using two large and one small capillary probe at three locations within the dissolution container. The large probes caused hydrodynamic changes which, when compared with results obtained through manual sampling, resulted in significant changes in dissolution rates at each location. With a capillary probe, the changes were less evident, with an insignificant difference between results of automated and manual sampling when the capillary probe was placed midway between the paddle shaft and the wall of the dissolution container.

USP/NF states that samples should be removed at approximately half the distance from the bottom of the basket or paddle to the surface of the dissolution medium and not closer than 1 cm to the side of the flask. These guidelines are based on tests run by employing multiple sampling probes at specific positions (99). The choice of a filter should be preceded by an investigation of the adsorption characteristics of the drug and the particular filter material. It should be noted that the filter material must be saturated with the drug by repeated passage to avoid losses that might go undetected during the test sampling. In the case of manual sampling, it is recommended that the sampling process be accomplished as rapidly as possible and that sampling time be carefully sequenced (99). The accumulation of particulate matter on the filter surface (clogging) may cause significant errors in dissolution testing and generating data. The best practice would be to purge the filter with a reversed flow of dissolution medium or air at the end of each sample interval.

Dosage Form Position

While employing one of the dissolution testing devices containing a basket, such as screen size and basket design, mechanical factors play an important role in dissolution testing, especially with nondisintegrating tablets. In tablet testing, hydrodynamic characterization is important to the establishment and understanding of procedures for optimal use of the device and to correct interpretation of the dissolution test results. Changes or modifications introduced in the mechanics (design) of any dissolution testing device can alter the position of the dosage form in the dissolution medium. Additionally, with these changes there will be significant changes in the fluid flow patterns introduced in the system. These can markedly influence the dissolution characteristics of the dosage form being tested.

Howard et al. (105) examined the influence of tablet position and basket-type effects in a spin-filter dissolution device. Dissolution experiments were conducted on nondisintegrating double-layered tablets containing salicylic acid as the dissolving layer and ethyl cellulose as an inert nondissolving layer. Visualization of flow and dissolution patterns was possible by testing nondisintegrating colored tablets. Visual observation revealed that color was drawn more rapidly from the tablet face resting on the bottom of the basket. Dissolution data from multilayered tablets revealed that when the salicylic acid face was resting on the bottom of the basket, the dissolution was appreciably more rapid than when it was facing up in the basket, as shown in Fig. 5.21. This observation was found for several stirring speeds.

In summary, the dissolution data show definite tablet-position dependency effects. This finding is potentially important in dissolution testing for tablets in general and for multilayered tablets in particular. Unfortunately, there is not enough literature that addresses this phenomenon.

Type of Device

One of the more prominent factors that can influence the dissolution performance of a dosage form that is being tested is the type of apparatus employed. It is well recognized that different dissolution testing devices offer different working conditions, depending on their mechanics. Consequently, parameters such as type and level of agitation, adequacy of mixing, and type of dissolution medium differ significantly from apparatus to apparatus. Also, the drawbacks associated with each type of apparatus as well as systematic errors associated with some of the official methods of dissolution can significantly alter the dissolution rate determinations (106,107). As a result, a large amount of effort is being focused on the characterization, comparison, and comprehensive understanding of various types of dissolution testing apparatus (108–110).

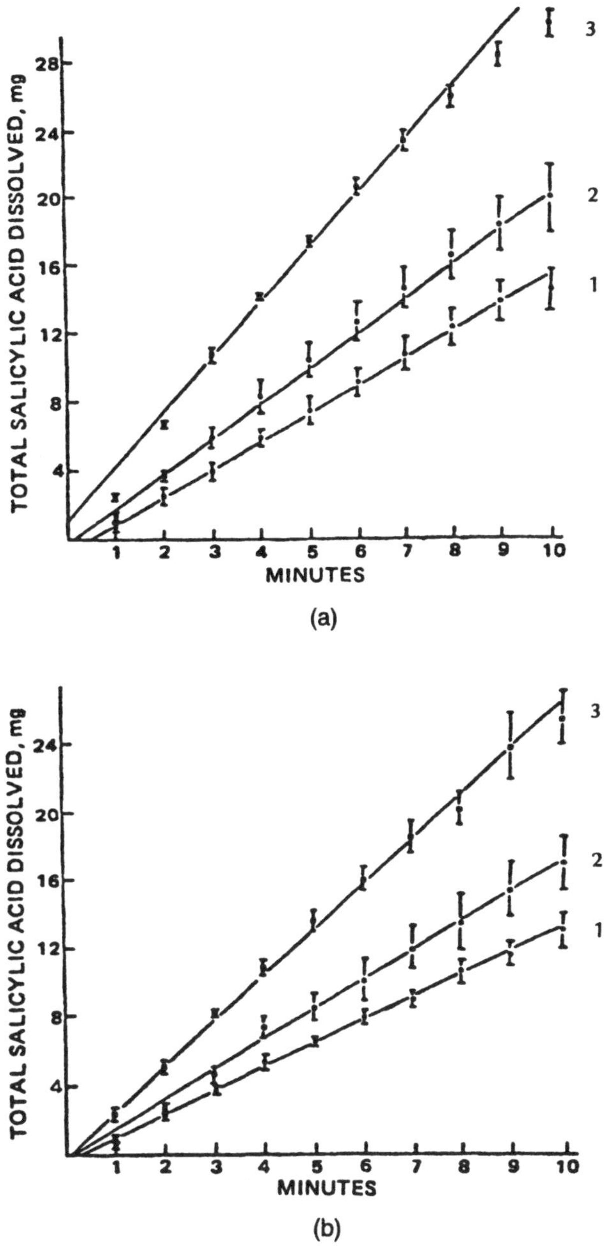

Fig. 5.21 Dissolution profiles of salicylic acid tablets demonstrating the effect of salicylic acid layer position on dissolution from basket at (a) 300 rpm, and at (b) 500 rpm. 1, Faced up; 2, faced down; 3, up–down. (From Ref. 105.)

Hardwidge et al. (108) compared three dissolution testing devices—the rotating basket, the rotating paddle, and the rotating filter–stationary basket—for their suitability as production control tools. The rotating basket and rotating basket assemblies were easier to use and less variable than the rotating filter–stationary basket. When the experimental conditions were held as similar as possible, all three types of apparatus correlated with each other and equally well with the serum drug levels from experimental formulations of an oral hypoglycemic drug after administration to dogs. None of these three types of apparatus gave substantially better correlations when other test conditions, such as relative agitation levels and dissolution medium, were kept constant. Such an observation suggests that the choice of one apparatus over another cannot be made a priori.

FACTORS RELATED TO DISSOLUTION TEST PARAMETERS

Several dissolution test parameters need to be assessed critically before a recommendation can be made by the authorities as a quality control requirement for a given dosage form. Several of these factors affect the dissolution characteristics of the drug as well as the drug product. Factors such as the nature and characteristics of the dissolution medium, pH environment, and ambient temperature have been shown to influence the dissolution performance of a product. Factors such as agitation were discussed in an earlier section. It must be noted, however, that to understand the dissolution characteristics more completely, a collective evaluation is warranted.

Temperature

USP/NF specifies that the dissolution medium must be held at 37°C (±0.5°). Although most commercial water baths can meet this standard of performance, failure to meet this requirement is not uncommon. It is often assumed that the water-bath temperature and the flask temperature are the same. Plastic flasks have a heat transfer coefficient approximately 3.5 times less than that of glass (1). As the temperature difference between the bath and the flask's medium is lowered, the amount of heat transferred into the flasks is reduced. In some environments it is impossible to hold the temperature of the flask at 37°C without implementing substantially higher bath temperatures (~40°C). Heat-up time for the last 1 or 2° of flask medium temperature may take almost 25% as much time as it takes to heat the flask medium up to 35°C from room temperature, as shown in Fig. 5.22. Additionally, the cooling effect of evaporation from the surface of the medium can exceed the rate of heat transfer through the plastic to the point at which stability cannot be maintained. It is vital to cover the flasks at least during dissolution testing. It is quite obvious that plas-

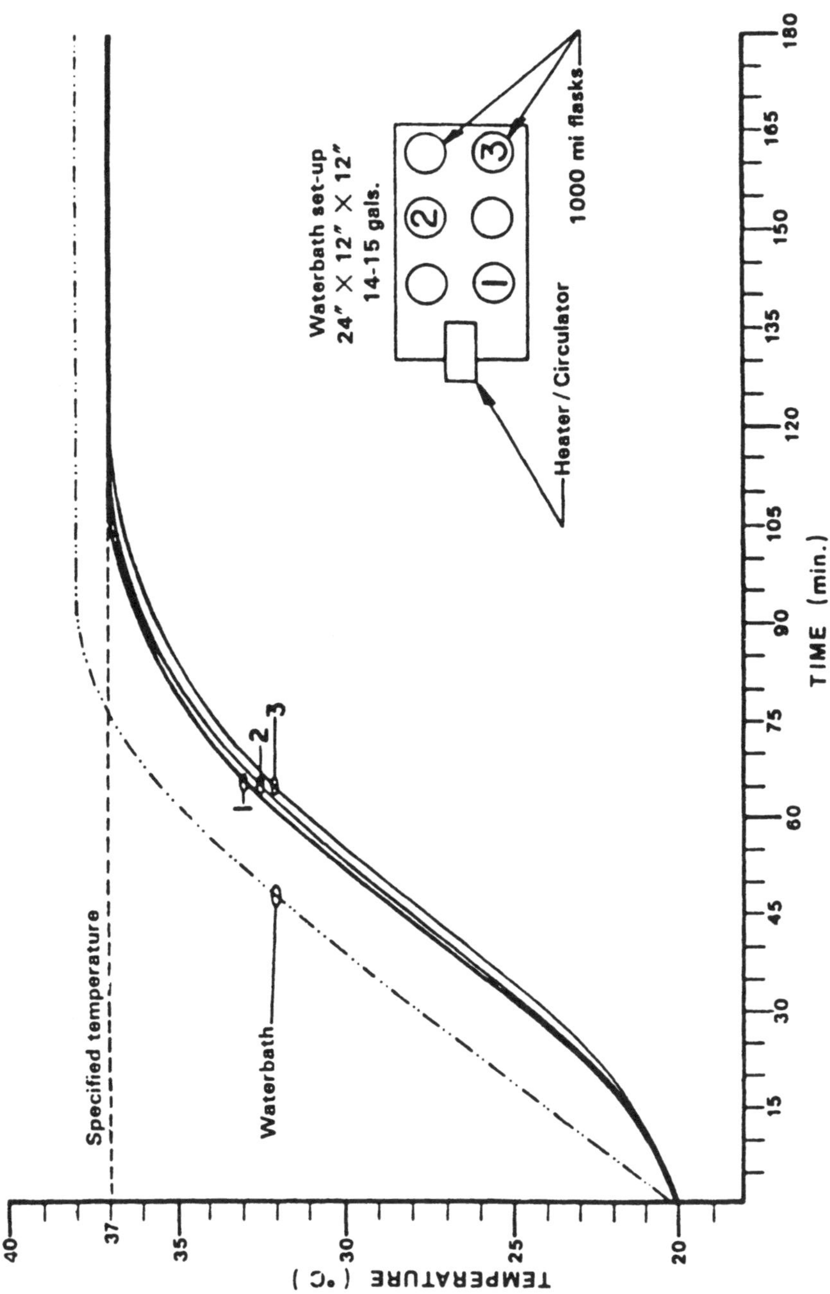

Fig. 5.22 Tests on temperature transfer into dissolution flasks employing standard commercial water bath with mounted circulator/heater. Note the time necessary for equilibrium from 35 to 37.5°C. (From Ref. 85.)

tic and glass flasks cannot be mixed in the same test if consistent results are to be obtained.

Since the drug solubility is temperature dependent, its careful control during the dissolution process is crucial. The effect of temperature variations of the dissolution medium depends mainly on the temperature–solubility curves of the drug and excipients in the formulation. Stokes' equation explains the temperature dependency of a dissolved molecule and diffusion coefficient:

$$D = \frac{kT}{6\pi\eta r} \tag{5.4}$$

where k is the Boltzmann constant and the denominator expresses the Stokes force for a spherical molecule, η is the viscosity, and r is the radius of the molecule.

Numerous reports have been published in the literature documenting the influence of temperature on dissolution of drug substances (111–114). Niebergall and Goyan (111), who were among the first investigators to develop an automatic recording apparatus for use in dissolution-rate studies, showed that the dissolution rate of benzoic acid increased as the temperature increased from 25°C to 40°C. Nogami (112) investigated the influence of temperature on the dissolution of phenobarbital anhydrate at various temperatures under a constant agitation rate of 300 rpm. Significant differences in the dissolution rate were noted, as shown in Fig. 5.23. Although the temperature range employed was below body temperature, it serves to demonstrate the influence of temperature on the solubilization of drug substances.

Dissolution Medium

The constituents, nature, and overall characteristics of the dissolution medium have a significant bearing on the dissolution performance of a drug substance. Also, selection of the proper dissolution medium for dissolution testing depends on the solubility of the drug as well as on economics and practicality. Factors such as dissolved gases, media pH, and viscosity of the medium have been shown to be significantly influential as far as dissolution rate is concerned.

Dissolved Gases–Air

All liquids are in equilibrium with the surrounding gas at the gas–liquid interface. At any given temperature and pressure, a portion of the gas is dissolved in the liquid. In the dissolution process, such an occurrence can interfere with reproducibility of the results in a number of ways. The dissolved gas–air can alter the pH of the medium (distilled water, pH 6; deareated distilled water, pH 7.2). With the change in temperature, the dissolved gases may be released in the form of bubbles. These bubbles can alter the flow patterns associated

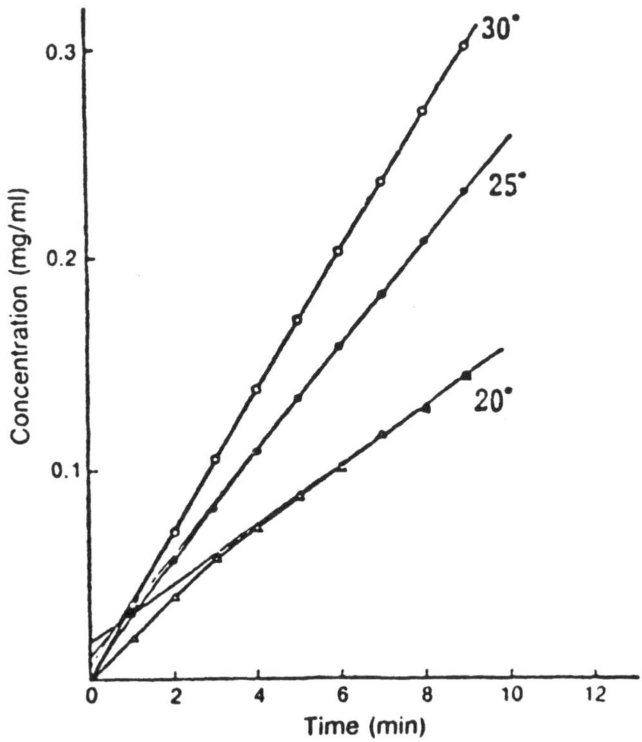

Fig. 5.23 Influence of temperature on the dissolution rate of tablets. (From Ref. 112.)

with particles or the dosage form itself, disturbing the boundary layer at the solid–liquid interface. Additionally, they can collect at the screen of the basket, changing the effective mesh porosity. In doing so, they interfere with the dissolution process.

In a study conducted by DRTL in 1978 (100), a 30% higher dissolution rate was observed for prednisone in deaerated distilled water. In this test this effect is described as "critical." It is suspected that variability in collaborative studies can be due to the presence of dissolved air–gas. Dissolved gases are less likely to influence pH in buffered media, but certainly the pH of distilled water media should be carefully checked and controlled.

Sometimes an air bubble fails to vent from the basket. This should not be confused with dissolved gas. In such cases the dissolution rate may be reduced as much as 50% (115). It is recommended that the test be aborted when such an air pocket develops.

Dissolution Media Composition and pH

Dissolution rates of drug products can be influenced by both the composition and pH of the dissolution medium. Parrott et al. (116) found that the dissolution rate of benzoic acid from tablets was decreased when various concentrations of sodium chloride, sodium sulfate, and dextrose were added to the dissolution medium. Sodium sulfate was most effective in decreasing the dissolution rate, whereas with the addition of urea, the dissolution rate increased. In most cases there is a change in pH of the dissolution medium associated with the addition or deletion of the constituents to the dissolution medium.

Early efforts were oriented toward simulating in vivo conditions, especially pH, surface tension, viscosity, and sink condition. These studies employed 0.1 *N* HCl or buffered solutions with a pH close to 1.2, similar to gastric media (38,39,96). Faster disintegration, and thus enhanced dissolution rates, were observed due to the higher acidity of the dissolution medium. Due to the corrosive action of the acidic fumes, however, it is currently a general practice to use distilled water unless investigative studies show a specific need for an acidic solution in order to generate meaningful dissolution data. Such deleterious effects can be avoided by replacing hydrochloric acid with acidic buffers, such as sodium acid phosphate, to maintain low pH. Yen (117) investigated the influence of pepsin in the dissolution medium on the dissolution rate of a tablet containing triametrene and hydrochlorothiazide. He noted that only the dissolution rate of hydrochlorothiazide was affected adversely. Numerous other studies have also examined the effect of changes in the composition of the dissolution medium, leading to changes in pH, on the dissolution characteristics of drug products over the pH range 2 to 7 (118,119). Figure 5.24 illustrates the effect of changes in the pH of the dissolution medium on the dissolution rate of papaverine hydrochloride.

Viscosity

Dissolution rate decreases with increased viscosity of the dissolution medium, especially in the case of diffusion-controlled dissolution processes. Viscosity can have very little effect, however, on interfacial-controlled dissolution processes. Kellaway and Najib (120) investigated dissolution-rate control by polymers through changes in properties of the bulk solution or the particle–medium interface. In doing so they evaluated the relationship between the bulk viscosity of the dissolution media and the dissolution-rate constants employing sulfadimidine as the test substance. They concluded that a predictable relationship exists between the dissolution rate and knowledge of the apparent viscosity of the dissolution medium.

Other studies addressing the influence of viscosity on the dissolution rate have been reported (121,122). In most instances, the dissolution rate decreases

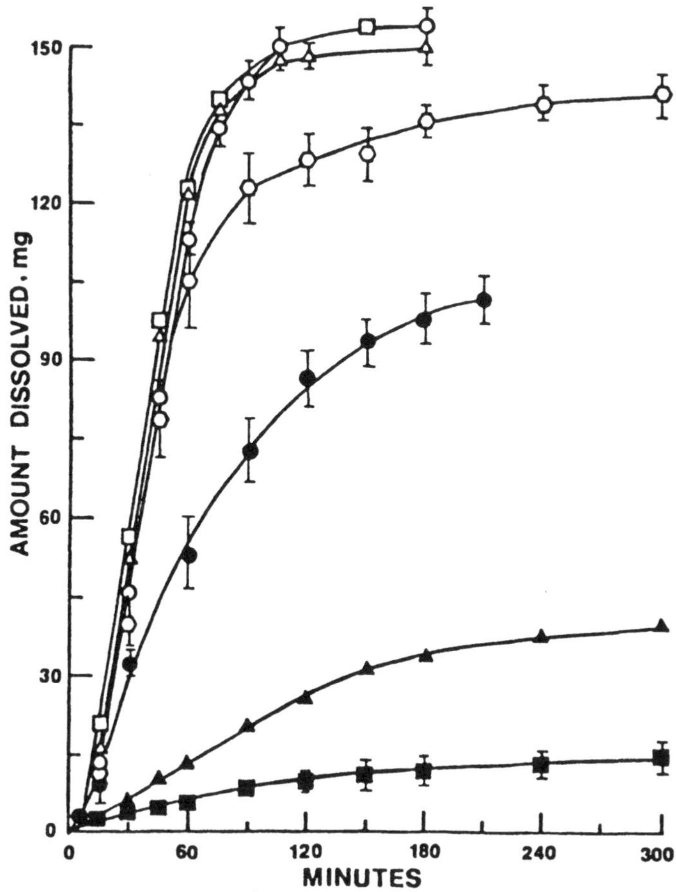

Fig. 5.24 Dissolution profiles of papaverine HCl from papaverine sustained-release pellets in citric acid–phosphate buffers at various pH values. ○, 2.2; △, 3; □, 4; ○, 5; ●, 5.4; ▲, 6; ■, 7. (From Ref. 118.)

rapidly for lower apparent viscosity values and then plateaus, as shown in Fig. 5.25.

Other Factors

Several other factors pertaining to dissolution media can markedly influence the dissolution characteristics of a dosage form. The most important ones that need to be recognized are the surface tension of the dissolution medium and unknown traces of ions or surfactants present in the dissolution medium.

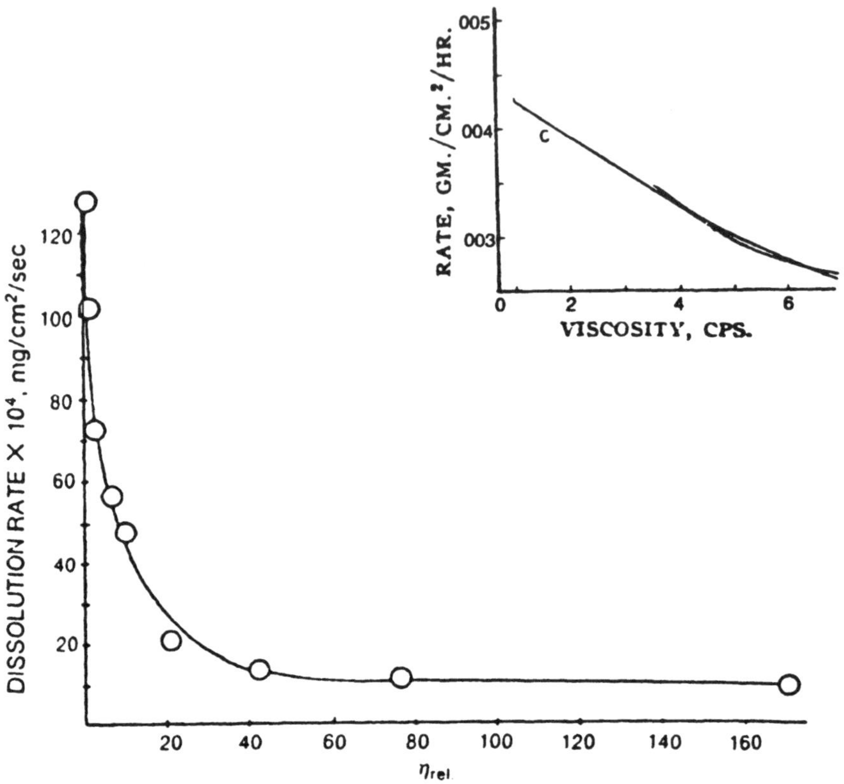

Fig. 5.25 Effect of viscosity on the dissolution rate of benzoic acid in methyl cellulose solutions (from Ref. 122); inset From Ref. 121.

The interfacial tension between a drug and the dissolution medium has been shown to have a significant effect on the dissolution rate of drugs and their release rates from solid dosage forms. Surface-active agents and wetting agents improve the penetrability of the dissolution medium into the matrix by lowering the contact angle, thereby enhancing the dissolution process (58,96,123–125).

If the dissolution media are stored, there are chances that ions from the walls of the container may migrate into the dissolution medium. These extraneous ions can interfere with the dissolution process. It is recommended that the presence of unknown traces of ions that may significantly influence dissolution be checked. Additionally, if the media are stored, the effects of evaporation accompanying pH changes should not be overlooked.

Very often, large volumes of dissolution medium are prepared and used after several hours. With relatively low humidity and at 37°C, substantial quantities can be lost due to evaporation. For example, a loss of 15 mL (not too uncommon) from a 900-mL flask produces a 1.6% error in the data.

The volume of the medium should be maintained. Volumes of dissolution medium withdrawn for analytical purposes or for any other purposes must be returned, replaced, or accounted for and included in calculations for generating dissolution data. Otherwise, the results are not only less meaningful but erroneous.

MISCELLANEOUS FACTORS

In addition to the factors discussed earlier, there are several miscellaneous factors that cannot be included in any given class but significantly influence the dissolution characteristics of drug products. We discuss them briefly below.

Adsorption

In an extremely large number of pharmaceutical dosage forms, including tablets, capsules, and suspensions, there exist drug(s) incorporated with other excipients. Since many of the active ingredients are capable of adsorbing drugs and since dissolution of drugs takes place following their introduction into the body, it is of interest to know the effect of adsorption on the dissolution rate. The contents of the gastrointestinal tract as well as stomach and intestinal walls can be considered as potential adsorption sites for the drug molecules. It has been shown that adsorption can significantly influence the dissolution characteristics of dosage forms (121,126–128).

Wurster and Polli (126) examined the influence of an adsorbent on the dissolution rate of a slightly soluble solid. They reported that the adsorbent was capable of increasing the dissolution rate observed in water under conditions of a decreased concentration gradient applying Nernst–Brunner film theory. The maximum dissolution rate was obtained when a constant-concentration gradient was maintained. Adsorption isotherms were employed to calculate the approximate amount of adsorbent required to increase the slower dissolution rate.

Sorption

Although the penetration capability of the dissolution medium has been addressed to a fair extent, very little attention has been given to changes in physical properties due to water penetration in compressed tablets. Nyqvist and Nicklasson (129) examined the effect of water sorption on the disintegration, and thus dissolution properties, among other physical properties, of tablets containing microcrystalline cellulose. They concluded that water sorption from the atmosphere into the tablets containing microcrystalline cellulose is a very rapid first-order process, resulting in substantial changes in the physical properties. These changes are attributed to the breaking of hydrogen bonds. The relative density of the tablets was found to decrease, resulting in increased disintegration time with increase in water sorption-rate constants. These changes were found to be irreversible. On the basis of these results, appropriate packaging materials can be recommended for tablets containing large amounts of microcrystalline cellulose because even a short-time exposure at high humidity can cause detrimental changes in the physical properties as well as dissolution characteristics of the dosage form.

Humidity

In relation to the dissolution rate of a drug substance, humidity is usually associated with storage effects. Moisture has been shown to influence the dissolution of many drugs from solid dosage forms (86,130,131). Taborsky-Urdinola et al. (130) reported decreases in the dissolution of prednisone tablets exposed to the environment with varying degrees of relative humidity. Hanson and Hanson (86) found that three of the four formulations of prednisone tablets showed drastic decreases in dissolution rate when the tablets were exposed to high humidity. Gupta and Gupta (131), however, did not find significant changes in dissolution behavior of two drugs, except weight gain. The environmental conditions to which the dosage forms are exposed, moisture content in particular, should be rigorously assessed if reproducible and reliable dissolution data are to be obtained. Additionally, humidity during the manufacture of the dosage form should be carefully controlled to guarantee the quality of the product from batch to batch.

Detection Errors

Cartwright (133) has pointed out that the two most common variables leading to interlaboratory disagreement are the failure to use standards during analysis, and external vibration. Care should also be exercised to ensure that excipients in the dosage form do not influence the analysis. It is advisable to withdraw standard as well as samples using the same equipment, to avoid interferences such as sorption of the active principle onto tubing or filters (e.g., nitroglycerin, digitoxin, etc).

Also, the introduction of minute amounts of nickel and chromium ions into dissolution media may interfere with fluorometric determinations. It is therefore imperative that analytical methods be checked carefully for each dissolution system. Extreme care must also be exercised when laboratory methods are introduced into quality control to ensure that no part of the equipment interferes with sensitive determinations. Such occurrences can lead to inappropriate determinations and interpretations of dissolution data.

FINAL COMMENTS

The in vitro dissolution tests imposed by pharmacopoeia and regulatory authorities are attempts to obtain a more reproducible in vitro product. The most significant random variables that influence the dissolution rates have been reviewed in this chapter. Some of these factors should be tolerated together with the expected changes in dissolution rates that have been reported in detailed studies. In many instances, hints on methods for controlling such variables have been included for ready reference.

It should be stressed that many of the foregoing factors are interdependent, often making quite complicated the situation in a given case (2). The literature is full of such examples. This chapter should serve as a guide for up-to-date appraisal by the pharmaceutical scientist in the field of drug product formulation and development.

Despite the fundamental relationship between bioavailability and dissolution rate, the present evidence suggests that no single dissolution-rate test can be applied to all drugs. The possibility that a single test may be applied to drugs having similar physicochemical properties remains to be established. These observations are attributable, primarily, to the inability to assess and control the many variables affecting the dissolution process of a drug substance.

After accounting for and overcoming the various factors influencing dissolution performance, properly designed in vitro tests can be implemented that will ensure product quality from batch to batch and lot to lot. Also, rigorous evaluation of these factors will provide information as to how closely these variables have to be controlled during routine production.

REFERENCES

1. W. A. Hanson, *Handbook of Dissolution Testing*, Pharmaceutical Technology Publications, Springfield, Oreg. (1982), p. 23.
2. J. G. Wagner, *Drug Intell. Clin. Pharm.*, *4*, 132 (70).
3. J. Piccolo and A. Sakr, *Pharm. Ind.*, *46*, 1277 (1984).
4. S. S. Al-Saier and G. S. Riley, *Pharm. Acta Helv.*, *57*, 8 (1982).
5. H. Ueda, N. Nambu, and T. Nagai, *Chem. Pharm. Bull.*, *32*, 244 (1984).
6. H. Ueda, N. Nambu, and T. Nagai, *Chem. Pharm. Bull.*, *30*, 2618 (1982).
7. M. D. Tuladhar, J. E. Carless, and M. P. Summers, *J. Pharm. Pharmacol.*, *35*, 269 (1983).
8. Y. Fukumori, T. Fukuda, Y. Yamamoto, Y. Shigitani, Y. Hanyu Y. Takeuchi, and N. Sato, *Chem. Pharm. Bull.*, *31*, 4029 (1983).
9. S. A. Hill, H. Seager, and C. B. Taskis, *J. Pharm. Pharmacol.*, *24*, 152P (1972).
10. S. A. Hill, K. H. Jones, H. Seager, and C. B. Taskis, *J. Pharm. Pharmacol.*, *27*, 594 (1975).

11. A. J. Aguir, J. Krc, Jr., A. W. Kinkel, and J. C. Samyu, *J. Pharm. Sci.*, *56*, 847 (1967).
12. T. R. Bates, H.-L. Fung, H. Lee, and A. V. Tembo, *Res. Commun. Chem. Pathol. Pharmacol.*, *11*, 233 (1975).
13. T. Tachibana and A. Nakmura, *Kolloid Z. Z. Polym.*, *203*, 130 (1965).
14. A. P. Simonelli, S. C. Mehta, and W. I. Higuchi, *J. Pharm. Sci.*, *58*, 538 (1969).
15. O. I. Corrigan and R. F. Timoney, *J. Pharm. Pharmacol.*, *27*, 759 (1975).
16. O. I. Corrigan, *Drug Dev. Ind. Pharm.*, *11*, 697 (1985).
17. A. P. Simonelli, S. C. Mehta, and W. I. Higuchi, *J. Pharm. Sci.*, *65*, 355 (1976).
18. O. I. Corrigon, M. A. Farvar, and W. I. Higuchi, *Int. J. Pharm.*, *5*, 229 (1980).
19. W. L. Chiou and S. Riegelman, *J. Pharm. Sci.*, *60*, 1281 (1971).
20. E. Shefter and K. C. Cheng, *Int. J. Pharm.*, *6*, 179 (1980).
21. H. Sekikawa, M. Nakano, and T. Arita, *Chem. Pharm. Bull.*, *27*, 1223 (1979).
22. A. A. Badawi and A. A. El-Sayed, *J. Pharm. Sci.*, *69*, 492 (1980).
23. O. I. Corrigan and E. M. Holohan, *J. Pharm. Pharmacol.*, *36*, 217 (1983).
24. A. Anwari and U. V. Banakar, *Abstracts of the APhA/APS*, San Francisco (1986).
25. P. Finholt, H. Kristiansen, O. C. Schmidt, and K. Wold, *Medd. Nor. Farm. Selsk.*, *28*, 17 (1966).
26. J. A. K. Lauwo, *Drug Dev. Ind. Pharm.*, *11*, 1565 (1985).
27. J. M. Newton and N. A. H. Muhammad, *J. Pharm. Pharmacol.*, *36*, 42 (1983).
28. H. M. Abdou, in *Remington's Pharmaceutical Sciences*, 17th ed., Mack Publishing, Easton, Pa. (1986), pp. 653–666.
29. G. Levy, J. Antlkowiak, J. Proknal, and D. White, *J. Pharm. Sci.*, *52*, 1047 (1963).
30. J. Yen, *Can. Pharm. J.*, *97*, 25 (1964).
31. E. Marlow and R. F. Shangraw, *J. Pharm. Sci.*, *56*, 498 (1967).
32. S. S. Kornblum and J. O. Hirschorn, *J. Pharm. Sci.*, *59*, 606 (1970).
33. J. O. Hirschorn and S. S. Kornblum, *J. Pharm. Sci.*, *60*, 445 (1971).
34. M. Wersterberg, B. Jonsson, and C. Nyström, *Int. J. Pharm.*, *28*, 23 (1986).
35. Z. T. Chowhan and L.-H. Chi, *Pharm. Technol. 9(3)*, 84 (1985).
36. P. Finholt, unpublished data (1972).
37. H. E. Johansen, *Arch. Pharm. Chem.*, *79*, 209 (1972).
38. P. Finholt and S. Solvong, *J. Pharm. Sci.*, *57*, 1968 (1968).
39. S. Solvong and P. Finholt, *J. Pharm. Sci.*, *59*, 49 (1970).
40. F. Jaminet, L. DeLattre, and J. P. Delporte, *Pharm. Acta Helv.*, *44*, 418 (1969).
41. J. T. Jacob and E. M. Plein, *J. Pharm. Sci.*, *57*, 802 (1968).
42. G. Suren, *Acta Pharm. Suec.*, *5*, 483 (1970).
43. A. S. Alam and E. L. Parrott, *J. Pharm. Sci.*, *60*, 263 (1971).
44. P. H. Cox and A. S. Mulders, *Pharm. Weekbl.*, *104*, 469 (1969).
45. *Problem Solver and Reference Manual*, FMC Corporation, Food and Pharmaceutical Products Division, Philadelphia (1984).
46. E. Graf, A. H. Ghanem, and A. Nada, *Pharm. Ind.*, *45*, 81 (1983).

47. E. Graf. A. H. Ghanem, and A. Nada, *Pharm. Ind.*, *44*, 317 (1982).
48. E. Graf, A. H. Ghanem, A. Sakr, and H. Mahmond, *Pharm. Ind.*, *43*, 576 (1981).
49. E. V. Vadas, G. R. B. Down, and R. A. Miller, *J. Pharm. Sci.*, *73*, 781 (1984).
50. G. Levy and R. H. Gumtow, *J. Pharm. Sci.*, 1139 (1963).
51. P. Finholt, R. H. Pedersen, S. Solvong, and K. Wold, *Medd. Nor. Farm. Selsk*, *28*, 238 (1966).
52. E. Graf, A. Sakr, and A. Nada, *Pharm. Ind.*, *43*, 282 (1981).
53. J. Rhodes, D. E. Bernardo, S. F. Phillips, A. Rovelstad, and A. F. Hoffman, *Gastroenterology*, *57*, 241 (1969).
54. H. Wientraub and M. Gibaldi, *J. Pharm. Sci.*, *58*, 1368 (1968).
55. P. Fucho, E. Schottky, and G. Schenk, *Pharm. Ind.*, *32*, 581 (1970).
56. M. Gibaldi, S. Feldman, and N. D. Weiner, *Chem. Pharm. Bull.*, *18*, 715 (1970).
57. R. N. Nasipuri, *J. Pharm. Pharmacol.*, *37*, 212 (1985).
58. B. Gander, K. Ventouras, R. Gurny, and E. Deolker, *Int. J. Pharm.*, *27*, 117 (1985).
59. P. O. Bremer, B. Kolstad, and P. Finholt, *Medd. Norsk. Farm. Selsk.* *31*, 67 (1969).
60. E. Sandell, K. Ericksson, and G. Mellstrom, *Farm. Notisbl.*, *80*, 118 (1971).
61. P. Finholt, in *Dissolution Technology*, L. J. Leeson and J. T. Carstensen, eds., Industrial Pharmaceuticals Technology Section, APhA, Washington, D.C. (1974), pp. 136–137.
62. J. L. Kanig and E. M. Rudnic, *Pharm. Technol.*, *8*(4), 50 (1984).
63. K. S. Murthy and J. C. Samyn, *J. Pharm. Sci.*, *66*, 1215 (1977).
64. E. Cid and F. Jaminet, *J. Pharm. Belg.*, *26*, 360 (1971).
65. G. Levy and R. H. Gumtow, *J. Pharm. Sci.*, *52*, 1139 (1963).
66. C. F. Lerk et al., *Pharm. Acta Helv.*, *57*, 282 (1982).
67. G. K. Bolhuis, A. J. Smallenbroek, and C. F. Lerk, *J. Pharm. Sci.*, *70*, 1382 (1981).
68. K. A. Khan, P. Musikabhumma, and M. H. Rubinstein, *Pharm. Acta Helv.*, *58*, 109 (1983).
69. T. Higuchi, A. N. Rao, L. W. Busse, and J. V. Swintosky, *J. Am. Pharm. Assoc. Sci. Ed.*, *42*, 194 (1953).
70. M. C. B. van Oudtshorn, F. J. Potgeiter, C. J. deBlaey, and J. Polderman, *J. Pharm. Pharmacol.*, *23*, 583 (1971).
71. H. E. Johansen and Wiese, *Arch. Pharm. Chem.*, *77*, 243 (1970).
72. D. Ganderton, J. W. Hadgraft, W. T. Rispin, and A. G. Thompson, *Pharm. Acta Helv.*, *42*, 1967 (1967).
73. H. L. Smith, C. A. Baker, and J. H. Wood, *J. Pharm. Pharmacol*, *23*, 536 (1971).
74. N. Kitamori and T. Makino, *J. Pharm. Pharmacol.*, *31*, 501 (1979).
75. K. A. Khan and C. T. Rhodes, *J. Am. Pharm. Assoc.*, *64*, 444 (1975).
76. J. E. Carless and A. Sheak, *J. Pharm. Pharmacol.*, *28*, 17 (1976).
77. A. R. Fassihi, *Int. J. Pharm.*, *32*, 93 (1986).

78. A. J. Aguiar, L. M. Wheeler, S. Fusari, and J. E. Zelmer, *J. Pharm. Pharmacol.*, *57*, 1844 (1968).
79. K. Arnold, N. Gerber, and G. Levy, *Can. J. Pharm. Sci.*, *5*, 89 (1970).
80. H. W. Gouda, M. A. Moustafa, and H. A. Al-Shora, *Int. J. Pharm.*, *18*, 213 (1984).
81. H. W. Gouda, M. A. Moustafa, and A. M. Molokhia, *Int. J. Pharm.*, *5*, 345 (1980).
82 P. York, *Pharmazie*, *32*, 101 (1977).
83. J. T. Rubino, L. M. Halterlein, and J. Blanchard, *Int. J. Pharm.*, *26*, 165 (1985).
84. S. Solvong and P. Finholt, *Medd. Norsk. Farm. Selsk.*, *31*, 101 (1969).
85. W. A. Hanson, *Pharm. Technol.*, *1*(5), 30 (1977).
86. W. Hanson and R. Hanson, *Pharm. Technol.*, *3*(3), 42 (1979).
87. W. Beyer and D. Smith, *J. Pharm. Sci.*, *60*, 1556 (1971).
88. W. Hanson, "Effect of vibration on dissolution testing," presented at the *Beckman Conference on Dissolution*, Mountainside, N.J. (1975).
89. A. Cartwright, *J. Pharm. Pharmacol.*, *31*, 434 (1979).
90. D. E. Wurster and P. W. Taylor, *J. Pharm. Sci.*, *54*, 169 (1965).
91. G. Levy, *Am. J. Pharm.*, *135*, 78 (1963).
92. F.I.P. Working Group 5, *Pharm. Ind.*, *43*, 334 (1981).
93. J. Carstensen, T. Lai, and V. K. Prasad, *J. Pharm. Sci.*, *67*, 1303 (1978).
94. G. Levy and J. A. Procknal, *J. Pharm. Sci.*, *51*, 58 (1964).
95. J. Tingstad, E. Gropper, L. Lachman, and E. Shami, *J. Pharm. Sci.*, *62*, 293 (1973).
96. J. M. Newton and N. A. H. Muhammad, *J. Pharm. Pharmacol.*, *36*, 42 (1984).
97. G. Levy, J. R. Leonards, and J. A. Procknal, *J. Pharm. Sci.*, *54*, 1719 (1965).
98. K. Thakker, N. Naik, V. Gary, and S. Sun, *Pharm. Forum*, *6*, 177 (1980).
99. D. Cox, C. Douglas, W. Furman, R. Kirchhoefer, J. Myrick, and C. Wells, *Pharm. Technol.*, *2(4)*, 40 (1978).
100. Drug Research and Testing Laboratory, *Report 77–535*, DRTL, (Jan. 1978).
101. F. L. Underwood and D. E. Cadwallader, *J. Pharm. Sci.*, *65*, 697 (1976).
102. M. Lagas and C. F. Lerk, *Pharm. Weekbl.*, *113*, 1277 (1978).
103. C. E. Wells, *J. Pharm. Sci.*, *70*, 232 (1981).
104. T. S. Savage and C. E. Wells, *J. Pharm. Sci.*, *71*, 670 (1982).
105. S. A. Howard, J. W. Manger, A. Khwangsopha, and D. A. Pasquerelli, *J. Pharm. Sci.*, *68*, 1542 (1979).
106. D. C. Cox, W. B. Furman, L. K. Thornton, T. W. Moore, and E. H. Jefferson, *J. Pharm. Sci.*, *72*, 910 (1983).
107. D. C. Cox, W. B. Furman, and D. P. Page, *J. Pharm. Sci.*, *72*, 1061 (1983).
108. E. A. Hardwidge, A. C. Sarapu, and W. C. Laughlin, *J. Pharm. Sci.*, *67*, 1732 (1978).
109. J. T. Carstensen, T. Lai, and V. K. Prasad, *J. Pharm. Sci.*, *66*, 607 (1977).
110. M. R. Baichwal, S. G. Deshpande, and U. C. Shetty, *Drug Dev. Ind. Pharm.*, *11*, 1639 (1985).
111. P. J. Niebergall and J. E. Goyan, *J. Pharm. Sci.*, *52*, 29 (1963).

112. H. Nogami, *Chem. Pharm. Bull.*, *17*, 499 (1969).
113. J. T. Carstensen, R. Kothari, V. K. Prasad, and J. Sheridan, *J. Pharm. Sci.*, *69*, 290 (1980).
114. D. J. W. Grant, M. Mehdizadeh, A. H.-L. Chow, and J. E. Fairbrother, *Int. J. Pharm.*, *18*, 25 (1984).
115. A. Sarapu and J. Clark, Jr., *J. Pharm. Sci.*, *69*, 129 (1980).
116. E. L. Parrott, D. E. Wurster, and T. Higuchi, *J. Pharm. Sci.*, *44*, 269 (1955).
117. J. K. C. Yen, *Can. J. Pharm. Sci.*, *5*, 112 (1970).
118. A. T. M. Serajuddin and M. Rosoff, *J. Pharm Sci.*, *73*, 1203 (1984).
119. A. T. M. Serajuddin and C. I. Jarowski, *J. Pharm. Sci.*, *74*, 148 (1985).
120. I. W. Kellaway and N. M. Najib, *Int. J. Pharm. Technol. Prod. Manuf.*, *4*(2), 37 (1983).
121. D. E. Wurster and G. P. Polli, *J. Pharm. Sci.*, *53*, 311 (1964).
122. R. Braun and E. Parrott, *J. Pharm. Sci.*, *61*, 175 (1972).
123. H. Mohamad, R. Renoux, and J. M. Aiache, *Labo-Pharm. Probl. Tech.*, *32*, 284 (1984).
124. P. Singh, S. Desai, A. P. Simonelli, and W. I. Higuchi, *J. Pharm. Sci.*, *57*, 959 (1968).
125. J. E. Hilton and M. P. Summers, *Int. J. Pharm.*, *31*, 157 (1986).
126. D. E. Wurster and G. P. Polli, *J. Pharm. Sci.*, *50*, 403 (1961).
127. S. A. H. Khalil, *J. Pharm. Pharmacol.*, *26*, 961 (1974).
128. G. Boman, P. Lundgren, and G. Stjernstrom, *Eur. J. Clin. Pharmacol.*, *8*, 293 (1975).
129. H. Nyqvist and M. Nicklasson, *Int. J. Pharm. Technol. Prod. Manuf.*, *4*, 67 (1983).
130. C. J. Taborsky-Urdinola, V. A. Gray, and L. T. Grady, *Am. J. Hosp. Pharm.*, *38*, 1322 (1981).
131. V. D. Gupta and A. Gupta, *Am. J. Hosp. Pharm.*, *38*, 1539 (1981).
132. G. G. Knapp and D. P. Page, *Am. J. Hosp. Pharm.* *40*, 623 (1983).
133. A. Cartwright, *J. Pharm. Pharmacol.*, *31*, 434 (1979).

ADDITIONAL READING

Ahmed, S. U. and P. L. Madan, *Drug Dev. Ind. Pharm.*, *15*, 1243 (1989).
Akbuga, J. and A. Gursoy, *Pharm. Ind.*, *51*, 1046 (1989).
Alonso, M. J., P. Maincent, T. Garcia Arias et al., *Int. J. Pharm.*, *42*, 27 (1988).
Aly, S. A. and E. O. Uwaeke, *Acta. Pharm. Jugosl.*, *38*, 131 (1988).
Anderberg, E. K., M. Bisrat, and C. Nystrom, *Int. J. Pharm.*, *47*, 67 (1988).
Anon., *Manuf. Chem.*, *59*, 57 (1988).
Asker, A. F. and C. W. Harris, *Drug Dev. Ind. Pharm.*, *16*, 165 (1990).
Augsburger, L. L. *S T P Pharma.*, *4*, 116, (1988).
Baveja, S. K., S. Singh, and A. Singh, *Pharma Times*, *20*, 11 (1988).
Bisrat, M. and C. Nystrom, *Int. J. Pharm.*, *47*, 223 (1988).
Botzolakis, J. E. and L. L. Augsburger, *Drug Dev. Ind. Pharm.*, *14*, 29 (1988).
Burger, A. and A. W. Ratz, *Pharm. Ind.*, *50*, 1186 (1988).

Carstensen, J. T., R. Jarecki, and C. Ertell, *Drug Dev. Ind. Pharm.*, *14*, 1971 (1988).
Chan, H. K. and D. J. Grant, *Int. J. Pharm.*, *57*, 117 (1989).
Chattaraj, S. C. and S. K. Das, *Drug Dev. Ind. Pharm.*, *16*, 283 (1990).
Chen, C. M., D. Alli, M. R. Igga et al., *Drug Dev. Ind. Pharm.*, *16*, 379 (1990).
Chowhan, Z. T. and A. A. Amaro, *Drug Dev. Ind. Pharm.*, *14*, 1079 (1988).
Chow, A. H. and D. J. Grant, *Int. J. Pharm.*, *51*, 129 (1989).
Chukwu, A. and P. Okpalaezinne, *Drug Dev. Ind. Pharm.*, *15*, 325 (1989).
Coulibaly, S., Y. D. Konan, A. J. Danho et al., *S T P Pharma.*, *4*, 21 (1988).
Dahlan, R., C. McDonald, and V. B. Sunderland, *Drug Dev. Ind. Pharm.*, *14*, 1125 (1988).
Das, S. K. and B. K. Gupta, *Drug Dev. Ind. Pharm.*, *14*, 537 (1988).
Dedhiya, M. G., C. W. Woodruff, F. A. Menard et al., *Drug Dev. Ind. Pharm.*, *14*, 53 (1988).
Doherty, C. and P. York, *J. Pharm. Pharmacol.*, *41*, 73 (1989).
Doherty, C. and P. York, *Int. J. Pharm.*, *50*, 223 (1989).
El Din, E. E., M. H. El Shaboury, and H. A. El Aleem, *Pharm. Ind.*, *51*, 694 (1989).
Esezobo, S., S. Zubair, and N. Pilpel, *J. Pharm. Pharmacol*, *41*, 7 (1989).
Fassishi, A. R., R. Dowse, and S. Daya, *Drug Dev. Ind. Pharm.*, *15*, 235 (1989).
Fassihi, A. R. and D. L. Munday, *J. Pharm. Pharmacol*, *41*, 369 (1989).
Fini, A., I. Orienti, and V. Zecchi, *Arch. Pharm. Weinheim Ger.*, 321, 209 (1988).
Gadalla, M. A., M. H. Abd El Hameed, and A. A. Ismail, *Drug Dev. Ind. Pharm.*, *14*, 1107 (1988).
Gadalla, M. A., M. H. Abd El Hameed, and A. A. Ismail, *Drug Dev. Ind. Pharm.*, *15*, 427 (1989).
El Gawad, A. H., E. El Din, and H. A. El Alim, *Pharmazie*, *43*, 624 (1988).
Georgarakis, M., P. Hatzipantou, and J. E. Kountourelis, *Drug Dev. Ind. Pharm.*, *14*, 915 (1988).
Georgarakis, M., *Pharmazie*, *44*, 209 (1989).
Giron, D., *S T P Pharma.*, *4*, 330 (1988).
Gordon, M. S., B. Chatterjee, and Z. T. Chowhan, *J. Pharm. Sci.*, *79*, 43 (1990).
Hannula, A. M., M. Marvola, and E. Aho, *Acta. Pharm. Fenn.*, *98* 131 (1989).
Hannula, A. M., M. Marvola, and T. Kopra, *Acta. Pharm. Fenn.*, *98*, 11 (1989).
Harland, R. S., A. Gazzaniga, M. E. Sangalli et al., *Pharm. Res.*, *5*, 488 (1988).
Hintz, R. J. and K. C. Johnson, *Int. J. Pharm.*, *51*, (1989).
Ibrahim, S. A., E. Hafez, T. H. El Faham et al., *Bull. Pharm. Sci. Assuit. Univ.*, *11*, 196 (1988).
Imai, T., Y. Saito, H. Matsumoto, et al., *Int. J. Pharm.*, *53*, 7 (1989).
Johansen, H., I. S. Andersen, and H. Leedgaard, *Drug Dev. Ind. Pharm.*, *15*, 477 (1989).
Keipert, S. and S. Hildebrandt, *Pharmazie*, *44*, 707 (1989).
Kikuchi, M. and K. Uekama, *Yakugaku Zasshi*, *108*, 156 (1988).
Klauschenz, E., V. Hagen, B. Gentsch et al., *Pharmazie*, *43*, 167 (1988).
Law, S. L. and C. H. Chiang, *Drug Dev. Ind. Pharm.*, *16*, 137 (1990).
Lin, S. Y., *J. Pharm. Sci.*, *77*, 229 (1988).
Lin, S. Y. and Y. H. Kao, *Int. J. Pharm.*, *56*, 249 (1989).

Lin, S. Y., Y. H. Kao, and J. C. Yang, *Drug Dev. Ind. Pharm.*, *14*, 99 (1988).
Marshall, K., *Drug Dev. Ind. Pharm*, *15*, 2153 (1989).
McNamara, D. P., G. L. Amidon, *J. Pharm. Sci.*, *77*, 511 (1988).
Mitra, A. K. and S. A. Gordziel, *Drug Dev. Ind. Pharm.*, *14*, 953 (1988).
Mitra, A. K. and S. A. Gordziel, *Drug Dev. Ind. Pharm.*, *14*, 953 (1988).
Morasso, M. I., J. Salas, and A. Arancibia, *Farmaco Ed. Prat.*, *43*, 177 (1988)
Murthy, K. S., N. A. Enders, and M. B. Fawzi, *Pharm. Tech.*, *13*, 72 (1989).
Naggar, V. F. and M. W. Samaha, *Pharm. Ind.*, *51*, 543 (1989).
Okor, R. S., *Pharm. World*, *5*, 106 (1988).
Okor, R. S., *Int. J. Pharm.*, *47*, 263 (1988).
Okor, R. S., *Int. J. Pharm.*, *47*, 263 (1988).
Ozturk, S. S., B. O. Palsson, and J. B. Dressman, *Pharm. Res.*, *5*, 272 (1988).
Pacheco, R. M., J. L. Vila Jato, A. Concheiro et al., *Int. J. Pharm.*, *47*, 37 (1988).
Padmadisastra, Y. and I. Gonda, *J. Pharm. Sci.*, *73*, 508 (1989).
Parrott, E. L., *Drug Dev. Ind. Pharm.*, *15*, 561 (1989).
Patel, N. K., N. R. Poola, A. Babar et al., *Drug Dev. Ind. Pharm*, *15*, 1175 (1989).
Pezoa, R., M. I. Morasso, B. Ludwig et al., *Drug Dev. Ind. Pharm.*, *14*, 475 (1988).
Pommier, A. M., C. Brossard, J. Ser et al., *S T P Pharma.*, *4*, 384 (1988).
Ramtoola, Z. and O. I. Corrigan, *Drug Dev. Ind. Pharm.*, *14*, 2241 (1988).
Richter, M., H. W. Rahn, and R. Voigt, *Pharmazie*, *44*, 43 (1989).
Sarisuta, N. and E. L. Parrott, *Drug Dev. Ind. Pharm.*, *14*, 1877 (1988).
Schafer, U., H. Oelschlager, and H. Stricker, *Pharm. Ind.*, *50*, 588 (1988).
Schoonen, A. J. and G. W. De Vries, *Int. J. Pharm.*, *49*, 261 (1989).
Schoonen, A. J. M., H. Grijseels, and G. W. DeVries Nijboer, *Int. J. Pharm.*, *47*, 249 (1988).
Serajuddin, A. T., P. C. Sheen, D. Mufson et al., *J. Pharm. Sci.*, *77*, 414 (1988).
Shah, V. P., J. J. Konecny, R. L. Everett, et al., *Pharm. Res.*, *6*, 612 (1989).
Shawky, S. and M. S. Mesiha, *S T P Pharma.*, *4*, 270 (1988).
Shukla, A. J. and J. C. Price, *Pharm. Res.*, *6*, 418 (1989).
Sjokvist, E. and C. Nystrom, Int. J. Pharm., 47, 51 (1988).
Sjokvist, E., C. Nystrom, and M. Alden, *Int. J. Pharm.*, *54*, 161 (1989).
Snaselova, M., J. Pokorny, and V. Hofschneider, *Farm Obz.*, *58*, 395 (1989).
Soltero, R. A., J. M. Hoover, and T. F. Jones, *J. Pharm. Sci.*, *78*, 35 (1989).
Szabo Revesz, P., K. Pintye Hodi, M. Miset et al., *Pharm. Ind.*, *50*, 981 (1988).
Szabo Revesz, P., K. Pintye Hodi, L. Kun et al., *Acta. Pharm. Hung.*, *59*, 99 (1989).
Takahashi, K., T. Katagi, and S. Tamagawa, *Int. J. Pharm.*, *49*, 179 (1989).
Tarimci, N. and N. Celebi, *Pharmazie*, *43*, 323 (1988).
Villiers, M. M. De and J. G. Van Der Watt, *Drug Dev. Ind. Pharm.*, *15*, 621 (1989).
Wan, L. S. and K. P. Prasad, *Int. J. Pharm.*, *41*, 159 (1988).
Wehrle, P., P. Nobelis, and A. Stamm, *S T P Pharma.*, *4*, 202 (1988).
Wu, P., F. Attarchi, N. Anderson et al., *Drug Dev. Ind. Pharm.*, *15*, 11 (1989).
Zhang, W. H., *Yaoxue Tongbao*, *24*, 135 (1989).
Zubair, S., S. Esezobo, and N. Pilpel, *J. Pharm. Pharmacol.*, *40*, 278 (1988).

SIX

Interpretation of Dissolution Rate Data and Techniques of In Vivo Dissolution

Umesh V. Banakar
St. Louis College of Pharmacy
St. Louis, Missouri

Chetan D. Lathia* and John H. Wood
Virginia Commonwealth University
Medical College of Virginia
Richmond, Virginia

INTRODUCTION

The rate at which a drug substance dissolves in a medium is commonly referred to as its rate of dissolution or dissolution rate. It is now well accepted that dissolution-rate data, when considered together with data on drug's solubility and other important parameters, such as partition characteristics and dissolution constant, can provide crucial information as to the drug's absorption potential following administration.

There is an abundance of literature on the theory of dissolution rate. Generally, dissolution rate studies have one of two purposes:

1. The employment of these studies to arrive at a kinetic scheme for the overall dissolution process (1)

* *Current affiliation*: Lederle Laboratories, Pearl River, New York

2. The treatment of the results of such studies with one of several distribution functions to enable the data to be expressed in terms of the parameters of the function chosen (2–7)

Several workers have proposed numerous ways of interpreting dissolution-rate data, the primary purpose being the determination of the kinetics of the dissolution process and supplementing the information by providing an insight into the dissolution process that could occur in vivo. This has resulted in analyzing and expressing dissolution-rate data in several ways. Most of the techniques employed to interpret as well as to express dissolution-rate data involve some type of mathematical treatment. Such techniques, when employed to determine as well as interpret dissolution of dosage forms, can be extremely beneficial to pharmaceutical dosage form development specialists. This is particularly true since dissolution is often the rate-limiting step for bioavailability. Additionally, dissolution testing can provide the direction for development of a dosage form for a drug substance under investigation. Consequently, it is imperative at this juncture to review some of the more prominent methods routinely employed for interpretation of dissolution-rate data.

Although there exists a plethora of information on theories and methodologies of dissolution of drugs and drug products, there is no single source which comprehensively presents the methods of interpreting data on dissolution rate. Furthermore, most of the reports revolve around the interpretation and analysis of in vitro dissolution test data. However, before becoming bioavailable, the dosage form has to undergo dissolution in vivo as well. The intention of this chapter is to present comprehensively methods reported in the literature on interpretation of in vitro dissolution-rate data of both drug substances and drug products (dosage forms). Additionally, we focus on the techniques employed in in vivo dissolution testing of dosage forms.

TABLET AND CAPSULE DISSOLUTION DATA

Despite the upsurge in the development and introduction of modified and so-called specialized drug delivery systems, tablets and capsules still rate among the most popular solid dosage forms. More than 52% of the various dosage forms available for drug entities comprise tablets or capsules. These dosage forms have been available since the mid-nineteenth century. The chronological age of these dosage forms is indicative of the amount of work invested to understand their working and behavior both in vitro and in the biological system. There is a superabundance of literature that attempts, directly or indirectly, to provide an insight into the mechanics of their dissolution and subsequent release of drug entity in the surrounding media: dissolution medium or biological fluids. Such data are still being generated and are frequently reported. In the attempt to determine the mechanics of dissolution of capsules and/or tablets, the resultant data have been collected, interpreted, and analyzed in numerous ways. This has resulted in a critical mass of information that when presented comprehensively can provide the scientist working in this discipline with numerous pathways for analyzing dissolution data. Such a treatment will be beneficial in the development of the dosage unit—tablet or capsule—for the drug entity under investigation. Consequently, it is crucial to present a comprehensive summary on interpretation of dissolution-rate data of tablets and capsules.

The common factor associated with dissolution of tablets and capsules is that they undergo disintegration prior to dissolution. The only exceptions to this are the nondisintegrating matrix tablets and some special dissolution-rate-modulated capsules. Numerous approaches have been attempted to determine the disintegration time, if not delineate it, from the overall dissolution performance of these dosage forms. Many studies concentrate on interpreting overall dissolution behavior in a way that distinguishes and differentiates these interrelated processes: disintegration followed by dissolution. Since, in general, ultimate dissolution of these dosage forms is dependent on the disintegration time and rate of disintegration, it is critical that the overall dissolution performance should account for both disintegration and dissolution.

Usually, the overall dissolution of tablet and capsule dosage forms has been presented in one of the following ways:

1. Cumulative amount of drug dissolved as a function of time
2. Cumulative percent of drug dissolved as a function of time
3. Amount of drug remaining to be dissolved as a function of time

Very seldom, the amount of drug dissolved per unit time as a function of time is reported. In addition, other approaches for interpreting dissolution data have been suggested. However, these depend primarily on the mathematical expressions derived to exemplify the mechanics and/or the kinetics of dissolution. In the following sections we describe some of the more prominent and noteworthy attempts to describe and interpret dissolution of tablet and/or capsule dosage forms.

Dissolution Efficiency Concept

The tremendous interest in drug availability has resulted in a proliferation of in vitro dissolution testing, now standard for many dosage forms. Usually, the method of evaluation involves the comparison of the time taken for given proportions of the active principle to be released into solution. Parameters such as $T_{20\%}$, $T_{50\%}$, and $T_{90\%}$ are frequently quoted. The fraction of drug in solution after a given time (e.g., 60% release in 30 min) is sometimes noted as well.

Khan and Rhodes (8) have suggested another parameter suitable for the evaluation of in vitro dissolution: *dissolution efficiency* (DE). DE is defined as the area under the dissolution curve up to a certain time *t*, expressed as a percentage of the area of the rectangle described by 100% dissolution in the same time (6,8). The evaluation of a tablet dosage form is depicted in Fig. 6.1, where

$$DE = \frac{\int_0^t y\,dt}{y_{100}\,t} \times 100 \tag{6.1}$$

It must be noted that DE can assume a range of values depending on the time intervals chosen for interpretation. This should preferably be greater than the $T_{90\%}$ value of the formulation, to ensure that most of the dissolution pattern has been accounted for. This is not always possible, however, for dosage forms that release the drug slowly. In any case. it is crucial that constant time intervals be chosen for comparison. DE_{50}, for example, would relate to the dissolution of drug from a particular formulation after 50 min and could only be compared with the DE_{50} of other formulations.

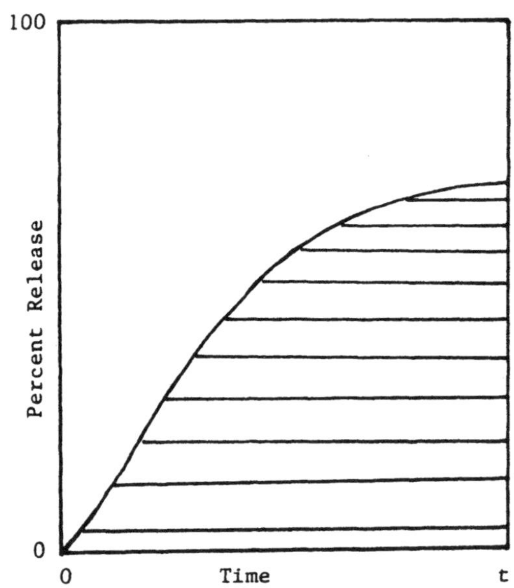

Fig. 6.1 Schematic representation of a dissolution profile of drug from a tablet:

$$DE(15) = \frac{\text{shaded area}}{\text{area of rectangle}} \times 100$$

In the case of dissolution of capsules as dosage forms, the presence or absence of lag time has a bearing on the determination of DE. Figure 6.2 illustrates schematically the dissolution of drug from a capsule. If a comparison of different capsule fills is desired, then assuming that there is no interaction between capsule contents and gelatin shell, the lag time could be excluded. However, if a final product is being tested (i.e., production or storage of test samples), the lag time should be included (8).

It is imperative to establish that the total content of drug in the formulation is available for release. Also, DE is a comparative parameter and should be quoted in conjunction with the $T_{50\%}$ or preferably $T_{90\%}$ value. Several advantages are offered by the concept of DE. The summation of drug release data into a single figure facilitates comparison of various formulations. Second, DE can theoretically be related to in vivo data. If it is assumed that the extent of absorption of drug is proportional to the concentration of the drug in solution and the time this solution is in contact with the absorptive surface, then DE as described is a function of these two variables. Consequently, since bioavaila-

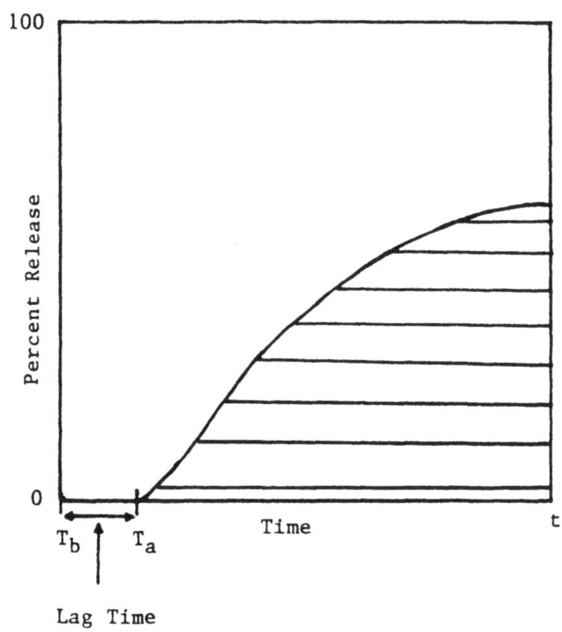

Fig. 6.2 Schematic representation of a dissolution profile of drug from a capsule ($Tb - Ta$ = lag time):

$$\underset{\text{without lag time}}{\text{DE(15)}} = \frac{\text{shaded area}}{\text{area of rectangle}} \times 100$$

bility can be estimated by integrating the area under the blood concentration curve, it seems reasonable to express in vitro dissolution results similarly. Furthermore, DE takes into account the entire dissolution profile as a whole, as opposed to $T_{50\%}$ or $T_{90\%}$ values. This approach employs a more realistic and meaningful method of comparison as well as interpretation of in vitro dissolution data for various formulations.

Surface Area Concept

Although there is extensive literature on the theory of rate of dissolution, it will be appropriate to review some of the equations in order to elicit relationships between some of the constants and to establish their dimensions. It has been shown that under sink conditions a percent-dissolved value at time t may simply be equivalent to the percent surface area generated to time t for dissolution to occur (9); see Fig. 6.3.

Under sink conditions, the amount of substance dissolved, C_1, is far less than the solubility of the substance in the dissolution medium, C_s. The dissolution process can thus be explained by

$$dW/dt = KSC_s \qquad C << C_s \tag{6.2}$$

where dW/dt is the rate of dissolution and K is the dissolution-rate constant with dimensions of length/time. The cumulative amount of substance dissolved, W, within a time interval $t = 0$ to $t = T$ can be determined by integrating Eq. (6.2):

$$W = KC_s\int_0^T s(t)\,dt \tag{6.3}$$

The integral also represents the cumulative surface area that has been made available for dissolution within the limits of the time interval. Thus for infinite time,

$$W = KC_s\int_0^\infty S(t)\,dt \tag{6.4}$$

where W represents the amount in solution at infinite time. Additionally, the integral represents the total surface area of drug that has been made available for dissolution during the test period.

The percent dissolved at time t can be calculated by dividing Eq. (6.3) by Eq. (6.4). Thus

$$\%W_t = W/W_\infty \times 100 = \frac{\int_0^T s(t)\,dt}{\int_0^\infty S(t)\,dt} \times 100 \tag{6.5}$$

Equation (6.5) essentially determines the percent surface area generated to time T of total surface area generated. Assuming the validity of Eq. (6.5), the

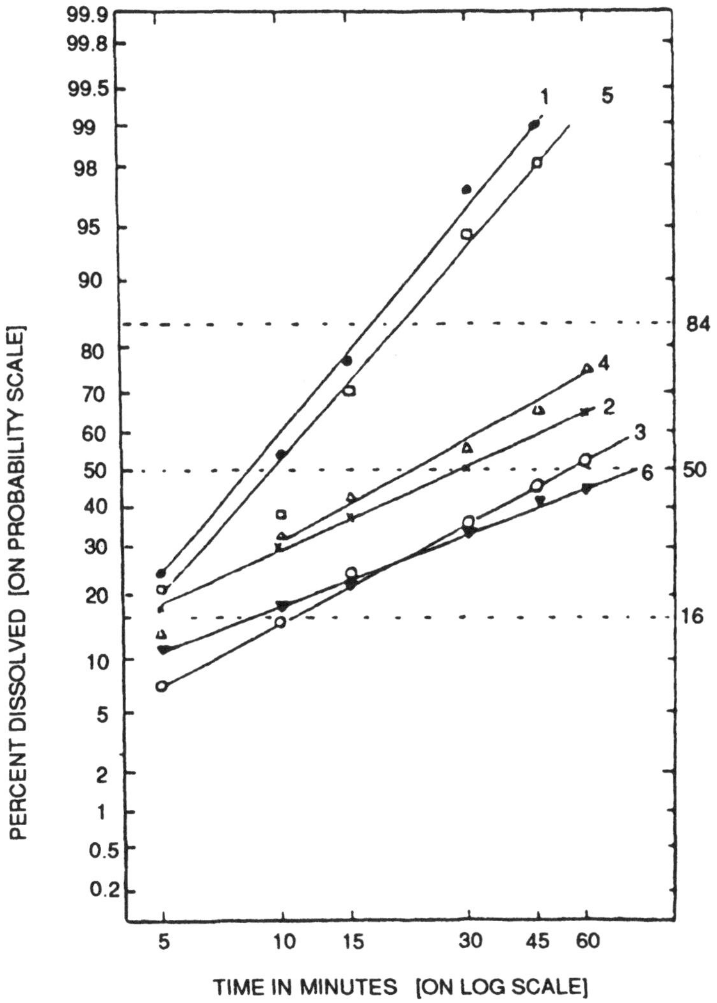

Fig. 6.3 In vitro dissolution of six griseofulvin formulations in simulated intestinal fluid as reported by Symchowicz and Katchen, treated according to the method by Wagner. (From Ref. 9.)

percent dissolved–time data derived from in vitro dissolution testing of tablets and capsules may best be described by a distribution function, such as the *logarithmic-normal* or *logarithmic-logistic* distribution functions (10). If dissolution data follow a log-normal distribution, one can expect a single linear trend when percent-dissolved values are plotted on the probability scale (ordinate) as a function of time values on the logarithmic scale (abscissa) of probit (log-normal) graph paper [refer to Eq. (6.4)].

Wagner (9) reported that data generated by the log-normal distribution function could be interpreted according to first-order kinetics. However, in such cases the first-order plots could be artifacts. Four percent dissolved–time plots were generated employing log-normal distribution function, as shown in Fig. 6.4. If the data were described by the corresponding distribution function, the points should fall randomly about a straight line that could be drawn through the points. In the case of log-normal graph paper, an estimate of the medium time may be obtained by reading the time corresponding to the 50% point. An estimate of the standard deviation may be obtained from the 16, 50, and 84% points by appropriate conversions of the time values to their logarithms, then taking differences.

When plotted in first-order kinetic fashion, the data of curves A and D of Fig. 6.4 yield Fig. 6.5. Semilogarithmic plots of percent not dissolved (100% dissolved) as a function of time yield an apparent linear plot in the range 72.5 to 1.4% not dissolved (curve A). Data from curve D of Fig. 6.4 appear to yield two apparently linear segments in Fig. 6.5. As indicated earlier, the real percent dissolved–time data sometimes yield two apparent first-order rates that are really artifacts (11). The data shown in Fig. 6.4 are best described by the

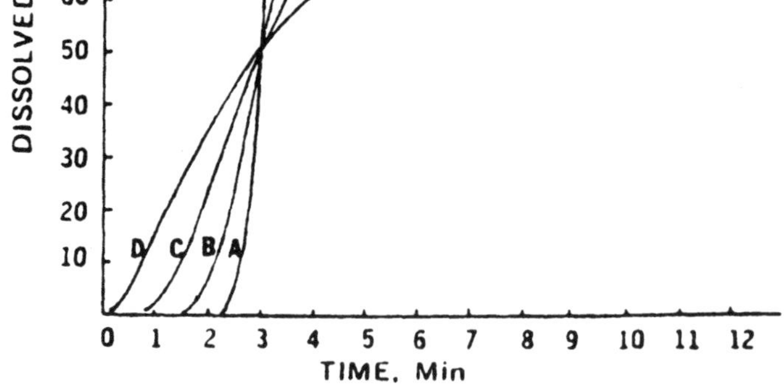

Fig. 6.4 Percent dissolved as a function of time plots for four hypothetical formulations generated with the log-normal distribution functions.

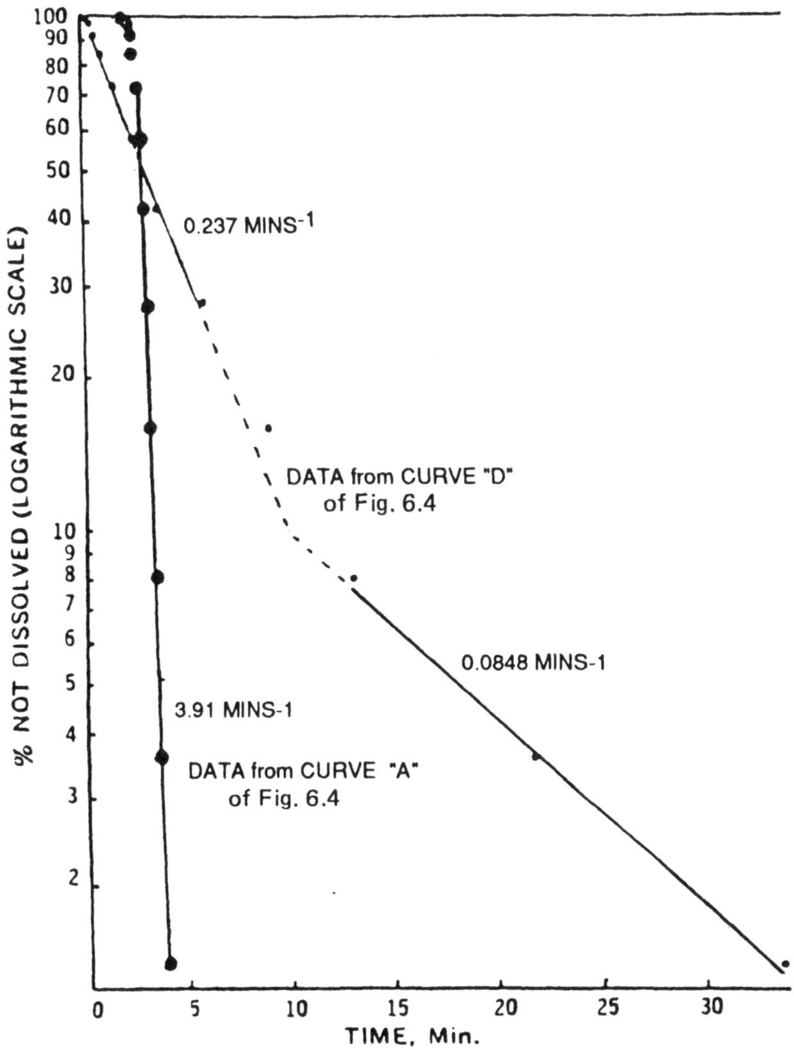

Fig. 6.5 Data of profiles A and D from Fig. 6.4 graphed in accordance with first-order kinetics.

medians and standard deviations, which are parameters of log-normal distributions, not by the apparent first-order rate constants (9,12–16).

The theoretical principles developed by Wagner (9,10) were employed by Weintraub and Gibaldi (17) while interpreting dissolution data for aspirin dosage forms. The percent dissolved–time data obtained for the various dosage forms, with and without surfactant in the dissolution medium, at an agitation intensity of 2.4 rpm were well described by log-normal probability plots, as shown in Fig. 6.6. The critical parameters used to describe the dissolution data for all dosage forms under various experimental conditions were also determined. As expected, for a given dosage form, both the median time and dissolution interval decrease with an increase in agitation intensity; with the exception of capsule data, the standard deviation increased with increasing agitation. Regardless of the agitation intensity, the median time increased in the following order: buffered tablet < plain tablet < capsule < timed-release tablet.

Estimation of Percent Disintegrated-Time

Since tablets and capsules undergo disintegration prior to dissolution, numerous investigations have been conducted either to estimate or clearly delineate and determine the time for disintegration along with percent disintegra-

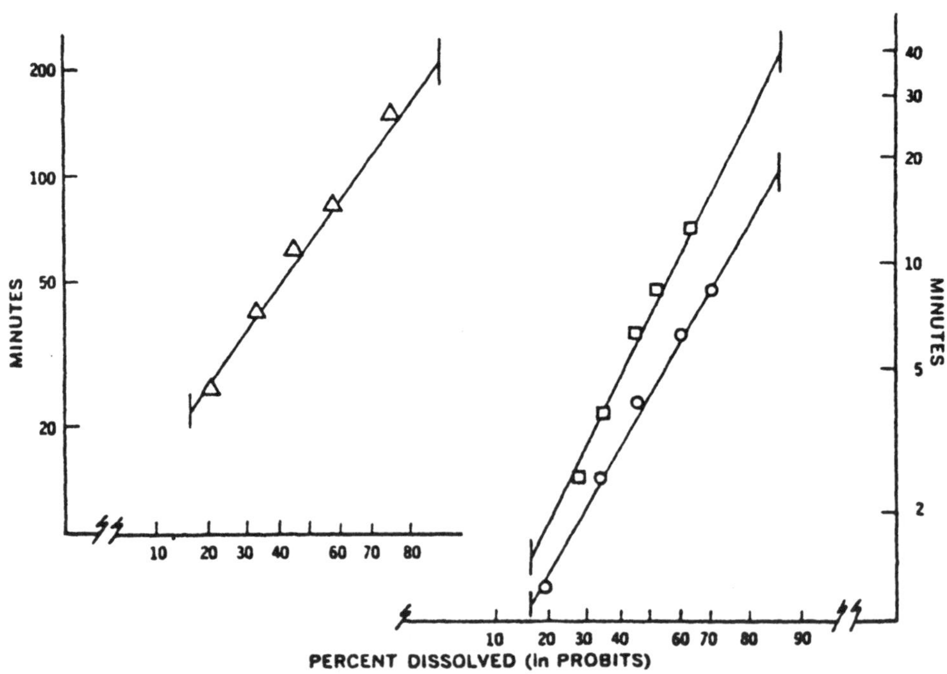

Fig. 6.6 Log-normal probability profiles of dissolution data from aspirin dosage forms in 0.1 *N* HCl at 2.4 rpm. ○, Buffered tablets; □, plain tablets; △, timed-release tablets. (From Ref. 17.)

tion. Few methods are available for utilizing dissolution rate data to estimate the fraction disintegrated as a function of time for tablets (18,19).

El-Yazigi (20) described two techniques for the treatment of dissolution rates to estimate the percent disintegrated—time data for tablets and capsules employing one of the two approaches described below. Both approaches are simple, rapid, and permit computations to be carried out manually.

Assuming first-order disintegration and dissolution processes, scheme I exemplifies the overall dissolution behavior of tablets and capsules (see Fig. 6.7). Assuming first-order disintegration as well as dissolution kinetics, scheme I can be represented mathematically as (21)

$$100 - f_s = \frac{100K_d}{K_d - K_s} e^{-K_s t} - \frac{100K_s}{K_d - K_s} e^{-K_d t} \tag{6.6}$$

where f_s is the cumulative percent dissolved at time t. The amount disintegrated at time t, A_d, which is equal to the amount of drug in the dosage form at $t = 0$, A_0, minus the amount of drug in dosage form at time t, A, is calculated as

$$A_d = A_0(1 - e^{-K_d t}) \tag{6.7}$$

Multiplying both sides of Eq. (6.7) by $100/A_0$ yields (20)

$$f_d = 100 - e^{-K_d t} \tag{6.8}$$

where $f_d = 100(A_d/A_0)$ and is the cumulative percent disintegrated at time t. The disintegration profile can be obtained by substituting for K_d in Eq. (6.8) the values determined graphically according to Eq. (6.6), where K_s can also be determined (20,21).

Theoretically, as Eq. (6.6) indicates, the disintegration time (DT) is equal to infinity. However, since the percent remaining for disintegration after six disintegration half-lives is equal to 1.56%, which is negligible, it may be assumed that the disintegration, $DT_{calc} = 6t_{0.5d}$, or (21)

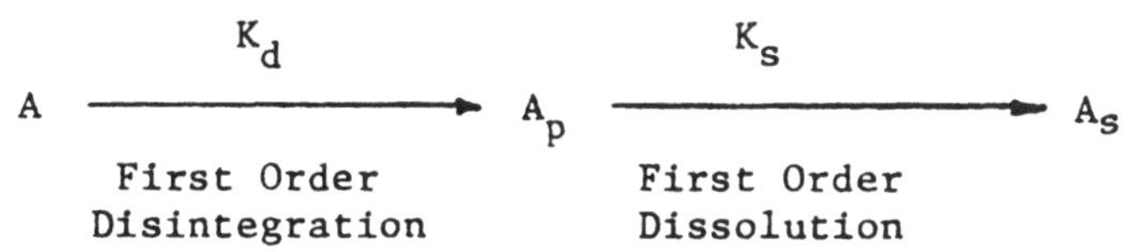

Fig. 6.7 Overall dissolution process of tablets and capsules assuming first-order disintegration and dissolution: A, A_p, and A_s represent amount of drug in dosage form, small particles, and solution, respectively. K_d and K_s represent apparent first-order rate constants for disintegration and dissolution, respectively.

$$\mathrm{DT_{calc}} = 6\left(\frac{0.693}{K_d}\right) = \frac{4.158}{K_d} \tag{6.9}$$

El-Yazigi (21) determined the dissolution of three commercial tablet formulations and three commercial capsule formulations. The dissolution data thus obtained adequately fit the equation developed. The apparent first-order rate constants and preexponential coefficients for dissolution and disintegration are shown in Table 6.1. Table 6.2 provides a comparison of experimental and calculated disintegration time values. While the dissolution profiles for the formulations tested are shown in Fig. 6.8, the semilogarithmic plot of $(100 - f_s)$ as a function of time for one of the formulations tested is shown in Fig. 6.9. This method is both simple and easy to implement.

The second approach assumes a first-order dissolution process, while disintegration is taken as a kinetics-independent process. A simple kinetic expression can describe this approach:

$$f_{d(t)} = \frac{(df_s/dt)t}{K_s} + f_{s(t)} \tag{6.10}$$

where $(df_s/dt)t$ is the dissolution rate at time t, and $f_{d(t)}$, $f_{s(t)}$, and K_s are as described earlier. A similar expression has been derived employing a convolution technique (19). Once $(df_s/dt)t$ is calculated and K_s determined, a direct calculation of the cumulative percent disintegrated–time data can be achieved. K_s can be determined from the terminal linear segment of $\ln(100 - f_s)$ as a function of the time plot.

Table 6.1 Apparent First-Order Rate Constants and Preexponentials

Formulation code	Dosage form	Q_s^a	k_s (min^{-1})	Q_d^a	k_d (min^{-1})
A	Tablet	160.0	0.089	69.2	0.321
B	Tablet	246.4	0.250	143.0	0.461
C	Tablet	168.6	0.165	81.1	0.456
D	Capsule	127.6	0.0859	25.0	0.365
E	Capsule	120.3	0.0619	22.1	0.413
F	Capsule	259.7	0.103	166.8	0.203

Source: Ref. 20.

[a] Q_s and Q_d are the preexponential coefficients for dissolution and disintegration, respectively [$Q_s = 100k_d/(k_d - k_s)$ and $Q_d = 100k_s/(k_d - k_s)$].

Table 6.2 Experimentally Determined Disintegration Times and Values Estimated according to Eq. (6.8)

Formulation	DT_{exp} (min)($n = 6$)	DT_{calc} (min)	DT_{exp}/DT_{calc}
A	14.0[a] (1.47)[b]	13.0	1.08
B	10.4 (0.55)	9.02	1.15
C	6.77 (2.9)	9.12	0.74
D	11.4 (1.09)	11.4	1.0
E	9.92 (5.6)	10.1	0.98
F	24.6 (2.09)	20.5	1.2

Source: Ref. 20.
[a] Mean.
[b] Standard deviation.

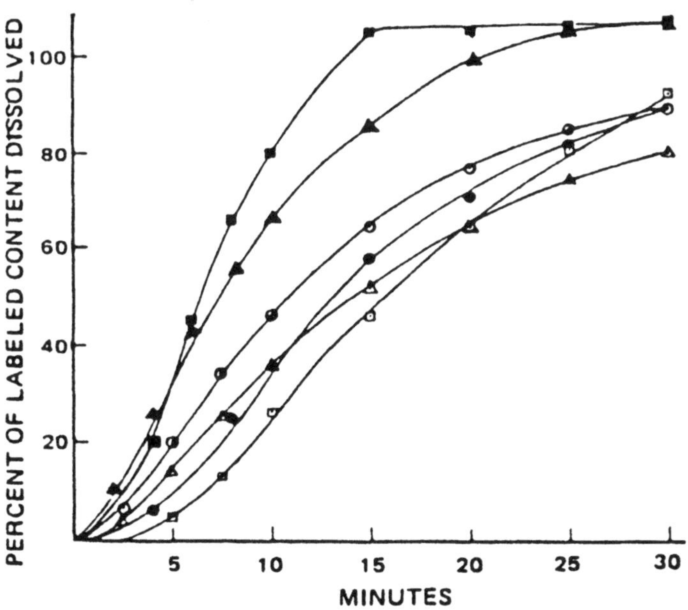

Fig. 6.8 Dissolution profiles for the formulations tested. Solid symbols, tablets; open symbols, capsules; ●, A; ■, B; ▲, C; ⊙, D; △, E; ⊡, F. (From Ref. 20.)

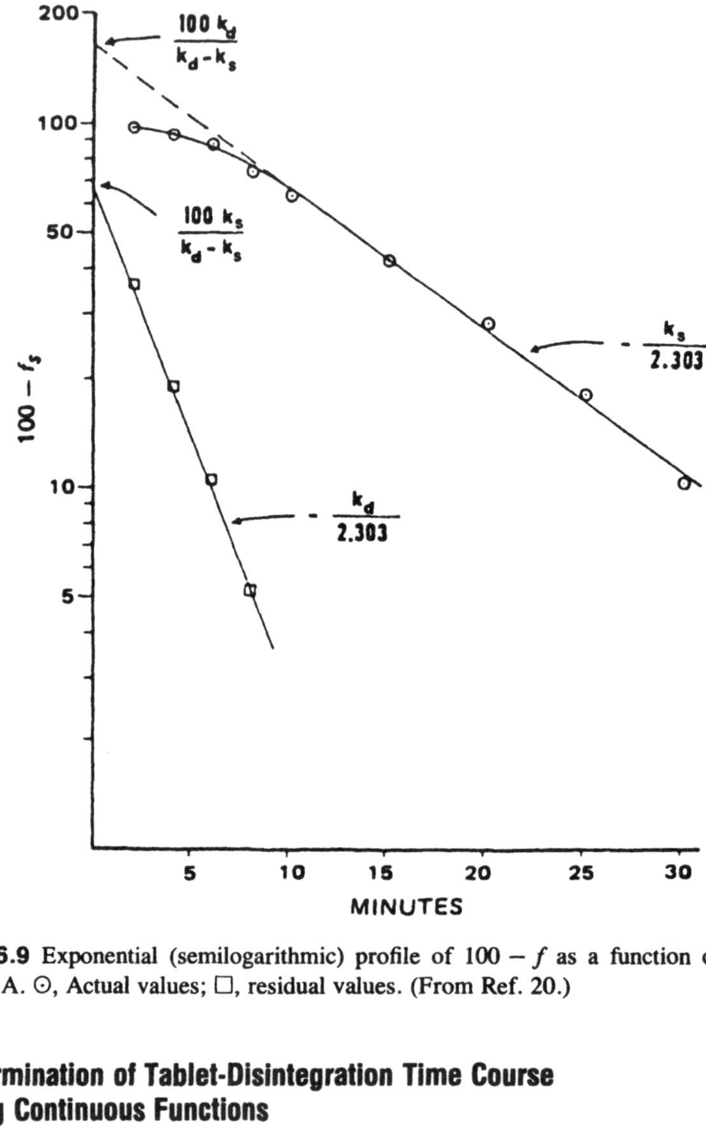

Fig. 6.9 Exponential (semilogarithmic) profile of $100 - f$ as a function of time for tablet A. ⊙, Actual values; □, residual values. (From Ref. 20.)

Determination of Tablet-Disintegration Time Course Using Continuous Functions

Nelson and Wang (18,19) have proposed an analysis of the disintegration–dissolution sequence of drug release from a tablet, leading to a mathematical expression relating disintegration to the dissolution profile of the tablet and the dissolution rate of the primary drug particles in the tablet. Initially, they proposed a method involving numerical analysis (17), following which they extended the method to provide a model based on continuum mathematics.

The principle underlying disintegration–dissolution analysis considers the processes of disintegration and dissolution as discrete events over many small, equal-time intervals (17). At any arbitrary interval, the fraction of drug in a tablet that has dissolved is considered to be the sum of the amounts dissolved from all disintegrated fractions, calculated employing the cube-root law for time periods between the disintegration intervals and the arbitrary interval. This process can be exemplified by

$$M_n = \sum_{i=0}^{n} W_i\{1 - [1 - K(t_n - t_i)]^3\} \tag{6.11}$$

where M_n is the fraction of drug dissolved after n time intervals corresponding to time t_n. The fraction disintegrated at the ith interval is W_i, and K is the cube-root law dissolution constant (18). The cumulative fraction of drug disintegrated from the tablet, W_n, up to time t_n, by setting the term in parentheses in Eq. (6.10) equal to 1, can be expressed by

$$W_n = \sum_{i=0}^{n} W_i \tag{6.12}$$

Employing numerical analysis followed by convolution and Laplace transformation, it can be shown that the function M is a continuous function that describes the fraction of drug in a tablet dissolved with time (18). An empirical equation such as the Weibull function can be fit to experimental tablet dissolution data to obtain a practical value for this function (18,22):

$$M(t) = 1 - e^{-(t^b/a)} \tag{6.13}$$

The scale factor a and shape factor b are adjustable parameters, and M is the continuous function at time t.

Applying Laplace transformations again, it can be shown that the cumulative fraction of the tablet disintegrated as a function of time, $W(t)$, is given by

$$W_{(t)} = 1 - \left(1 - \frac{bt^{b-1}}{Ka}\right) e^{-(t^b/a)} \tag{6.14}$$

Equation (6.14) now represents the disintegration profile for a tablet whose dissolution curve is represented by the Weibull function with parameters a and b, and whose particles dissolve in accordance with the parameter K (18). Dissolution of an acetaminophen tablet in accordance with Weibull function is illustrated in Fig. 6.10. The disintegration profile determined employing Eq. (6.14) is shown in Fig. 6.11. Although this method provides a means to determine dissolution and disintegration profiles simultaneously, the mathematics involved is complicated and cannot readily be adopted.

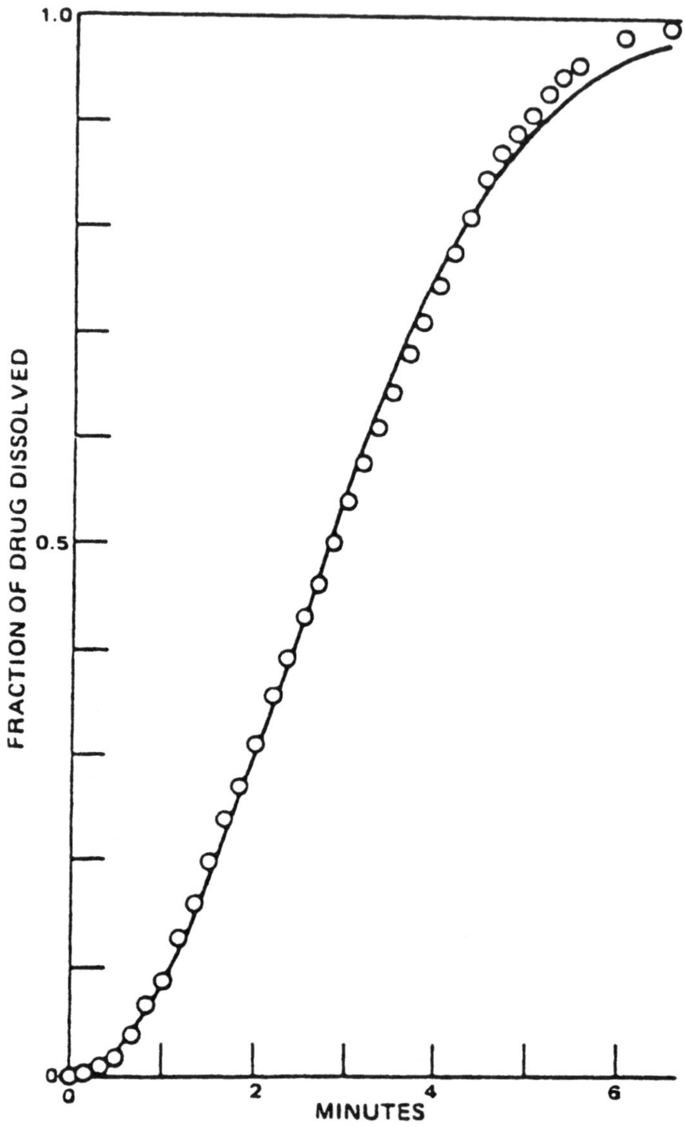

Fig. 6.10 Dissolution data for acetaminophen tablet (Ref. 19). The profile is the Weibull function with $a = 11.15$ and $b = 1.996$.

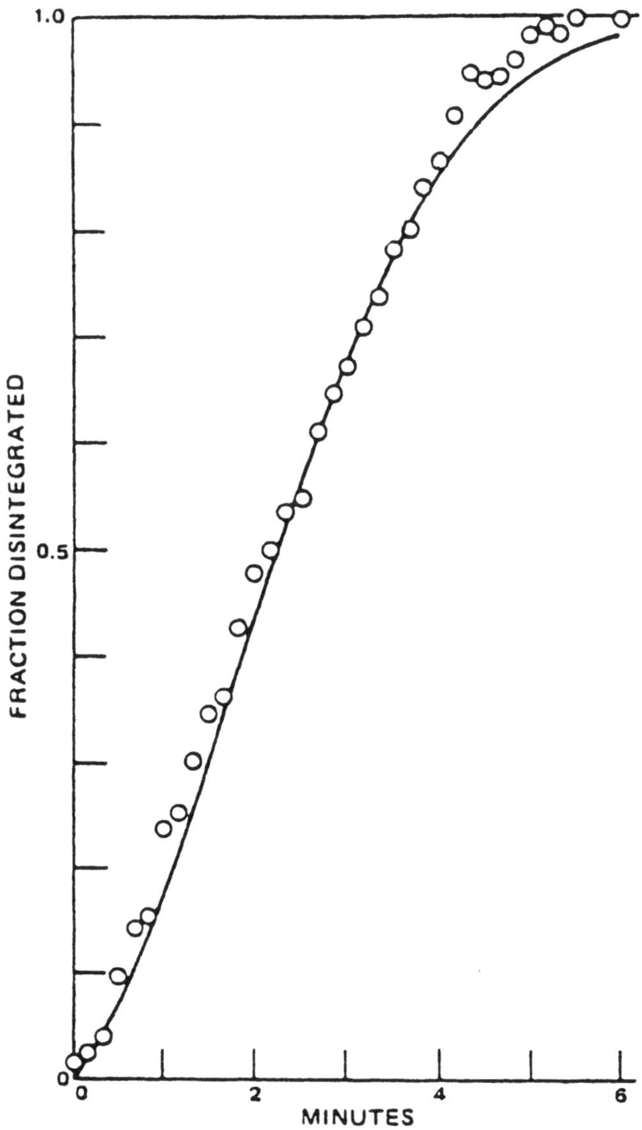

Fig. 6.11 Disintegration profile for acetaminophen determined employing Eq. (6.13). The data points result from a numerical method employing an exponential function. (From Ref. 19.)

Mathematical Expression of Tablet Dissolution: Method of Forward Differences

When the process of tablet dissolution is observed in a suitable apparatus, one can see that for a short time nothing happens to the tablet. After this brief period, the tablet starts to disintegrate into granules. The disintegration process accelerates until a time is reached when the tablet apparently loses its original form. The first process of tablet dissolution can be represented by a reaction resulting in a curve, as shown in Fig. 6.12. Three schemes giving curves of the required shape are (23)

$$\frac{d(A)}{dt} = -K[Ad_0 - (A)] \tag{6.15}$$

$$\frac{d(A)}{dt} = \frac{-K}{A} \tag{6.16}$$

$$\frac{d(A)}{dt} = -Kt \tag{6.17}$$

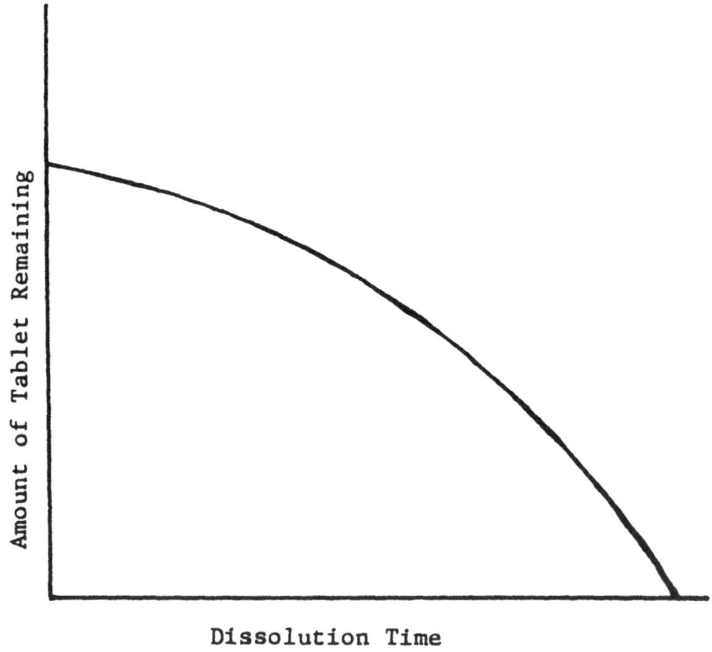

Fig. 6.12 Schemation representation of the physical process of dissolution of a tablet.

where A and K represent the amount of tablet remaining and the reaction (dissolution) rate constant, respectively. Equation (6.15), which relates the rate of disappearance of tablet to the amount of tablet that has dissolved, is somewhat difficult to use since initially $A = 0$. The rate of disappearance of the tablet, which is inversely proportional to the amount of tablet remaining, is represented by Eq. (6.16). The rate of disappearance of the tablet increases linearly with time [Eq. (6.15)], and combining this first stage with other processes yields relatively simple expressions for the amount of tablet in solution, P (23). The use of Eq. (6.17) additionally permits the determination of rate constants for forward differences.

Tablet dissolution can be explained adequately as a two-step process: an initial time-dependent breakup, followed by faster stages, which constitute the production of fine particles and their ultimate dissolution. The latter step can be described by a first-order process (24). Integration of these differential equations yields

$$P = \frac{1}{2}Kt^2 - \frac{K}{K_1^2}(K_1{}^t + e^{-K_1 t} - 1) \tag{6.18}$$

where K and K_1 are rate constants. Until $t = (2/K)^{0.5}$, this equation holds true, following which

$$P = 1 - B_L e^{-K_1 Z} \tag{6.19}$$

where B_L represents the concentration of large particles and $Z = t - t_L$. The first and second differentials of these expressions can be employed to determine K and K_1 from experimental data. From Eqs. (6.19) and (6.21), we can determine

$$\frac{d^2P}{dt^2} = K(1 - e^{-K_1 t}) \tag{6.20}$$

and

$$\frac{d^2P}{dt^2} = -K_1^2 B_L e^{-K_1 Z} \tag{6.21}$$

Inspecting Eqs. (6.20) and (6.21), it is seen that the second differential changes sign at time t_L. Hence K can be calculated as

$$K = \frac{2}{t_L^2} \tag{6.22}$$

At any time post t_L, we can calculate K_1 as

$$K_1 = \frac{dP/dt}{1 - P} \tag{6.23}$$

Thus both rate constants can be determined and interpreted easily. This method is simple to apply, as the two parameters of the model can easily be determined directly from experimental data. The regenerated traces have been shown to agree closely with the originals (23).

Statistical Analyses of Dissolution Data

Dissolution profiles of solid dosage forms represent several observations over time on an experimental unit such as a capsule or tablet. Comparison of these profiles under a variety of conditions relating to formulation characteristics and other variations is usually conducted employing statistical tools. Recently, two approaches have been reported for statistical analysis of dissolution data (25,26). Basic knowledge of statistical principles is needed to appreciate these methods fully. However, an introduction to statistical principles is beyond the scope of this book. Consequently, a brief discussion of the nature of statistical tools employed during analysis and of their utility in the analysis of dissolution profiles is provided. Interested readers are urged to refer to the original literature for details.

Gueurten (25) has described a multivariate approach to the analysis of dissolution profiles. This approach is very useful in the analysis of the drug release rate for sustained-release dosage forms since it permits us to analyze the data on the basis of two criteria: the level and the shape of the curve. This kind of analysis also permits construction of a regression model to predict dissolution from arbitrary fixed values of parameters such as formulation factors.

Mauger and co-workers (26) discuss the analysis of dissolution profiles employing an analysis of variance (ANOVA) approach. The dissolution profiles are tested for differences in level and shape, in particular. The shape characteristic is potentially important to a knowledge of differences in the mechanism of dissolution. Alternative conservative analysis methods with an arbitrary *F* test, together with the possibility of an arbitrary covariance matrix, are also described (26).

The use of ANOVA to compare typical dissolution data has numerous features. First, the analysis is independent of curve-fitting procedures. Second, the data can be analyzed employing variables such as fraction dissolved values (e.g., $T_{50\%}$). Additionally, ANOVA is capable of showing differences between profiles where a realistic variation exists, as well as among profiles.

A particular ANOVA approach described and employed by Mauger et al. (26) emphasizes the shape of the dissolution profile since it allows appreciation of the process over time and indicates whether or not different formulations are dissolving according to similar dissolution mechanisms. The authors claim that the calculation procedure for the analysis is relatively simple and can be carried out using a hand-held calculator.

TECHNIQUES OF IN VIVO DISSOLUTION

Products that generate equal areas under the plasma concentration–time curve (AUC) are by simple definition equally bioavailable but not necessarily bioequivalent or therefore therapeutically equivalent. When the plasma concentration–time curves are identical within accepted statistical criteria, the products are stated to be *bioequivalent*. Bioequivalent products are considered to be therapeutically equivalent since their pharmacodynamic driving forces are thought to be identical.

Dissolution-rate data have become the compendial standard for ensuring continuing therapeutic equivalence among the various products available to the pharmacist. Ensuring uniformity among different batches of the same manufacturer's product is thus a very important consideration in the pharmaceutical industry. The importance of this issue is reflected in the amount of attention accorded to it. This in vitro standard should be employed for the development of high-quality sustained-release formulations. If the pharmaceutical scientist has some understanding of the in vivo release kinetics of a drug in the GI tract, delivery of the drug from the dosage form can be designed accordingly. Such prior knowledge should improve the quality of formulations available in the marketplace and should help optimize the concentration–time profile and ultimate response of the drug.

In vivo studies in human beings must, by their nature, be limited in the scope and degree of information obtainable. Such studies must therefore impart the maximum information to correlate with and thus justify in vitro testing. There has been a continuing need to evaluate adequate fundamental in vivo parameters. This is exemplified by the voluminous literature in this area since 1955. Correlation of in vitro data with an in vivo parameter is critical in ensuring bioequivalence predictability. However, this is more easily said than done, chiefly because of the lack of adequate tools or techniques to obtain fundamental in vivo parameters. In fact, most bioequivalence problems are due to nonpredictive in vitro dissolution tests, which do not lend themselves to adequate correlatability with the phenomena occurring in the body.

Recently, several articles describing methods of obtaining in vivo dissolution rate have been published. The process of in vivo dissolution for controlled-release dosage forms is by definition time intensive. For these dosage forms, in vitro dissolution tests need to be designed such that adequate correlation can be established with in vivo data.

Correlation of in vivo dissolution parameters for oral dosage forms with some in vitro parameter is thus of prime significance to the pharmaceutical industry. The in vivo release-rate constant, K_r, would be an adequate parameter to compare and correlate with in vitro data. Once an adequate correlation is established, reproducibility of the in vitro parameter should suffice as an indicator for batch-to-batch bioequivalence.

The purpose of the following sections is to review, reassess, and make recommendations for using the present techniques of in vivo dissolution measurement. We also discuss advantages and disadvantages associated with each technique.

In Vivo Dissolution Factors

A number of factors affect the in vitro dissolution of pharmaceutical dosage forms. These have been reviewed elsewhere and are beyond the purview of this chapter, except as they are relevant to observed in vivo performance (27,28). A comprehensive discussion of the factors affecting the process of absorption and dissolution in vivo exists in the literature (29–32). The processes of disintegration, dissolution, and absorption occur in tandem, and thus an exact delineation between the factors affecting these processes cannot easily be achieved.

The following aspects as they affect drug release from the dosage form will be examined briefly in the next few pages: (a) gastrointestinal motility and presence of food, (b) gastrointestinal pH and fluid present, (c) physicochemical nature of the drug, and (d) pharmacological effect of drug on GI motility.

Gastrointestinal Motility and Presence of Food

Generally, the dosage form dissolves in the segment of the GI tract where the milieu is conducive for that process. It is important to understand the differences in GI motility in that state produced by the intake of food and that when no food is present (i.e., the fasted state). The digestive pattern of motility persists in the fasted state, and the interdigestive pattern is initiated after the ingestion of food (33).

The interdigestive pattern has four phases of motility which are repeated cyclically until the next meal is ingested.

Phase I: Resting phase of about 30 to 40 min.

Phase II: Contractions that cause mixing of the contents. Strength of contractions increases as time elapses and ends in 60 to 90 contractions of maximum strength.

Phase III: Circular contractions that travel distally. They form a length of bowel over which peristaltic contractions pass. The band starts in the duodenum and reaches the ileum in 90 to 120 min. This is also referred to as the *housekeeper*.

Phase IV: Segmental and peristaltic contractions eventually diminish in magnitude and strength and the cycle is repeated. The GI tract goes back to the resting phase, I.

When a meal is ingested the digestive pattern starts. At this point the peristaltic wave stops and mixing starts, during which the contents of the stomach are emulsified. Particles greater than 5 mm in diameter will rarely leave the stomach during digestion. This is particularly applicable to solid dosage forms since disintegration of most drugs occurs in the stomach unless the dosage form has an enteric coating. The disintegration time for the full dosage form and for major pieces of it may be retarded significantly by endogenous mucoids and by soluble viscous components of the food intake. Solid particles 1 to 3 mm in diameter will then enter the intestine, where the majority of dissolution might occur. If the drug is sparingly soluble in the GI contents, absorption of drug through the duodenum will shift the solubility equilibrium, causing more of the solid particles to go into solution.

Food, of course, is a major determinant of the in vivo dissolution process. Besides affecting GI motility, it will also affect the process of dissolution (e.g., by complexation). It could also physically obstruct the dosage form from coming in contact with the gastric fluid, thereby decreasing the dissolution rate. Food invariably alters the pH of the stomach. This would also have an effect on the dissolution rate, as explained later. A meal with a high fat content could prolong the motility pattern of the digestive cycle.

Gastrointestinal pH

The pH of the GI tract varies from one segment to another. As a general rule the pH increases down the length of the GI tract. In general, one can say that as one proceeds farther down the GI tract, the pH increases. An acidic drug would therefore dissolve more rapidly in the intestine, whereas a basic drug would dissolve efficiently in the stomach. In addition, the pH of the stomach is a variable critically dependent on the host. A truly resting stomach has a pH of 5 to 7 (34). However, any stress initiates acid secretion and the conventionally assumed low pH. In the presence of a food bolus, the mass tends to be buffered at a pH of about 4.5.

The volume of fluid available in the stomach is a variable depending on food residue, tilt of the lower portion (a significant variable within a population), posture and general body activity, and individual mobility after fluid intake. Also of importance is the pH of the diffusion layer around the dosage form, which differs from the pH of the bulk solution (35,36). Obviously, the nature of this layer and the drug flux through it will be critically dependent on the nature of the fluid present and on general motility.

Physicochemical Nature of the Drug

Molecular size and shape, pK_a, and lipophilicity are the most important properties affecting dissolution of the drug in vitro, and these in vitro factors may become more significant in vivo. In particular, the change in lipophilicity as evidenced by octanol–water partition is dependent on the nature of the drug species present. Hence the pH profile of the drug milieu becomes a critical interactant with the drug pK_a, not just to effect drug dissolution at an adequate rate but also the pH gradient across the diffusion layer and the degree of ionization of the drug. In this regard, the formulator must consider whether the pH environment controlling the drug diffusion layer for dissolution will allow the use of a free-base or free-acid drug or whether the use of a salt becomes essential to ensure an optimal drug flux to the intestinal surface.

Pharmacological Effect of Drug on GI Motility

Certain drugs or food habits affect the motility of the GI tract. Anticholinergics reduce the GI motility, whereas cholinergics increase it. If the mixing and propelling actions slow down, the dissolution process might also decelerate. This factor is particularly important for drugs absorbed in the *absorption window*. Thus controlled-release dosage forms that are otherwise incompletely bioavailable because they release drug past the absorption window could be reformulated to augment their bioavailability. A classic example of such enhancement in bioavailability is of triethanolamine myristate, a GI motility retardant which when incorporated with riboflavin enhances riboflavin bioavailability (37). This is a major investigational area where pharmaceutical researchers can combine their skills with gastroenterologists to improve drug delivery and bioavailability.

In Vivo Dissolution Measurement

The techniques available for evaluating in vivo dissolution rate could be divided in two categories: indirect and direct. The indirect techniques involve the mathematical treatment of observed conventional plasma, blood, and urine drug concentrations with time. The conclusions drawn depend on the assumptions made for the mathematical model. Among the direct techniques are external scintigraphy and its modifications. Classically, intubation techniques have been used extensively to appraise the absorption rate in the stomach, duodenum, jejunum, ileum, and colon (38–41). These methods can also be used to evaluate the dissolution rate in different segments of the GI tract.

Indirect Techniques

Indirect techniques discussed here are (a) Loo–Riegelman analysis, (b) statistical moments, and (c) deconvolution.

Loo–Riegelman analysis. Loo and Riegelman derived an equation to determine the input function. This could be obtained accurately after intravenous and oral administration. For a two-compartment model as shown in Fig. 6.13, the following equation applies:

$$\frac{(X_A)_T}{(X_A)_\infty} = \frac{C_T + K_{10}\int_0^T C\,dt + (X_2)_T/V_c}{K_{10}\int_0^\infty C\,dt} = \mathrm{INPUT}_T \qquad (6.24)$$

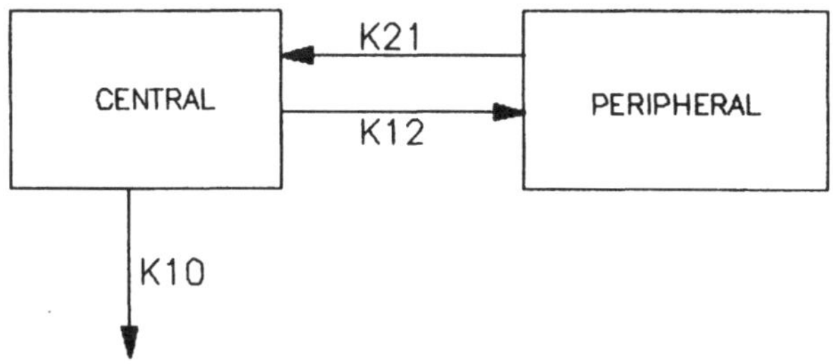

Fig. 6.13 Schematic representation of a two-compartment open model.

The left-hand side of the equation changes continuously as a function of time, where $(X_A)_T/(X_A)_\infty$ = fraction of drug absorbed at time T, C_T = plasma concentration at time T, $\int_0^T C\,dt$ = area under the curve from time 0 to T, and $\int_0^\infty C\,dt$ = area under the curve from time 0 to ∞:

$$\frac{(X_2)_T}{V_C} = K_{12}e^{-(K_{21}t)}\int_0^t C(t)e^{-(k_{21}t)}\,dt \tag{6.25}$$

where K_{21}, K_{12}, and K_{10} are intercompartmental microrate constants.

A plot of the fraction remaining to be absorbed versus time would yield the absorption rate constant K_a. The Loo–Riegelman technique used for investigating the absorption phenomenon can give an estimate of the first-order absorption-rate constant. The absorption-rate constant K_a so obtained would be a composite of K absorption and K degradation. This would lead to an erroneous estimation of the absorption-rate constant (42). For a detailed derivation and understanding of this technique, the reader is referred to the original publications (43,44).

To get an estimate of the release-rate constant K_r, Chan and Gibaldi modified the Loo–Riegelman techniques for situations where intravenous (IV) reference data are not available (45). If plasma concentration–time data are available for solution and solid dosage form, it is valid to analyze the data with the Loo–Riegelman technique. This is true only when the assumption of linearity is not violated. The microrate constants are obtained after administration of the solution. These constants would then be used for analysis of the solid dosage form pharmacokinetic data.

In a Loo–Riegelman analysis ($1 - \text{INPUT}_T$), the fraction remaining to be absorbed is plotted against time on a semilog scale to get a plot as shown in Fig. 6.14. Thus if the release-rate constant is first order and sufficiently different in magnitude from the absorption-rate constant, the two constants can be obtained by the method of residuals.

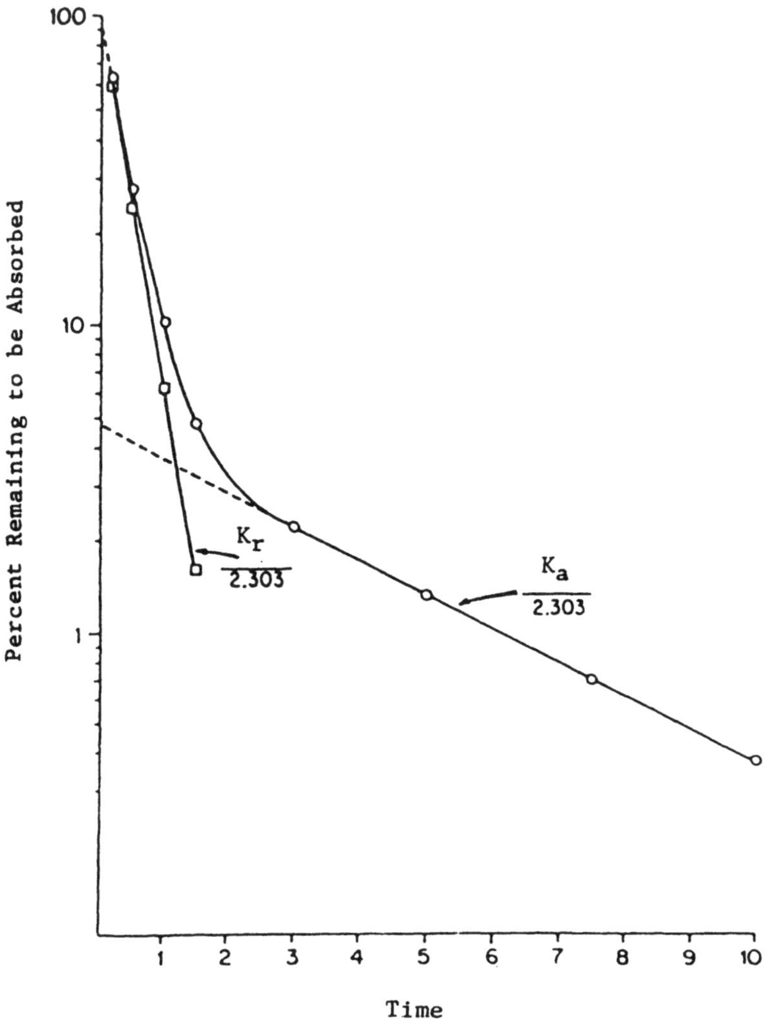

Fig. 6.14 Semilogarithmic plot of percent not absorbed as a function of time. Two processes can be quantified from the graph. If $K_r > K_a$, the plot will look as above. If $K_a > K_r$, the terminal rate constant will be K_r and stripping will yield K_a. If $K_a \cong K_r$, the two rate constants cannot be resolved. (Modified from Ref. 46.)

Chan and Gibaldi performed several simulations with the scheme shown in Fig. 6.15, wherein the value of these rate constants were varied (46). All calculations were performed after the addition of 10% random error to the simulated data. In all simulations, microrate constants were determined from solu-

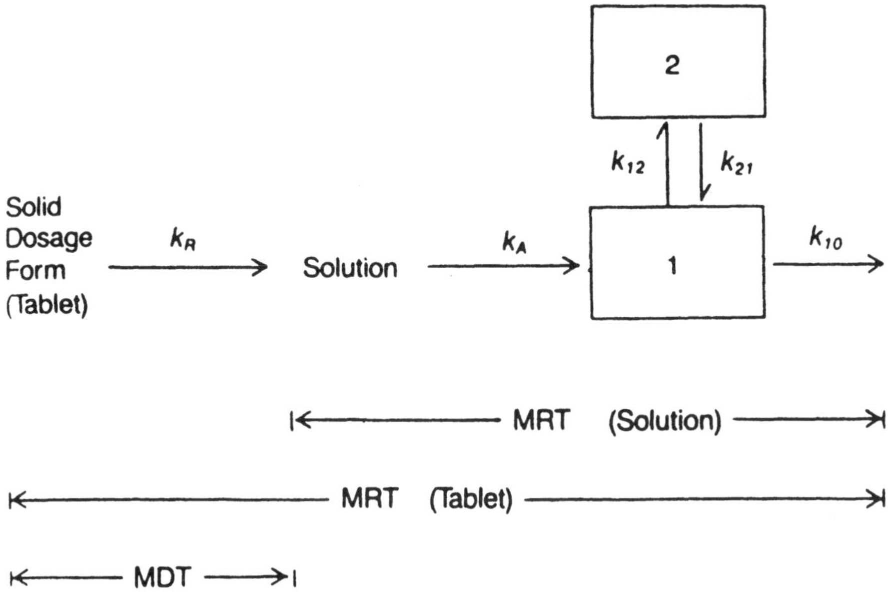

Fig. 6.15 Two-compartment open model with a first-order release and absorption rate constants. It also emphasizes that MDT = $MRT_{tablet} - MRT_{solution}$. (From Ref. 45; reproduced with permission of the copyright owner, the American Pharmaceutical Association.)

tion data, and the results remained unaffected, regardless of the magnitudes of α and K_a (α is the macrorate constant of the initial distribution phase obtained by residual analysis of multicompartment pharmacokinetic data). The results are shown in Table 6.3. For cases in which K_r approached K_a, the method yielded inaccurate estimates of the terminal rate constant. When K_r approached the value of the terminal elimination-rate constant, the method of residuals could not separate the rate constants using the plots shown above.

Patel et al. described the use of simultaneous fitting for estimating the release-rate constant K_r of the solid dosage form (47). Employing the model shown in Fig. 6.14, they derived pharmacokinetic equations to describe the solution and the solid dosage form data (45). The rate constants K_r and K_a were obtained by the method of residual analysis. These were used as initial estimates for fitting the data simultaneously to both equations by a nonlinear regression program, NONLIN (48). The same could be done by using the SAS NLIN program (49). The authors found that simultaneous fitting of data leads to a better estimation of the release-rate constant of the drug than can be obtained using the Loo–Riegelman technique. This was especially true for data

Table 6.3 Micromate Constants Determined from Solution Data

	Solution	Tablet			Solution	Tablet	
Data set	MRT[a]	MRT[a]	MDT[a]	k_r^a	k_a^b	k_1^b	k_2^b
1. $k_a = 7.5$	2.121 (−0.66%)	—	—	—	7.209 (−3.8%)	—	—
4. $k_a = 7.5$, $k_r = 8.0$	—	2.236 (−1.1%)	0.115 (−8.0%)	8.696 (+8.7%)	—	5.33 (−28.9%)	17.33[c] (+116.6%)
5. $k_a = 7.5$, $k_r = 3.1$	—	2.417 (−1.7%)	0.296 (−8.2%)	3.378 (+9.0%)	—	2.77 (−10.7%)	8.56 (+14.1%)
6. $k_a = 7.5$, $k_r = 1.1$	—	3.003 (−1.4%)	0.882 (−3.0%)	1.134 (+3.1%)	—	1.07 (−2.7%)	7.29 (−2.8%)
7. $k_a = 7.5$, $k_r = 0.4$	—	4.676 (+0.9%)	2.555 (+2.2%)	0.371 (−2.3%)	—	0.37 (−7.5%)	—[d]
2. $k_a = 3.05$	2.309 (−0.90%)	—	—	—	2.927 (−4.0%)	—	—
8. $k_a = 3.05$, $k_r = 8.0$	—	2.415 (−1.6%)	0.106 (−15.2%)	9.434 (+17.9%)	—	2.83 (−7.2%)	8.88 (+11.0%)
9. $k_a = 3.05$, $k_r = 3.1$	—	2.622 (−1.2%)	0.313 (−3.0%)	3.195 (+3.1%)	—	1.95 (−36.1%)	6.54[d] (+111.1%)

10. $k_a = 3.05$	—	3.215	0.906	1.104	—	1.3	3.47
$k_r = 1.1$		(−0.7%)	(−0.3%)	(+0.4%)		(−6.4%)	(+13.8%)
11. $k_a = 3.05$	—	4.903	2.594	0.386	—	0.36	—[c]
$k_r = 0.4$		(+1.5%)	(+3.8%)	(−3.6%)		(−10.0%)	
3. $k_a = 1.05$	2.925	—	—	—	1.044	—	—
	(−0.98%)				(−0.6%)		
12. $k_a = 1.05$	—	3.056	0.131	7.634	—	1.11	5.54
$k_r = 8.0$		(−0.8%)	(+4.8%)	(−4.6%)		(+5.7%)	(−30.8%)
13. $k_a = 1.05$	—	3.250	0.325	3.077	—	1.05	3.15
$k_r = 3.1$		(−0.8%)	(+0.7%)	(−0.7%)		(0%)	(+1.6%)
14. $k_a = 1.05$	—	3.831	0.906	1.104	—	0.77	2.17[d]
$k_r = 1.1$		(−0.8%)	(−0.3%)	(+0.4%)		(−26.7%)	(+97.3%)
15. $k_a = 1.05$	—	5.531	2.606	0.384	—	0.36	1.61
$k_r = 0.4$		(+1.4%)	(+4.2%)	(−4.1%)		(−10.0%)	(+53.3%)

Source: Ref. 45; reproduced with permission of the copyright owner, the American Pharmaceutical Association.

[a] Parameters calculated with statistical moments.

[b] Parameters calculated by the Loo–Riegelman technique.

[c] Two rate constants not resolved by residual analysis.

[d] When $K_r = K_a$, the estimates of the rate constants obtained deviated by more than 25%. Numbers in parentheses represent percent error or percent deviation from the actual values as shown in the first column.

to which random error was added with a relative standard deviation of $\pm 10\%$. These authors also found that an extended sampling schedule during the absorption phase of the drug improved the estimates of K_r obtained by the Loo–Riegelman method.

Obviously, the coherence of the parameters obtained depends on the quality of the nonlinear fitting to the series of exponentials. If the curve cannot be truly fitted in shape, the magnitude of error function in the derived microrate constants becomes extreme.

Statistical moments. Statistical moments have been used to determine the release-rate constant K_r and the absorption-rate constant K_a (50,51). The term *mean absorption time* (MAT), the mean time for the drug molecule to be absorbed, was proposed by Cutler in 1978 (50). Using the convolution integral he derived the mean absorption time. This was subsequently generalized by Riegelman and Collier for noninstantaneous input (51). The *mean residence time* (MRT) is defined as the average time a drug molecule takes to travel through the body. This is a composite of all kinetic processes of absorption, distribution, and elimination. Thus the MRT after a noninstantaneous input would be equal to the sum of the MRT after IV administration and the MRT of the input of the drug. If this is applied to oral data after the administration of a solid dosage form, the following equation would apply:

$$\mathrm{MRT}_{\text{solid dosage form}} = \mathrm{MDT}_{\text{solid dosage form}} + \mathrm{MAT}_{\text{solution}} + \mathrm{MRT}_{\text{intravenous bolus}} \qquad (6.26)$$

where MRT is mean residence time, MDT is mean dissolution time, and MAT is mean absorption time. Thus if a drug is administered orally as a tablet or capsule, the average time the drug molecule spends in the body will be the sum of the average time a molecule requires to dissolve, the average time a molecule takes to be absorbed, and the average time for the disposition. Pure disposition is described after an intravenous (IV) bolus administration of drug. Thus $\mathrm{MRT}_{\mathrm{IV}}$ after bolus administration represents the mean time for a composite of all kinetic processes involved in the disposition of the drug. This could include distribution, biotransformation, biliary excretion and recycling, and excretion of unchanged drug in the urine (52).

Using the principles of statistical moments explained above, the input rate for two different nonintravenous routes can be compared provided that the same drug is administered and the disposition parameters do not change during the period between two studies. Thus if a drug is administered as a solution and as a solid dosage form such as a tablet or capsule, $\mathrm{MRT}_{\text{solution}}$ is a known quantity.

$$\mathrm{MRT}_{\text{solution}} = \mathrm{MAT}_{\text{solution}} + \mathrm{MRT}_{\mathrm{IV}} \qquad (6.27)$$

Combining Eqs. (6.26) and (6.27), we get

$$MDT_{\text{solid dosage form}} = MRT_{\text{solid dosage form}} - MRT_{\text{solution}} \tag{6.28}$$

Equation (6.28) thus yields the parameter of interest.

Mean disintegration time in vivo (MDIT) could be estimated in a similar manner (53). If a drug is administered as a solid dosage form and as a powder, MDIT could be calculated by the following equation:

$$MDIT_{\text{tablet}} = MDT_{\text{tablet}} - MDT_{\text{powder}} = MRT_{\text{tablet}} - MRT_{\text{powder}} \tag{6.29}$$

The same equation could also be used for capsule dosage forms. In vivo disintegration is also a useful parameter and should be correlated with in vitro disintegration time. Disintegration time was considered a standard in the earlier pharmacopoeia. Several models have been proposed for describing the dissolution phenomenon. The major drawback of these models is the difficulty in comparing dissolution parameters of two dosage forms whose profiles are explained by different models. This can be resolved by the use of mean dissolution time obtained using the model-independent method of statistical moments. At this point it is important to mention the assumptions involved in using statistical moments. The input, sampling, and elimination of a drug should be from the central compartment of a multicompartmental pharmacokinetic model describing the disposition of the drug. The disposition kinetics of the drug should be characterized by first-order processes.

For simplicity and ease of calculation, a computer program was written in BASICA version 3.10, the advanced basic compiler of IBM PC. This program calculates the mean dissolution time for the solid dosage form in question. It also calculates the area under the curve (AUC) and the area under the moment curve (AUMC) for the solution and solid dosage forms. The program finds out the maximum concentration (C_{max}) and the time required to reach the maximum concentration (T_{max}) from the data provided. It has a user-determined option to calculate area under the curve up to a certain time point by the trapezoidal rule and from that point on by the log trapezoidal rule. The reader is referred to the appendix to this chapter for the program code, input file and format, and output file that the program produces.

The program calculates the mean dissolution time based on the following equation:

$$MDT = \left(\frac{AUMC}{AUC}\right)_{\text{solid dosage form}} - \left(\frac{AUMC}{AUC}\right)_{\text{solution}} \tag{6.30}$$

The program calculates the area under the curve and the area under the moment curve by a combination linear and log trapezoidal rule (54). The linear trapezoidal rule overestimates the area during the declining exponential phase, especially when the number of data points are small. The log trapezoidal rule yields a better estimate of the area in the terminal exponential phase. It should be borne in mind that when the log trapezoidal rule is used in the ascending portion, near the peak or in the distribution phase of the plasma time profile, erroneous estimates of the area may be obtained. The area under the curve and the area under the moment curve are calculated by the linear and the log trapezoidal rule where applicable. The same program could be used for calculating the mean absorption time. In this case the input file "Data.in" is modified to enter intravenous bolus data in place of solution data and oral data in place of solid dosage form data. [The term *oral data* means administration of any dosage form (i.e., solid, semisolid, or liquid) by the peroral route.] This program will thus simplify the rate calculations required for the analysis of linear pharmacokinetic data. Although statistical moments provide a useful tool for the noncompartmental analysis of pharmacokinetic data, particularly mean dissolution time, one should be aware of the assumptions and drawbacks of employing this method for data analysis.

The mean dissolution time, Eq. (6.30), calculated by the program would be only an estimate of the complex process in vivo. This depends on the GI transit time and GI motility. Correlation of MDT in vivo data with in vitro data might then be obscured. It is thus up to the judgment, pharmacokinetic knowledge, and formulation skills of the pharmaceutical scientist to resolve whether the dosage form under test needs reformulation.

The risk of error in moment analysis increases with the magnitude of extrapolation required. The precision and accuracy of the assay used for analysis at low drug concentrations becomes important. Also, if one is not assured of being in the terminal exponential phase at the last sampling time, the use of moment analysis is highly erroneous and is not recommended.

Real oral data are always confounded with lag-time and analytical errors. It necessitates an accurate estimate of the time from when the dissolution starts to the appearance of drug in blood. Thus frequent sampling, at least every 15 min in the absorption phase, is necessary to estimate the lag time and AUMC and MRT values correctly. MRT will be overestimated without the lag-time correction. It should be noted here that the MDT calculated by the program will hold regardless of whether dissolution is a first- or zero-order process.

Brazell and Kaplan evaluated the ability of statistical moment analysis to provide accurate estimates of absorption and dissolution rates and the effects of sampling schedule, random error, and the estimate of the terminal elimination-rate constant on the accuracy of these estimates (55). They found that the accuracy of the MDT value tended to decrease as the absorption-rate constant and elimination-rate constant increased in magnitude and as the two-compartment characteristics of the concentration–time curve became more pronounced. Increased sampling during the absorptive phase tended to increase the accuracy of the MDT value. Inaccuracy in the estimation of the terminal elimination-rate constant could cause large errors in calculation of the mean dissolution time. They concluded that MAT and MDT values calculated from data generated by a less than rigorous experimental design may yield poor estimate of the actual values and thus misleading conclusions.

Chan and Gibaldi were the first workers who evaluated MAT using both statistical moments and conventional techniques (56). They approached the problem with simulations. The authors simulated concentration–time profiles and tried to determine the absorption rate constant. It was found that statistical moments exhibited a smaller percentage error in estimating the absorption-rate constant than did the Loo–Riegelman method.

In a later publication, Chan and Gibaldi reassessed and compared statistical moments with Loo–Riegelman analysis as applied to the flip-flop model and a variety of other situations (45). They looked at the effect of random error on the MDT and K_r values determined using the Loo–Riegelman technique. The important modification here was to use an oral solution as the reference dosage form and then to evaluate the release rate. The Loo–Riegelman method was described earlier in the chapter. The mean dissolution time was calculated using techniques similar to those just described. Chan and Gibaldi looked at a two-compartment model where the release-rate constant approached the absorption-rate constant. They also considered cases where K_r approached β, the terminal elimination-rate constant in a two-compartment open model. Data analysis revealed that statistical moments resulted in accurate estimates of the mean dissolution time with smaller confidence intervals than those with the Loo–Riegelman method. Residual analysis of the plot of fraction remaining to be absorbed versus time yielded incorrect estimates of the two rate constants, K_r and K_a, when they approached each other. The results obtained by statistical moments can be compared with those obtained by the Loo–Riegelman technique presented in Table 6.3. It suggests that statistical moments consistently provided superior estimates of MDT over the Loo–Riegelman method. The statistical moments gave an accurate estimate of K_r which is equal to 1/MDT. Patel et al. reported that simultaneous fitting of the data by nonlinear regression analysis would yield more accurate estimates (47). Chan and Gibaldi concluded that this is true only if the correct pharmacokinetic model is known. Without an IV bolus reference curve the true model is seldom known. Although nonlinear regression is a powerful statistical tool, it does not select models. Model selection is done by the user. If a wrong model is assigned, this results in incorrect estimates of the rate constant in question. Also, the order of the parameter $K_r = 1/\text{MDT}$ cannot be known using statistical moments.

Khoo et al. compared C_{max} and T_{max}, conventional bioavailability parameters, with MDT and other parameters calculated by statistical moments (57). (Reminder: C_{max} and T_{max} are parameters related to the in vivo dissolution process.) These authors reached the following conclusions:

1. The time required to reach the maximum concentration, T_{max}, and MDT were adequate as dissolution parameters only in some instances. The sensitivity of T_{max} and MDT to discern dissolution-rate differences decreases with an increase in the multicompartment characteristic of the data.
2. They also found that the accuracy of MDT depends on its magnitude relative to the MRT of the solid dosage form. As the MRT of the solid dosage form increases relative to MDT, so does the standard deviation of the mean MDT values obtained after several simulations. Mean MDT has also been referred to as $MDT_{average}$ by Riegelman and Collier (51).
3. They found that C_{max} was superior not only to MDT but also to T_{max} in evaluating in vivo dissolution differences. They concluded that under the conditions they had simulated mean dissolution time may be an insensitive measure for bioequivalence comparison.

Thus while statistical moments may yield good estimates of dissolution rate, one should be aware of the inherent problems in using statistical moments. This technique can only be used when all the aforementioned assumptions are satisfied. The errors involved in the extrapolation of a terminal exponential phase should be kept at a minimum, and an accurate estimate of the first-order terminal elimination-rate constant is necessary. In addition, the MDT would not provide the time course of release of the drug in the GI tract from the dosage form. Above all, we should always bear in mind that we are dealing with averages. The estimates obtained will reflect the average time required for all molecules to be dissolved. Thus a single number is obtained to describe the pharmacokinetic data, in contrast to the compartmental analysis, wherein a few rate constants are obtained that would allow us to reproduce the entire plasma concentration–time profile as the model would best predict it.

Deconvolution. The last of the indirect techniques of evaluating the release rate of drug from the dosage form that we discuss is the technique of numerical deconvolution. Numerical deconvolution not only provides the release-rate constant but also the release profile of the drug in the GI tract from the solid dosage form. To obtain the release profile, one must have available the plasma concentration–time data for the solution and solid dosage form.

The use of numerical deconvolution was first discussed by Rescigno and Segre for use in tracer and compartmental kinetics (58). It was first described in the pharmacokinetic literature by Benet and Chiang and later by Wagner (59,60). Gillespie and Veng-Pedersen were the first to calculate the in vivo release of the drug from the dosage form as a function of time (61).

Laplace transforms relate statistical moments to the convolution integral (50). A few simple mathematical relationships are presented here to familiarize the reader with these concepts and their mathematical existence.

$$L\{f(t)\} = \int_0^\infty f(t)e^{-st}\,dt = F(s) \tag{6.31}$$

where $L\{f(t)\}$ is the Laplace transform of function $f(t)$. The inverse transform

$$L^{-1}\{F(s)\} = f(t) \tag{6.32}$$

Similarly,

$$L\{g(t)\} = \int_0^\infty g(t)e^{-st}\,dt = G(s) \tag{6.33}$$

where $f(t)$ and $g(t)$ are any two functions of time and $F(s)$ and $G(s)$ are defined in the Laplace domain and the Laplace variable is a dummy variable. The convolution integral is thus defined as

$$L^{-1}\{F(s)G(s)\} = C(t) = \int_0^t f(t-T)g(T)\,dt \tag{6.34}$$

$$C(s) = F(s)G(s) \tag{6.35}$$

In Eq. (6.34), $C(t)$ describes the plasma concentration–time data after the administration of a solid dosage form such as a tablet or a capsule. The unit impulse response is represented by $f(t)$. This is the response observed after injecting a unit of drug by the intravenous bolus route or that observed after administering 1 unit of solution orally. Thus if D (dose) units of solution are administered, the response would be $Df(t)$. This applies only when the pharmacokinetic system is linear. Continuous in vivo release of drug in the GI tract is represented by $g(t)$.

If the unit impulse response is independent of the time at which the response is measured, the response after input $g(t)$ between time T and $T + dT$ is $F(t - T)g(T)\,dT$ for $0 \leqslant T \leqslant t$. Here $t - T$ is the time elapsed after the amount $g(T)\,dT$ is introduced, the measured response is expressed by the convolution integral [Eq. (6.34)]. An excellent explanation of this has been provided by Cutler (62). Equation (6.34) is as explained by Benet (63). Here the Laplace-transformed input function is multiplied by the Laplace-transformed disposition function to get the Laplace transform function describing the concentration–time profile.

This process of deconvolution for use in obtaining in vivo release profiles is described well by Gillespie and Veng-Pedersen (61,64). They have also provided a FORTRAN algorithm to calculate the fraction released as a function of time and to calculate MDT and relative bioavailability.

The cube-root law has been used to describe the process of dissolution from the tablet (65). Cutler has described the use of the cube-root law to describe dissolution in vivo (62). Interested readers who want to follow analytic deconvolution using the cube-root dissolution model may find pertinent information in the references cited. Since a thorough discussion is provided in the literature, it will not be discussed here in detail. Suffice to say that two parameters are evaluated: fraction of dose reaching the systemic circulation and the time of dissolution. The advantage of using deconvolution is that the dissolution profile can be obtained even if no model is assumed. This is done with the help of polynominals (66). Deconvolution and its allied technique, statistical moments, have the advantage of being applicable without assuming a pharmacokinetic model, provided that the inherent assumptions are not violated.

Direct Techniques

Historical aspects. It will be of interest to mention the historical aspects of the study of in vivo dissolution. Initially, these investigations were aimed at finding the in vivo disintegration time. Later, pharmaceutical researchers started realizing the importance of in vivo dissolution. Wagner has provided a concise account of the work done in the past (67). Fluoroscopy and roentgenography have been used in conjunction with radiopaque substances such as barium sulfate to determine the in vivo disintegration time. Wagner studied the disintegration of tablets in vivo in dogs using roentgenography (68,69). Tablets were fed to dogs after overnight fasting. X-ray photographs were taken after tablet administration. Disintegration time of the tablets was thus measured and correlated with in vitro disintegration times. Gruber et al. demonstrated the dissolution of core tablets by serial roentgenography (70). This was performed by incorporating potassium iodide in the tablets. They tested for iodide in saliva. They also employed a "yo-yo" technique in which tablets attached to a string were administered to human volunteers. Immediately following that process the tablets were withdrawn. This provided an idea of the in vivo disintegration times and was compared to the external characteristics of tablets. Steinberg et al. used the same yo-yo technique as Gruber et al. They also employed the use of fiberscope and biosonar to investigate disintegration of antacid tablets (71). Fiberscope consists of a flexible tube with 250,000 coated glass fibers which transport the image from the distal end to the ocular eyepiece at the proximal end. A camera attached to the eyepiece permitted color cinematography. This yields a profile of sequential in vivo disintegration. Biosonar was based on the principle of detecting the tablet by sound-wave deflection. It did not function adequately because it was difficult to distinguish the tablet from food, muscles, and bones.

Levy proposed the use of in vitro dissolution instead of in vitro disintegration as a compendial test for solid dosage forms. He was the first to realize that disintegration has little relationship to bioavailability (72). Dissolution rate, on the other hand, has a distinct correlation to biovailability. In 1963, Levy proposed the use of low agitation intensities for in vitro dissolution testing (73). He employed x-ray pictures to view the agitation of gastric contents during normal contractions of the GI tract. The disintegrated tablet thus remains as an aggregate and is not dispersed throughout the stomach.

Direct techniques of investigating in vivo dissolution could be classified as either invasive or noninvasive. Intubation of the GI tract is an invasive technique, while external scintigraphy is noninvasive but involves exposing the subject to radiation.

Intubation. The process of intubation has been used routinely in digestive physiology for feeding patients. Basically, with the use of multiple points of entry or removal, absorption from different segments of the GI tract can be evaluated. Since this is a relatively new technique, it will be explained in detail. For a more complete explanation of the method, the reader is referred to Refs. 38–41.

Normal healthy human volunteers selected for these studies are screened for GI and cardiovascular function. The normal exclusion protocol required in any drug study is followed. Subjects are thus required to abstain from medication, alcohol, and other specific items as stipulated for an appropriate period. Subjects are fasted overnight.

The direct method of intubation could be used either to deliver a liquid dose of drugs to a particular site in the GI tract, or it could be used to aspirate samples from any site in the GI tract. Solid dosage forms cannot be delivered at a particular site into the GI tract through the tube.

The intubation tubes used for these purposes are made of latex or plastic impregnated with a barium salt to make them radiopaque. They are moderately pliable in nature. These tubes have either one lumen or fused multiple lumens. The average length of these tubes could be between 10 and 15 ft. The tubes have a rigid end with a metal plate or an inflatable balloon to guide them through the GI tract. The inflatable balloon can be filled with a radiopaque marker. A thin metallic wire could be used to position the tube in the right place. With a multilumen tube, each tip is placed in an area to be investigated. Thus the lumens could, for example, be placed in the stomach, pylorus, duodenum, jejunum, colon, and so on. The radiopaque marker in the balloon facilitates identifying its location by the use of fluoroscopy. Usually, a gastroenterologist is required to insert these tubes. Intubation is usually nasogastric, but it may also be done through the oral cavity. The tube is inserted a day prior to the administration of the drug. The position of the tip of tube is confirmed under fluoroscopy prior to dosing and positioned at the region of interest. This is done to make sure that the tip reaches the desired site in the GI tract. It also helps the subject get acquainted to the presence of tubing. GI motility will then propel the tube down the GI tract. Particular care must be taken to avoid convoluting the tube in the stomach.

Since the volume of the GI contents is in a dynamic state, it is necessary to have a nonabsorbable marker such as polyethylene glycol (PEG) 4000 introduced in the GI tract with the drug. Marker concentration will be an indication of the volume of GI fluids at any time. Thus suitable corrections can be made to account for fluid fluxes.

Jobin et al. introduced two tubes in the GI tract to study the absorption of metoprolol from stomach, duodenum, and jejunum (38). Two markers were used in the study. Drug and [^{14}C]PEG 4000 were introduced in the stomach with a homogenized meal through a double lumen tube. Another triple lumen tube was positioned with perfusion of the unlabeled marker at the ampulla of Vater, angle of Treitz, and jejunum. This is shown in Fig. 6.16. The gastric contents were aspirated with a syringe, and the duodenal and jejunal contents were aspirated using intermittent negative pressure of 40 mm of mercury. Jobin et al. claim that this pressure would not alter GI motility. After 4 h the gastric contents were aspirated and the stomach was rinsed with 200 mL of normal saline containing 5 g of PEG 4000. Blood samples were collected over a 4-h period. The samples were analyzed by gas chromatography.

By using mass balance equations and perfusing the marker at a prespecified rate, they (38) were able to calculate the output of drug from stomach to duodenum and jejunum and also calculate the rate of absorption of the drug. Sampling of stomach contents led them to believe that drug was not absorbed from there. The profile of metoprolol concentration in the stomach as a function of time is shown in Fig. 6.17. Similarly, the amount of metoprolol in duodenum and jejunum were calculated as a function of time.

In the future, studies could be done to evaluate the dissolution of a solid dosage form in the GI tract. A tube with four lumens can be inserted with sites in stomach, duodenum, jejunum, and colon. After the insertion of tube, a solid dosage form might be administered orally. The solid dosage form will pass through the GI tract. There is adequate space between the tube and the GI walls. Although normal passage might be somewhat impaired, there appears to be no reason why such a study could not be done. Samples could be aspirated using negative pressures and analyzed in each segment as a function of time. Absorption of drug would tend to obfuscate the profile obtained. This is because the concentration at any point after the passage through the stomach will be increased due to dissolution of dosage form but decrease because of absorption. Although this process might complicate the evaluation of dissolution, it may be thought to be physiologic in its entirety. To study the dissolution of the drug in the intestine, one would need to deliver the dosage form to the duodenum. This can be accomplished by administering an enteric-coated

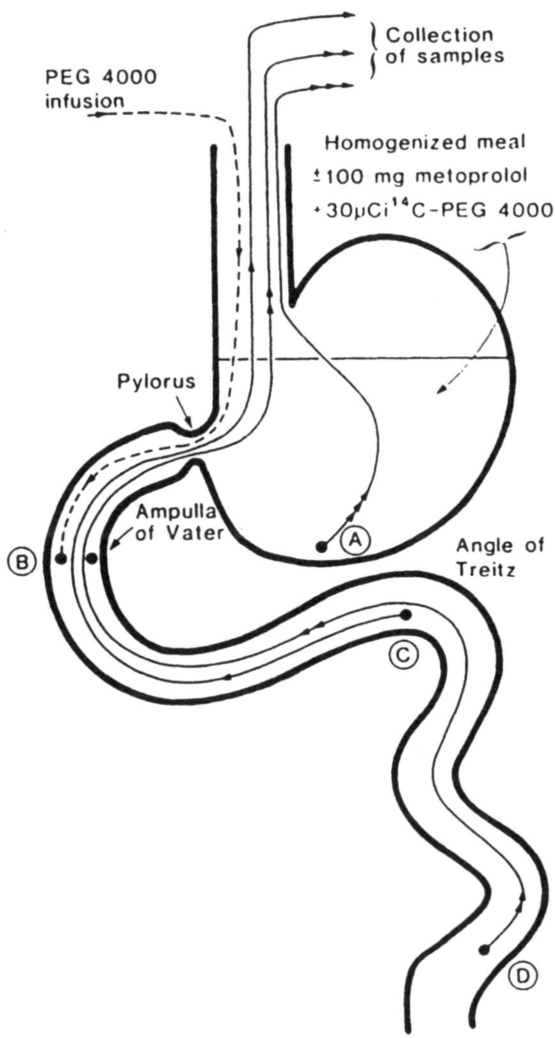

Fig. 6.16 Schematic representation of the positioning of tubes at different sites in the GI tract. A is stomach, B is ampulla of Vater, C is angle of Trietz, D is jejunum. Distance from B to C is 20 cm; distance from C to D is 30 cm. (From Ref. 38.)

dosage form. Perhaps dissolution properties of small beads or microcapsules, which are used in the manufacture of sustained-release dosage forms, may be studied by delivering them through the tubes used to aspirate the samples.

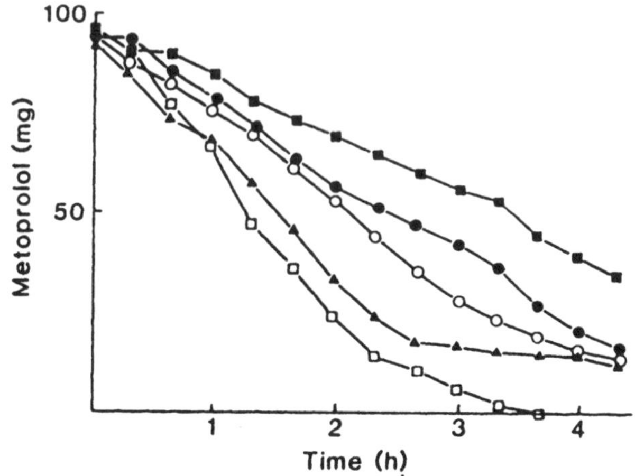

Fig. 6.17 Plot of amount of metoprolol remaining in the stomach as a function of time. Samples were drawn every 20 min for 4 h. Data for five subjects as shown. (From Ref. 38.)

One should realize the drawbacks associated with the use of this technique. A complete picture of the amount released from the dosage form as a function of time cannot be obtained. This will give a limited idea of the dissolution in individual segments of the GI tract. The investigator should also make sure that there is no adsorption of drug onto the tubes used for aspirating samples of delivering the drug. Besides, the intubation methodology is unphysiologic. Introduction of a tube in the GI tract may disturb GI motility. It may also affect the path of the dosage form under investigation in the GI tract. However, regardless of any differences induced by the presence of the lumen, conclusions regarding relative differences in absorption for segments of the GI tract should be valid.

Gamma scintigraphy. External scintigraphy using one gamma camera, perturbed angular correlation, summation peak ratio, and neutron activation are the techniques used commonly to study in vivo disintegration and dissolution. Gamma scintigraphy is a process of measuring the gamma rays emitted from radionuclide. Perhaps the technique that provides maximum information is direct assessment by gamma scintigraphy. Scintigraphy entails the inclusion of a gamma-emitting radionuclide in the formulation and its observation using a gamma camera. The camera is connected to a computer for data storage and subsequent analysis. A typical gamma camera system would appear as shown in Fig. 6.18 (74). In most of these systems, two radionuclides with different peak energies can be monitored simultaneously and independently. Nuclides such as indium-111 or indium-113m could be used to outline the GI tract while

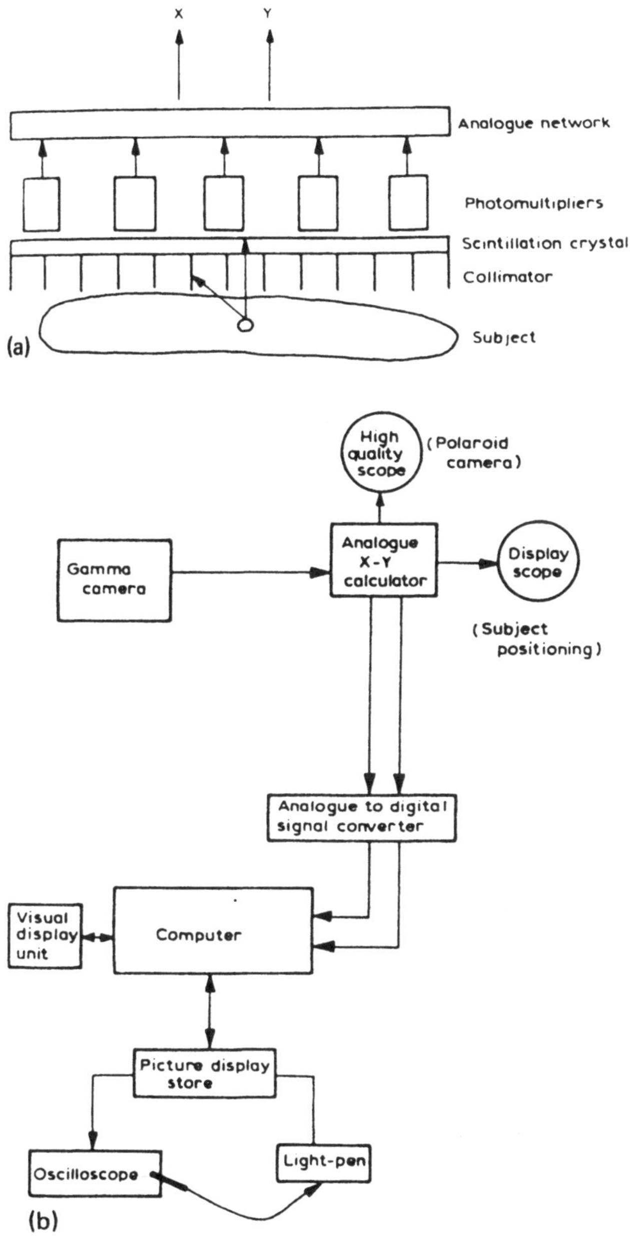

Fig. 6.18 Typical gamma camera system. (a) Photons pass through a collimator and strike a sodium iodide crystal. This resultant flash is multiplied by a photomultiplier. (b) Computerized data collection from the gamma camera and data display on a cathode ray oscilloscope. (From Ref. 74.)

other nuclides such as technetium-99m are incorporated by chelation with one of the dosage form excipients. To avoid systematic absorption of these radionuclides, they are chelated to compounds such as diethylenetriaminepentacetic acid or tagged to resins. These radionuclides will have different emission energies and do not interfere with the detection of the other.

The basic working of a gamma camera is simple (Fig. 6.18). The gamma rays emanating from the source pass through the collimators and come in contact with the sodium iodide crystals. The sodium iodide crystals contain 1% thallium iodide. When the gamma ray strikes the sodium iodide crystal, its energy is converted to light energy, resulting in a flash of light. These crystals convert chemical energy to light energy. The flash of light emitted is then detected by the photomultiplier tube. The signal is thus multiplied and the analog signal is then digitized by an analog-to-digital converter. The digitized information is stored in the computer and used for later analyses. The analog signal can also be displayed on a CRT tube.

Several radionuclides are available to the pharmaceutical researcher. The radionuclide of choice would depend on the kind of measurements the investigator needs to make. Selection criteria for radionuclides are reviewed thoroughly in the literature (75). An ideal radionuclide should have:

1. A detectable photon yield.
2. Radiation that is minimally absorbed by the subject.
3. Minimal particulate radiation. Therefore, nuclides emitting particles are totally excluded.
4. Gamma energies above 30 keV, preferably around 150 keV.
5. A physical half-life of $0.693T$, where T is the time after administration at which measurements are made.
6. The ability to label the drug or a desired excipient of the formulation.
7. The potential to be firmly attached to the component of the formulation it is to be in contact with. If the radionuclide is detached from that component, misleading results may be obtained.

Two types of labels are used in external scintigraphy. Covalent labels such as iodine-123 or iodine-131 and mercury-197 are used in research studies. However, labels used in external scintigraphy for the purposes of GI studies are restricted mostly to foreign metal-ion labels which are chelated to some entity in the formulation. Of the foreign metal-ion nuclides, technetium-99m is the most useful, along with indium-111 and indium-113m. Technetium-99m is an ideal nuclide because of its optimal decay energy, short half-life of 6 h, ease of manufacture, and ease of incorporation in a range of radio-imaging agents. Kits are available commercially for preparing technetium-99m labels as imaging agents. Indium-111 with a half-life of 2.8 days is frequently coupled with technetium-99m in external scintigraphy. Daly et al. and Wilson et al.

incorporated technetium-99m in their solid dosage forms and administered indium-113m in solution to image the GI tract (76,77). This helped identify the position of dosage form in the GI tract. Jay et al. have used indium-111 to measure in vivo dissolution (78).

It should be noted in external scintigraphy that it is not possible to detect the drug directly. Rather, its fate is presumed from the extent of integrity of the emitters. Disintegration is determined by recording the diameter of the solid dosage form. Once the diameter recorded by imaging exceeds a prespecified number, the solid dosage form is considered to be disintegrated. This is because the gamma camera cannot detect if the drug molecule is in solid state or in solution. This problem was overcome by Beihn and Digenis using perturbed angular correlation studies (79). Jay et al. reported the use of summation peak ratios of indium-111 to determine the dissolution rate (78).

Several other articles have been published where scintigraphy has been used to detect in vivo disintegration. Alpsten et al., using capsules loaded with insoluble polystyrene resin, studied disintegration in fasting versus fed states (80). They found that disintegration was delayed after food intake. Alpsten et al. did some classic work in Sweden to study the release and absorption from ferrous-59-labeled tablets (81). The determination of in vivo disintegration and that of in vivo dissolution using perturbed angular correlation in conjunction with gamma scintigraphy will also be reviewed. Determination of in vivo dissolution using summation peak ratios will be briefly discussed.

Disintegration of tablets was studied by Digenis in human (82). Technetium-99m and indium-113m were used for formulations *A* and *B*, which varied in the disintegrant used. These tablets were made up of lactose 88.75%, microcrystalline cellulose or polyvinyl pyrrolidone 10%, magnesium stearate 1%, and cabosil 0.25%. A gamma camera was used to measure the counts per minute and the data were stored on a computer. Two areas were monitored for radioactivity, the tablet itself, and the pylorus. Increase in activity at the pylorus corresponded to a decrease in activity around the tablet. The results are shown in Fig. 6.19 for three subjects. As is evident, formulation *A* disintegrates more rapidly than formulation *B*. The graphs give an idea of the disintegration behavior of the dosage forms.

Perturbed angular correlation. To get a quantitative assessment of in vivo dissolution in contrast to disintegration, Beihn and Digenis recommended the use of perturbed angular correlation in conjunction with external scintigraphy (79). Indium-111 decays with a delay in γ-cascade, as shown by the scheme in Fig. 6.20. The 85-ns delay is used advantageously to perform coincidence counting of both photopeaks. Interaction with the environment (i.e., with solid or liquid state) would cause the gamma rays from indium-111 to exhibit perturbance in angular correlation. This perturbance is due to the environment (solid or liquid state), electric and magnetic fields, and viscosity. In molecular

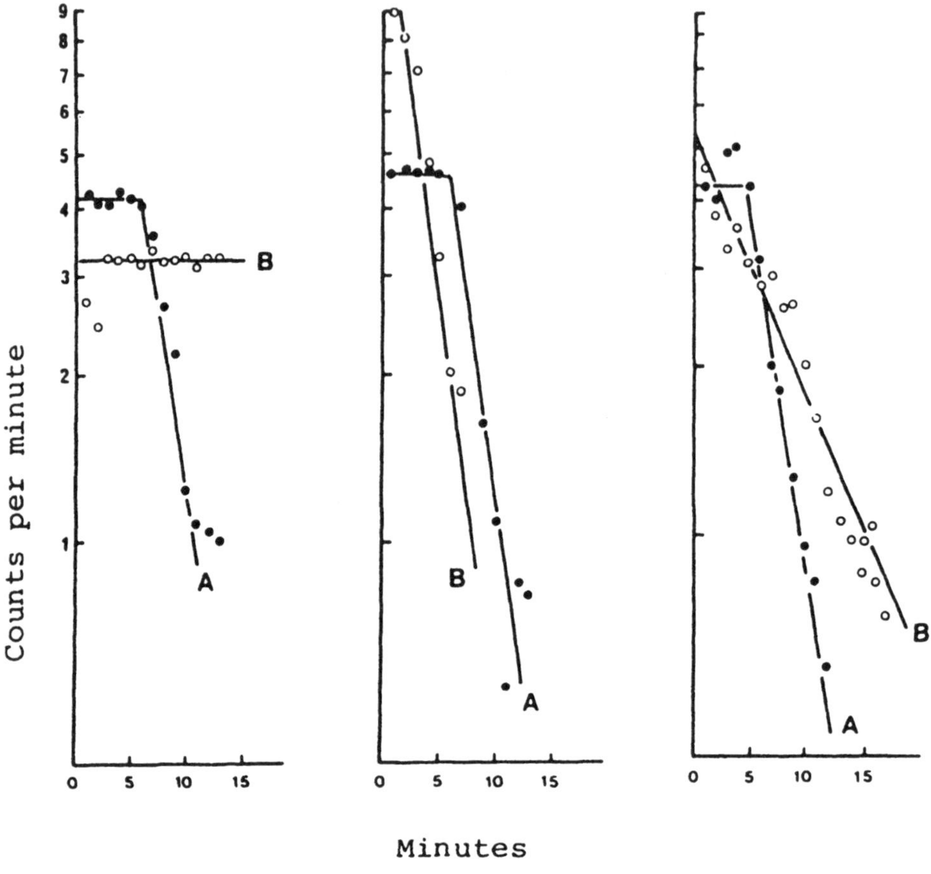

Fig. 6.19 Disintegration profiles of tablets A and B with different disintegrants in three human subjects. Formulation A disintegrates more rapidly than formulation B. (From Ref. 82.)

terms this could be described as the reorientation of nucleus because of the interaction with the environment. This perturbance is quantified using the following equation:

$$A = 1 - \frac{w(180°, t)}{w(90°, t)} \tag{6.36}$$

where A represents anisotropy and $w(180°, t)$ and $w(90°, t)$ are coincident counting rates at angles of 180° and 90°, respectively.

A plot of anisotropy as a function of time is shown for two formulations in Fig. 6.21. Figure 6.21(a) shows the correlation of anisotropy to in vitro disso-

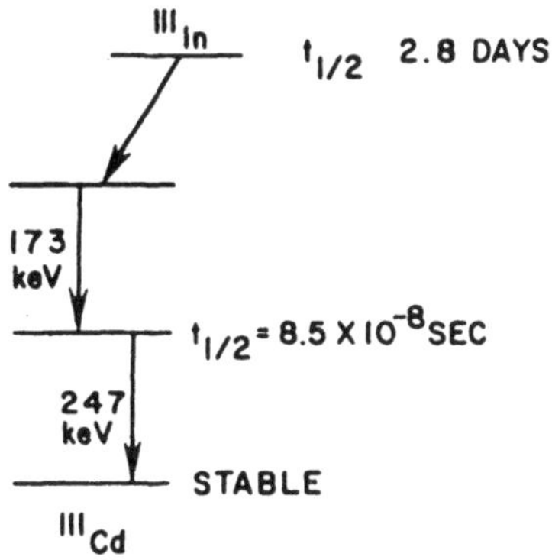

Fig. 6.20 Decay scheme of indium-111. (From Ref. 79.)

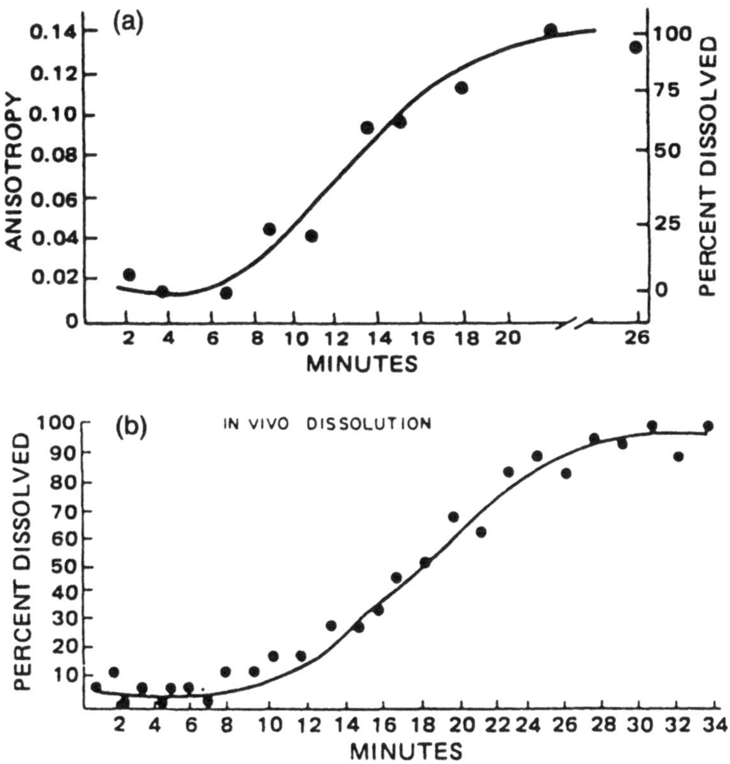

Fig. 6.21 (a) In vitro dissolution and correlation with anisotropy of an indium-111-labeled sucrose tablet. (b) In vivo dissolution of indium-111-labeled lactose tablet. There was an 8-min lag time before dissolution began. (From Ref. 79.)

lution. Figure 6.21(b) represents in vivo dissolution as a function of time. Thus anisotropy was used to measure the percent dissolved in vivo. Low values of anisotropy correspond to the solid state, and high values to the liquid state. In this figure, intermediate anisotropy values represent varying numbers of indium-111 passing from solid state to solution. There was an 8-min delay prior to the onset of dissolution.

Summation peak ratio. Jay et al. have described the use of summation peak ratios for determining in vivo dissolution (78). The intensity of the summation peak (i.e., the sum total of energies of two peaks) from two gamma photons emitted successively from a radionuclide is related to the physical and chemical environment experienced by the intermediate state of the nucleus.

In vitro dissolution was performed on a tablet containing salicylate and indium-111 as indium chloride. Figure 6.20 describes the decay scheme for indium-111. Indium shows photopeaks at 173 and 247 keV with an 85-ns delay between them. Radioactive counts at γ_{173} and γ_{247} and γ_{420} ($420 = 173 + 247$) were obtained by a gamma camera positioned beneath the dissolution beaker (γ = gamma). Both salicylic acid and indium-111 release were monitored separately, as shown in Fig. 6.22. Excellent correlations were obtained between the release of salicylic acid in vitro and that of indium-111 in vitro. This correlation was used to measure the dissolution of salicylic acid in vivo by actually monitoring the peak ratio as shown in Fig. 6.23.

The summation peak ratio method is much simpler than perturbed angular correlation because (a) it does not require the use of complex coincidence counting systems, and (b) it requires only one-half to one-fifth of the radioactivity needed for perturbed angular correlation. One of its drawbacks compared to perturbed angular correlation is that it can provide reliable data only when dissolution is occurring in an anatomical segment of GI tract such as stomach. It may thus not be applicable for controlled-release dosage forms such as OROS, the oral osmotic pump by ALZA Corporation, which releases drug slowly throughout the length of the GI tract.

Neutron activation. Neutron activation of inert excipients in the tablet is another method to study disintegration in vivo. Parr et al. studied radiolabeled intact tablets (83,84). The labeling was done in situ after the tablet was manufactured. They produced barium-139 and erbium-170 by irradiating the enteric-coated tablet with a neutron flux. Barium sulfate was incorporated in a small quantity (10 mg in a 300-mg tablet) in the dosage form. Irradiation by neutrons converted barium-138 to barium-139 with a yield of 91 μCi per tablet (83). Similarly, in another study, Parr et al. incorporated 2.1 mg of 96% pure erbium oxide in a 300-mg tablet (84). Once the tablets were prepared they

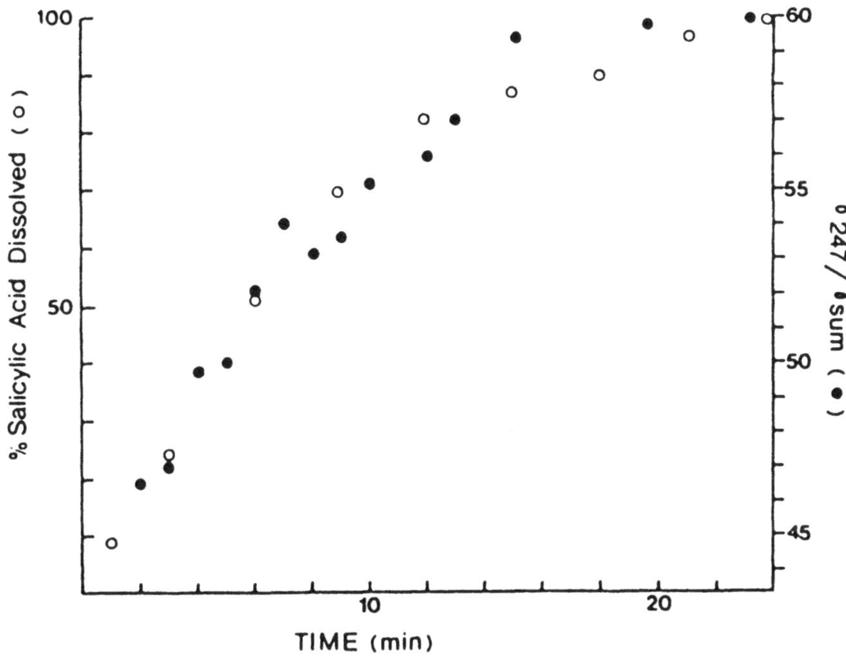

Fig. 6.22 In vitro dissolution of salicylic acid (O). In vitro dissolution of indium-111 chloride from the same tablet (●) as measured by its summation peak ratio. Good correlations exist between the in vitro dissolution of these two compounds from the same tablet. This indicates that indium-111 chloride can be used to monitor dissolution in vivo. (From Ref. 78.)

were placed in a flux trap for 15 min in a neutron flux of 4.4×10^{13} neutron/cm^2 per second. At the end of this treatment, the tablet had 800 μCi of erbium-171. The tablet was enteric coated before it was placed in the reactor. A high-resolution Ge(Li) detector was used for imaging. Figure 6.24 shows the images taken at various times. The tablet was in the stomach for 68 min and it disintegrated 12 min after it was ejected from the pyloric region. This provided a good idea of the disintegration of these tablets and an indication of the gastric emptying pattern. Neutron activation resolves several disadvantages of using conventional radiolabeling techniques.

1. Production time may be very long and not suitable for using short-lived nuclides. Here the nuclide of interest is prepared in situ, thus diminishing the time between the preparation of isotope and administration.

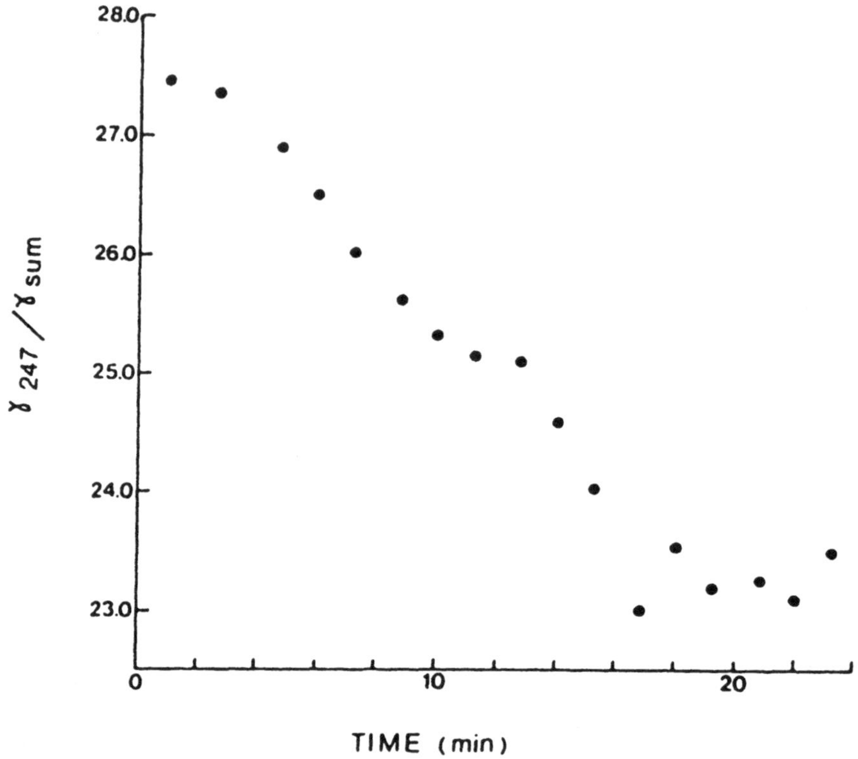

Fig. 6.23 In vivo dissolution of salicylic acid in humans as measured by indium-111 chloride summation peak ratios. (From Ref. 78.)

2. Special equipment may be required that may not be decontaminated easily after use. With neutron activation, the tablet prepared by regular means is placed in a reactor. Thus contamination is avoided.
3. Labeling may not be applicable to special dosage forms with enteric coating, inert drug delivery devices, or multiparticulate dosage forms. This is facilitated in neutron activation.
4. On-site preparation of radiolabeled dosage forms is limited to the handling of a small volume of material. This may not be representative of industrial-scale conditions. Industrially prepared dosage forms can be irradiated to produce radiolabels provided that the precursor of the radionuclide is incorporated in the dosage form.

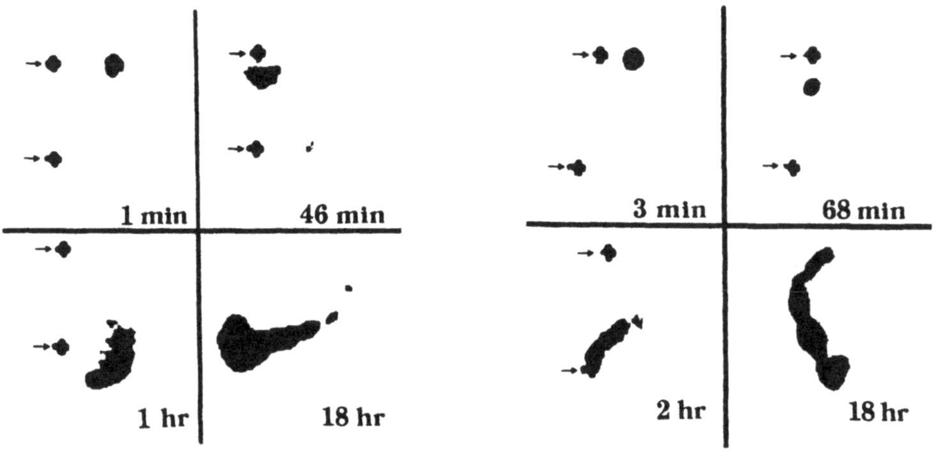

Fig. 6.24 Scintigraphic images of erbium-171 tablets labeled by neutron activation, at different times. The figure on the left is for uncoated tablets, that on the right is for enteric-coated tablets. Enteric-coated tablets are in the stomach for 68 min. Disintegration of uncoated tablet occurs within 46 min in the stomach. Arrows indicate external body location marker. (From Ref. 84.)

CONCLUSIONS

Indirect techniques such as statistical moments could be used with ease as long as solution data and solid dosage form data are available to determine the MDT. The evaluation requires no assumption of a model except that the system should exhibit first-order kinetics and elimination in vivo should occur from the central pool. The BASIC program "MOMENTS" should make this calculation easy. The more commonly used Loo–Riegelman analysis yields the same rate constants, but its ability to do so when the absorption rate constant K_a approaches the release-rate constant K_r, is doubtful. It is critically dependent on the model adequately fitting the data. Deconvolution is a powerful mathematical tool used to obtain the in vivo dissolution profile but is mathematically more complex relative to the two preceding methods.

The direct technique of intubation will not yield a continuous profile of the amount dissolved as a function of time. It exposes the subject to high radiation because of the use of x-rays to detect the position of the lumen of the tube. Nevertheless, it is useful in evaluating drug absorption from the dosage form in individual segments of the GI tract. Because of the intensive experimental demand and inherent risk, use of this technique is restricted to research studies.

External scintigraphy and its modifications are the only direct techniques available to determine the dissolution profile of drugs in vivo. The subject will be exposed to radiation here, but it will be much less compared to conventional x-rays. The dosage forms used for these studies require special manufacturing techniques.

The reader will hopefully be able to use one or more of these techniques to obtain the highly sought in vivo dissolution parameter, mean dissolution time. This in vivo parameter should be used for in vivo–in vitro correlations. Many bioavailability and bioequivalence problems can be resolved if strong correlations exist between in vivo and in vitro parameters. In vivo dissolution is an expensive and time-consuming process. Thus it may not be employed routinely. But the parameters once obtained for a spectrum of population in normal and diseased states could be employed for improving in vivo–in vitro correlations.

APPENDIX

The raw plasma concentration–time data for a solution and a solid dosage form would be tabulated in a manner similar to that shown in Table A.1. If it is a study on several subjects, data for each subject are tabulated accordingly.

The BASIC program "MOMENTS.BAS" in Table A.2 calculates mean dissolution time from data similar to those in Table A.1. It calculates the area under the curve and the area under the moment curve by trapezoidal rule up to the beginning of the terminal elimination phase. A log-trapezoidal rule is used to calculate the area under the curve once the terminal elimination phase begins. This is exemplified by Fig. A.1, where the log-trapezoidal rule should be started from observation 17 (i.e., 3 h). Thus the user should plot the data on a semilog scale and determine where the concentrations start declining linearly on a semilog plot. Once these points are determined for both the solution and solid dosage form data, one can proceed to create the input file. (For the solid dosage form it was found that the concentrations start declining in a log-linear fashion from observation 17.) As random error was not added to the data in Table A.1, Fig. A.1 has a perfect fit (i.e., all the data points lie on the fitted curve). Also, the sampling was done at the same time that points for the solution and solid dosage form data. This may not be true for actual bioavailability data. In real data, there is also bound to be some scatter. The sampling for the two dosage forms may not be performed at the same times. Despite these factors, once the concentrations are in the terminal (log-linear) elimination phase, this program can be used. Extrapolation of the area under the curve and the area under the moment curve are calculated by appropriate equations.

The user should transfer the BASIC program in the BASICA mode or using FRED or EDLIN. EDLIN is available as an executable file along with the disk

Table A.1 Concentration-Time Data

Observation number	Solid dosage form		Solution	
	Time	Concentration	Time	Concentration
1	0.0166	3.1004	0.0166	47.5439
2	0.0333	11.3512	0.0333	88.9677
3	0.05	23.3868	0.05	125.91
4	0.0666	38.0879	0.0666	155.9472
5	0.0833	54.5435	0.0833	162.6002
6	0.1666	142.0695	0.1666	265.0280
7	0.25	210.7084	0.25	291.709
8	0.3333	250.1689	0.3333	288.8703
9	0.4166	264.7288	0.4166	271.7129
10	0.5	262.0566	0.5	248.8149
11	0.5833	249.1153	0.5833	224.8231
12	0.6666	231.0748	0.6666	202.0881
13	0.75	211.3466	0.75	181.6494
14	1.0	158.0576	1	135.5947
15	1.5	99.1211	1.5	90.1957
16	2	74.3764	2	70.0226
17	3	50.1138	3	47.8449
18	4	35.0734	4	33.5189
19	5	24.6124	5	23.5231
20	6.5	14.4723	6.5	13.8318
21	8.0	8.5099	8	8.1334
22	10	4.1922	10	4.0067
23	12	2.065	12	1.9738

Source: Ref. 18, Fig. 3.

Table A.2 Program MOMENTS.BAS

```
10 REM THIS PROGRAM SHOULD BE TITLED AND SAVED AS "MOMENTS.BAS"
20 REM THE INPUT FILE SHOULD BE TITLED AS "DATA.IN"
30 REM THE OUTPUT FILE CREATED BY THE PROGRAM WILL BE SAVED AS "DATA.OUT"
40 REM IF THE BATCH FILE "INVIVO.BAT" IS USED THEN:
50 REM CONTINUED A) BOTH THE INPUT AND OUTPUT FILES WILL BE PRINTED OUT
60 REM CONTINUED B) THE INPUT FILE WILL BE RENAMED AS "LASTPR.IN"
70 REM CONTINUED C) THE OUTPUT FILE WILL BE RENAMED "LASTPR.OUT"
80 DEFDBL A,M
90 OPTION BASE 1
100 DIM TIMES(50),SOLUTION(50),TIMET(50),TABLET(50),TCONCS(50),TCONCT(50)
110  AUCS=0:AUCT=0:AUMCS=0:AUMCT=0
120 LOGAUCS=0:LOGAUCT=0:LOGAUMCS=0:LOGAUMCT=0
130 REM ALL VARIABLES IN PROGRAM ENDING WITH "T" REFER TO TABLET WHILE THOSE    ENDING WITH "S"
 REFER TO SOLUTION.
140 OPEN "DATA.IN" FOR INPUT AS #1
150 OPEN "DATA.OUT" FOR OUTPUT AS #2
```

```
160 INPUT #1,N,NSLOPE,W
170 FOR L=1 TO N
180 INPUT #1,TIMES(L),SOLUTION(L)
190 TCONCS(L)=TIMES(L)*SOLUTION(L)
200 NEXT L
210 INPUT #1,M,MSLOPE,X
220 FOR J=1 TO M
230 INPUT #1,TIMET(J),TABLET(J)
240 TCONCT(J)=TIMET(J)*TABLET(J)
250 NEXT J
260 CMAXSOLN=SOLUTION(1)
270 'THESE VARIABLES ARE INTRODUCED TO CALCULATE THE CMAX IN THE DATA.
280 CMAXTAB=TABLET(1)
290 Z=1
300 FOR G=1 TO N-1
310 IF SOLUTION(G)<SOLUTION(G+1) THEN B=SOLUTION(G+1) ELSE B=SOLUTION(G)
320 IF CMAXSOLN<B THEN CMAXSOLN=B:Z=G+1
330 NEXT G
340 Y=1
350 FOR H=1 TO M-1
360 IF TABLET(H)<TABLET(H+1) THEN D=TABLET(H+1) ELSE D=TABLET(H)
370 IF CMAXTAB<D THEN CMAXTAB=D:Y=H+1
380 NEXT H
390 FOR E=1 TO W-1
400 SUMS=1/2*(SOLUTION(E)+SOLUTION(E+1))*(TIMES(E+1)-TIMES(E))
410 AUCS=AUCS+SUMS
420 NUMS=1/2*(TCONCS(E)+TCONCS(E+1))*(TIMES(E+1)-TIMES(E))
430 AUMCS=AUMCS+NUMS
440 NEXT E
450 FOR P=W TO N-1
460 NUMERS=(SOLUTION(P+1)-SOLUTION(P))
470 DENOMS=(LOG(SOLUTION(P+1)/SOLUTION(P)))/(TIMES(P+1)-TIMES(P))
480 TOTAUCS=NUMERS/DENOMS
490 LOGAUCS=LOGAUCS+TOTAUCS
500 NUMLEFTS=TCONCS(P+1)-TCONCS(P)
510 TOTAUMCS=(NUMLEFTS/DENOMS)-((NUMERS)/(DENOMS^2))
520 LOGAUMCS=LOGAUMCS+TOTAUMCS
530 NEXT P
540 FOR F=1 TO X-1
550 SUMT=1/2*(TABLET(F)+TABLET(F+1))*(TIMET(F+1)-TIMET(F))
560 AUCT=AUCT+SUMT
570 NUMT=1/2*(TCONCT(F+1)+TCONCT(F))*(TIMET(F+1)-TIMET(F))
580 AUMCT=AUMCT+NUMT
590 NEXT F
600 FOR Q=X TO M-1
610 NUMERT=TABLET(Q+1)-TABLET(Q)
620 DENOMT=(LOG(TABLET(Q+1)/TABLET(Q)))/(TIMET(Q+1)-TIMET(Q))
630 TOTAUCT=NUMERT/DENOMT
640 LOGAUCT=LOGAUCT+TOTAUCT
650 NUMLEFTT=TCONCT(Q+1)-TCONCT(Q)
660 TOTAUMCT=(NUMLEFTT/DENOMT)-(NUMERT/(DENOMT^2))
670 LOGAUMCT=LOGAUMCT+TOTAUMCT
680 NEXT Q
690  AUCTAB=AUCT+LOGAUCT+(TABLET(M)/MSLOPE)
700 AUCSOLN=AUCS+LOGAUCS+(SOLUTION(N)/NSLOPE)
710 AUMCTAB=AUMCT+LOGAUMCT+(TIMET(M)*TABLET(M)/MSLOPE)+(TABLET(M)/(MSLOPE^2))
720 AUMCSOLN=AUMCS+LOGAUMCS+(TIMES(N)*SOLUTION(N)/NSLOPE)+(SOLUTION(N)/(NSLOPE^2))
730 MRTTAB=AUMCTAB/AUCTAB
740 MRTSOLN=AUMCSOLN/AUCSOLN
750 MDT=MRTTAB-MRTSOLN
760 PRINT #2,TAB(50) DATE$
770 PRINT #2, TAB(50) TIME$
780 PRINT #2,:PRINT #2,
790 PRINT #2,TAB(8) "MOMENT ANALYSIS OF LINEAR PHARMACOKINETIC DATA"
800 PRINT #2,: PRINT #2,
```

```
810 PRINT #2,TAB(7)"  TIME  "TAB(18)" TABLET "TAB(31)"  TIME  "TAB(41)"SOLUTION"
820 PRINT #2,TAB(16) "CONCENTRATION" TAB(39) "CONCENTRATION"
830 F$= "    #####.##"
840 IF N>M THEN A=M ELSE A=N
850 FOR R=1 TO A
860 PRINT #2,USING F$; TIMET(R),TABLET(R),TIMES(R),SOLUTION(R)
870 NEXT R
880 IF M-A=0 THEN LAST=N ELSE LAST=M
890 FOR T=A+1 TO LAST
900 IF LAST=M THEN PRINT #2, USING F$; TIMET(T),TABLET(T) ELSE PRINT #2, TAB(24) USING F$;TIMES
(T),SOLUTION(T)
910 NEXT T
920 PRINT #2,
930 PRINT #2,:PRINT #2, USING "CMAX OF THE SOLUTION IS =    #########.##";CMAXSOLN
940 PRINT #2,
950 PRINT #2, USING "TMAX OF THE SOLUTION IS =    #########.##";TIMES(Z)
960 PRINT #2,
970 PRINT #2,USING "AUC OF SOLUTION =     #########.##";AUCSOLN
980 PRINT #2,
990 PRINT #2, USING  "AUMC OF SOLUTION =     #########.##";AUMCSOLN
1000 PRINT #2,
1010 PRINT #2, USING "MRT OF SOLUTION =     #########.##";MRTSOLN
1020 PRINT #2,
1030 PRINT #2, USING "CMAX OF THE TABLET IS =     #########.##";CMAXTAB
1040 PRINT #2,
1050 PRINT #2,USING "TMAX OF THE TABLET IS =    #########.##";TIMET(Y)
1060 PRINT #2,
1070 PRINT #2, USING "AUC OF TABLET =     #########.##";AUCTAB
1080 PRINT #2,
1090 PRINT #2, USING "AUMC OF TABLET =     #########.##";AUMCTAB
1100 PRINT #2,
1110 PRINT #2, USING  "MRT OF TABLET =      ##########.##"; MRTTAB
1120 PRINT #2,
1130 PRINT #2, USING  "MDT OF TABLET = MRT OF TABLET - MRT OF SOLUTION =     #########.##";MDT
1140 CLOSE
1150 SYSTEM
```

operating system. For further information on this readers should consult the DOS manuals of their microcomputers. To enter the BASICA mode the user needs a file BASICA.COM on the disk. Once in BASICA, the user can transcribe the program as provided, with the line numbers on the screen. Then it should be saved under the title "MOMENTS.BAS". The program requires an input file "DATA.IN" in which the data are stored as shown in Table A.3.

To create the input file from the data in Table A.1, the following steps should be used:

1. An editor such as FRED or EDLIN should be invoked.
2. The first line of the input file contains parameters for the *solution data set*:
   a. The first entry is the total number of observations for the solution data set. In the data set provided in Table A.1, there are 23 observations.
   b. The second entry is the slope of the terminal elimination phase. It is 0.354 for the solution data set.

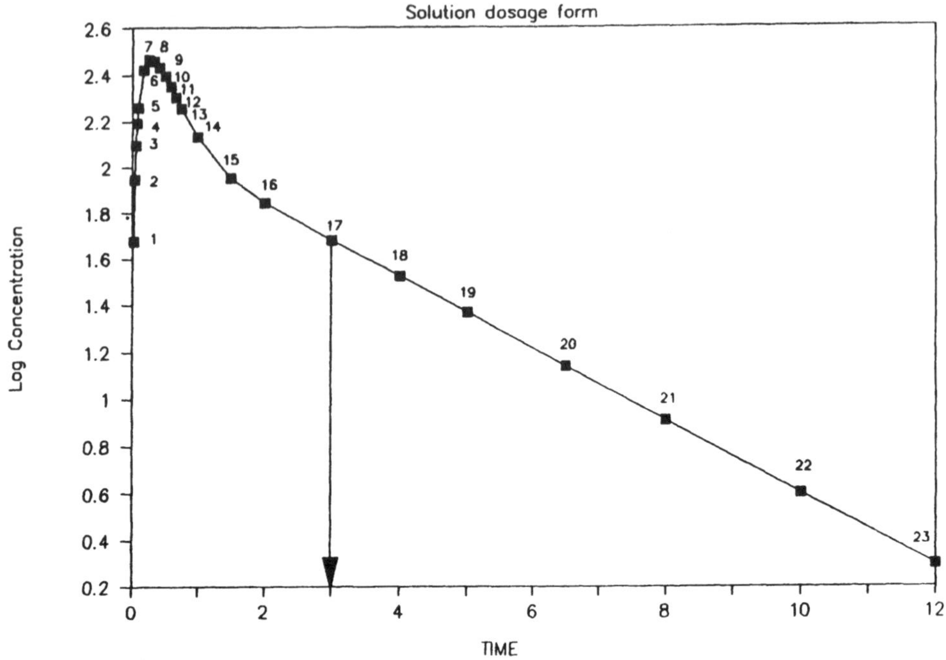

Fig. A.1. This exemplifies that the log-trapezoidal rule should be used from 3 h (i.e., data point 17) to 12 h (i.e., point 23). This is because the concentration declines in a log-linear fashion in that region of the plasma concentration–time curve.

   c. The third entry is the observation number from which the log-trapezoidal rule is started. It is 17 for this data set.
3. Lines 2 to 24 of the input file represent the time and concentration for the 23 data points of the solution data set.
4. Line 25 of the input file describes the parameters for the solid dosage form data.
   a. The first entry is the total number of observations for the solid dosage form data. Incidentally, solid dosage form data also has 23 observations. The observations for the solid dosage form data need not be the same as the solution data to use this program.
   b. The second entry is the terminal elimination rate constant. This is 0.354 for the solid dosage form data. This rate constant should be identical to the terminal rate constant of the solution data. Only then

Table A.3 Input File

```
23     ,   0.354     ,    17
0.0166 ,   47.5439
0.0333 ,   88.9677
0.05   ,   124.91
0.0666 ,   155.9472
0.0833 ,   162.6002
0.1666 ,   265.028
0.25   ,   291.709
0.3333 ,   288.8703
0.4166 ,   271.7129
0.5    ,   248.8149
0.5833 ,   224.8231
0.6666 ,   202.0881
0.75   ,   181.6494
1      ,   135.5947
1.5    ,   90.1957
2      ,   70.0226
3      ,   47.8449
4      ,   33.5189
5      ,   23.5231
6.5    ,   13.8318
8      ,   8.1334
10     ,   4.0067
12     ,   1.9738
23     ,   0.354     ,    17
0.0166 ,   3.10045
0.0333 ,   11.3512
0.05   ,   23.3868
0.0666 ,   38.0879
0.0833 ,   54.5435
0.1666 ,   142.0695
0.25   ,   210.7084
0.3333 ,   250.1689
0.4166 ,   264.7288
0.5    ,   262.0556
0.5833 ,   249.1153
0.6666 ,   231.0748
0.75   ,   211.3466
1.0    ,   158.0576
1.5    ,   99.1211
2.0    ,   74.3764
3.0    ,   50.1138
4      ,   35.0734
5      ,   24.6124
6.5    ,   14.4723
8.0    ,   8.5099
10     ,   4.1922
12     ,   2.065
```

can one be assured that concentrations are in the terminal elimination phase.

c. The third entry on line 25 of the input file is the point from which the log-trapezoidal rule should be used for the solid dosage form data. Coincidentally, it is the same as the solution data, which is data point

17. For controlled-release dosage forms this would be expected to be at later times since the dosage form would release the drug slowly for the first several hours.

5. Lines 26 to 48 are the times and concentrations for the solid dosage form data.
6. Although not necessary, all entries are separated by commas for convenience.
7. The first data set has to be for solution and the one that follows has to be for solid dosage form. *This order should not be reversed.*
8. For conventional bioavailability studies one can use the same program to calculate the mean absorption time. In that case the IV bolus data are entered in place of solution data and the oral data in place of solid dosage form data in the input file. This has to be input with appropriate parameters for those data sets. In such a case, the mean dissolution time in the output file actually represents the mean absorption time.
9. The input file should be stored as "DATA.IN". No files titled "DATA.IN", "DATA.OUT", "LASTPR.IN" and "LASTPR.OUT" should be present in the directory.

If the user wants to use the program without going into BASICA, the steps detailed in the following batch file will be useful. This batch file should be created by using EDLIN or FRED editors and saved under the name "INVIVO.BAT". It will take the input file "DATA.IN" and run it on the BASICA interpreter. Then the input file is renamed to "LASTPR.IN" and the output file "DATA.OUT" is renamed "LASTPR.OUT". It also prints on the attached printer the input and output files as shown in Tables A.3 and A.4, respectively. To run the program the user must type "INVIVO" at the DOS prompt. The batch file "INVIVO.BAT" is as follows:

```
BASICA MOMENTS. BAS
RENAME DATA.IN LASTPR.IN
RENAME DATA.OUT LASTPR.OUT
PRINT LASTPR.*
```

If the program is to be run again, the files "LASTPR.IN" and "LASTPR.OUT" should be renamed. If for some reason this batch file does not work on the DOS system of the available microcomputer, the program can be run in the basic mode. This is done by entering the BASICA mode, loading, and running the program. The output will then be stored in "DATA.OUT".

Table A.4 Output File

08-10-1987
15:16:39

MOMENT ANALYSIS OF LINEAR PHARMACOKINETIC DATA

TIME	TABLET CONCENTRATION	TIME	SOLUTION CONCENTRATION
0.02	3.10	0.02	47.54
0.03	11.35	0.03	88.97
0.05	23.39	0.05	124.91
0.07	38.09	0.07	155.95
0.08	54.54	0.08	162.60
0.17	142.07	0.17	265.03
0.25	210.71	0.25	291.71
0.33	250.17	0.33	288.87
0.42	264.73	0.42	271.71
0.50	262.06	0.50	248.81
0.58	249.12	0.58	224.82
0.67	231.07	0.67	202.09
0.75	211.35	0.75	181.65
1.00	158.06	1.00	135.59
1.50	99.12	1.50	90.20
2.00	74.38	2.00	70.02
3.00	50.11	3.00	47.84
4.00	35.07	4.00	33.52
5.00	24.61	5.00	23.52
6.50	14.47	6.50	13.83
8.00	8.51	8.00	8.13
10.00	4.19	10.00	4.01
12.00	2.07	12.00	1.97

CMAX OF THE SOLUTION IS = 291.71

TMAX OF THE SOLUTION IS = 0.25

AUC OF SOLUTION = 501.71

AUMC OF SOLUTION = 1164.60

MRT OF SOLUTION = 2.3213

CMAX OF THE TABLET IS = 264.73

TMAX OF THE TABLET IS = 0.42

AUC OF TABLET = 504.24

AUMC OF TABLET = 1227.75

MRT OF TABLET = 2.4349

MDT OF TABLET = MRT OF TABLET - MRT OF SOLUTION = 0.1136

REFERENCES

1. M. Gibaldi and S. Feldman, *J. Pharm. Sci.*, *56*, 1238 (1967).
2. F. Langenbucher, *J. Pharm. Pharmacol.*, *24*, 979 (1972).
3. J. G. Wagner, *J. Pharm. Sci.*, *58*, 1253 (1969).
4. J. G. Wagner, *Drug Intell. Clin. Pharm.*, *4*, 77 (1970).
5. J. G. Wagner, *Drug Intell. Clin. Pharm.*, *4*, 132 (1970).
6. K. A. Khan, *J. Pharm. Pharmacol.*, *27*, 48 (1975).
7. J. A. Goldsmith, N. Randall, and S. D. Ross, *J. Pharm. Pharmacol.*, *30*, 347 (1978).
8. K. A. Khan and C. T. Rhodes, *Pharm. Acta Helv.*, *47*, 594 (1972).
9. J. G. Wagner, *J. Pharm. Sci.*, *58*, 1953 (1969).
10. J. G. Wagner, *Biopharmaceutics and Relevant Pharmacokinetics*, Drug Intelligence Publications, Hamilton, Ill. (1974), pp. 115–120.
11. M. Gibaldi, *5th APhA/APS National Meeting Symposium*, Washington, D.C. (1968).
12. J. H. Gaddum, *Nature*, *156*, 143 (1945).
13. J. Moshonan, *J. Am. Stat. Assoc.*, *48*, 600 (1953).
14. C. Orr, Jr., *Particulate Technology*, Macmillan, New York (1966), pp. 12–18.
15. J. Berkson, *J. Am. Stat. Assoc.*, *48*, 565 (1953).
16. B. W. Lindgreen, *Statistical Theory*, Macmillan, New York (1962), pp. 89, 392.
17. H. Weintraub and M. Gibaldi, *J. Pharm. Sci.*, *59*, 1792 (1970).
18. K. G. Nelson and L. Y. Wang, *J. Pharm. Sci.*, *66*, 1758 (1977).
19. K. G. Nelson and L. Y. Wang, *J. Pharm. Sci.*, *67*, 86 (1978).
20. A. El-Yazigi, *J. Pharm. Sci.*, *71*, 1408 (1982).
21. A. El-Yazigi, *J. Pharm. Sci.*, *70*, 535 (1981).
22. F. Langenbucher, *J. Pharm. Pharmacol.*, *24*, 979 (1972).
23. J. R. Leary and S. D. Ross, *Int. J. Pharm.*, *17*, 193 (1983).
24. J. R. Leary, N. Randall, and S. D. Ross, *Int. J. Pharm.*, *15*, 1 (1983).
25. D. Gueurten, *Pharm. Acta Helv.*, *59*(9/10), 267 (1984).
26. J. W. Mauger, D. Chilko, and S. Howard, *Drug Dev. Ind. Pharm.*, *12*, 969 (1986).
27. J. G. Wagner, *Biopharmaceutics and Relevant Pharmacokinetics*, Drug Intelligence Publications, Hamilton, Ill. (1971), p. 89.
28. J. H. Wood, *Pharm. Acta Helv.*, *42*, 129 (1967).
29. R. M. J. Ings, in *Bioavailability Methodology and Regulation*, V. F. Smolen and L. Ball, eds., Wiley, New York (1984), p. 45
30. W. H. Barr, *Pharmacology*, *8*, 55 (1972).
31. H. Boxenbaum, *Drug Dev. Ind. Pharm.*, *8*, 1 (1982).
32. W. I. Higuchi, N. F. H. Ho, J. Y. Park, and I. Komiya, in *Proc. Edinburgh International Conference*, L. F. Prescott and W. S. Nimmo, eds., Adis Press, New York (1981), Ch. 5.

33. A. F. Hoffman, J. H. Pressman, and C. F. Code, *Drug Dev. Ind.* Pharm., *9*, 1077 (1983).
34. S. Kuna, *Arch. Int. Pharmacodyn. Ther.*, *152*, 79 (1964).
35. A. T. M. Serrajuddin and C. I. Jarowski, *J. Pharm. Sci.*, *74*, 142 (1985).
36. A. T. M. Serrajuddin and C. I. Jarowski, *J. Pharm. Sci.*, *74*, 148 (1985).
37. R. Groning and G. Heun, *Drug Dev. Ind. Pharm.*, *10*, 527 (1984).
38. G. Jobin, A. Cortot, J. Godbillon, M. Duval, J. P. Schoeller, J. Hirtz, and J. J. Bernier, *Br. J. Clin. Pharmacol.*, *19*, 97S (1985).
39. N. Vidon, D. Evard, J. Godbillon, M. Rongier, M. Duval, J. P. Scoeller, J. J. Bernier, and J. Hirtz, *Br. J. Clin. Pharmacol.*, *19*, 107S (1985).
40. J. Godbillon, D. Evard, N. Vidon, M. Duval, J. P. Schoeller, J. J. Bernier, and J. Hirtz, *Br. J. Clin. Pharmacol.*, *19*, 113S (1985).
41. A. B. Buch, W. H. Barr, N. L. Crocker, A. Lee, and H. L. Smith, in *Abstracts, 7th Annual Meeting, Graduate Research Association Students in Pharmaceutics*, Morgantown, W.Va. (1987), p. 3.
42. R. E. Notari, J. L. DeYoung, and R. H. Reunning, *J. Pharm. Sci.*, *61*, 135 (1972).
43. J. C. K. Loo and S. Riegelman, *J. Pharm. Sci.*, *57*, 918 (1968).
44. J. G. Wagner, *J. Pharm. Sci.*, *72*, 838 (1983).
45. K. K. H. Chan and M. Gibaldi, *J. Pharm. Sci.*, *74*, 388 (1985).
46. M. Gibaldi and D. Perrier, *Pharmacokinetics*, 2nd ed., Marcel Dekker, New York (1982), p. 433.
47. I. H. Patel, L. Bornemann, and W. A. Colburn, *J. Pharm. Sci.*, *74*, 359 (1985).
48. C. M. Metzler, G. L. Elfring, and A. J. McEwen, *Biometrics*, *30*, 562 (1974).
49. *SAS Users Guide*, SAS Institute, Cary, N.C. (1985).
50. D. J. Cutler, *J. Pharm. Pharmacol.*, *30*, 470 (1978).
51. S. Riegelman and P. Collier, *J. Pharmacokinet. Biopharm.*, *8*, 509 (1980).
52. K. Yamoaka, T. Nakagawa, and T. Uno, *J. Pharmacokinet. Biopharm.*, *6*, 547 (1978).
53. Y. Tanigawara, K. Yamoaka, T. Nakagawa, and T. Uno, *Chem. Pharm. Bull.*, *30*, 1088 (1982).
54. K. C. Yeh and K. C. Kwan, *J. Pharmacokinet. Biopharm.* *6*, 79 (1978).
55. R. K. Brazell and S. A. Kaplan, *J. Pharm. Sci.*, *72*, 713 (1983).
56. K. K. H. Chan and M. Gibaldi, *Eur. J. Clin. Pharmacol.*, *26*, 255 (1984).
57. K. Khoo, M. Gibaldi, and R. K. Brazell, *J. Pharm. Sci.*, *72*, 6 (1983).
58. A. Rescigno and G. Segre, *Drug and Tracer Kinetics*, Blaisdell/Wiley, New York (1966), p. 102.
59. L. Z. Benet and C. W. N. Chiang, in *Abstracts, 13th National Meeting APhA/APS*, Chicago (1972), vol. 2, no. 2, p. 169.
60. J. G. Wagner, *J. Pharmacokinet. Biopharm.*, *3*, 457 (1975).
61. W. R. Gillespie and P. Veng-Pedersen, *J. Pharmacokinet. Biopharm.*, *13*, 239 (1985).

62. D. J. Cutler, *J. Pharmacokinet. Biopharm.*, *6*, 265 (1978).
63. L. Z. Benet, *J. Pharm. Sci.*, *61*, 536 (1972).
64. W. R. Gillespie and P. Veng-Pedersen, *Biopharm. Drug Dispos.*, *6*, 351 (1985).
65. J. G. Wagner, *Biopharmaceutics and Relevant Pharmacokinetics*, Drug Intelligence Publications, Hamilton, Ill. (1971), p. 108.
66. D. J. Cutler, *J. Pharmacokinet. Biopharm.*, *6*, 243 (1977).
67. J. G. Wagner, *Biopharmaceutics and Relevant Pharmacokinetics*, Drug Intelligence Publications, Hamilton, Ill. (1971), p. 72.
68. J. G. Wagner, W. Veldkamp, and S. Long, *J. Am. Pharm. Assoc. Sci. Ed.*, *47*, 681 (1958).
69. J. G. Wagner, *J. Am. Pharm. Assoc. Sci. Ed.*, *49*, 179 (1960).
70. C. M. Gruber, A. S. Ridolfo, and W. A. Tosick, *J. Am. Pharm. Assoc. Sci. Ed.*, *47*, 862 (1958).
71. W. H. Steinberg, G. H. Frey, J. N. Masci, and H. H. Hutchins, *J. Pharm. Sci.*, *54*, 747 (1965).
72. G. Levy, *J. Pharm. Sci.*, *50*, 388 (1961).
73. G. Levy, *J. Pharm. Sci.*, *52*, 1039 (1963).
74. J. T. Fell and G. A. Digenis, *Int. J. Pharm.*, *22*, 1 (1984).
75. J. D. Kelly, in *Radionuclide Imaging in Drug Research*, C. G. Wilson and J. G. Hardy, eds., Croom Helm, London (1982), p. 39.
76. P. B. Daly, S. S. Davis, M. Frier, J. G. Hardy, J. W. Kennerly, and C. G. Wilson, *Int. J. Pharm.*, *10*, 17 (1982).
77. C. G. Wilson, G. D. Parr, J. W. Kennerly, M. J. Taylor, S. S. Davis, J. G. Hardy, and J. Rees, *Int. J. Pharm.*, *18*, 1 (1984).
78. M. Jay, M. A. Woodward, and K. R. Brouwer, *J. Pharm. Sci.*, *74*, 1131 (1985).
79. R. M. Beihn and G. A. Digenis, *J. Pharm. Sci.*, *70*, 1325 (1981).
80. D. L. Casey, R. M. Beihn, G. A. Digenis, and M. B. Shambhu, *J. Pharm. Sci.*, *65*, 1412 (1976).
81. M. Alpsten, G. Ekenved, and L. Solvell, *Acta Pharm. Suec.*, *13*, 107 (1976).
82. G. A. Digenis, in *Radionuclide Imaging in Drug Research*, C. G. Wilson and J. G. Hardy, eds., Croom Helm, London (1982), p. 103.
83. A. Parr, M. Jay, G. A. Digenis, and R. M. Beihn, *J. Pharm. Sci.*, *74*, 590 (1985).
84. A. Parr, R. M. Beihn, and M. Jay, *Int. J. Pharm.*, *32*, 251 (1986).

ADDITIONAL READING

Aiache, J. M., J. C. Maublant, M. Dopogny et al., *S T P Pharma.*, *4*, 215 (1988).

Baumann, T. J., M. A. Smythe, K. Kaufmann et al., *Am. J. Hosp. Pharm.*, *45*, 1667 (1988).

Block L. H. and U. V. Banakar, *Drug Dev. Ind. Pharm.*, *14*, 2143 (1988).

Graffner, C., *Manuf. Chem.*, *60*, 50 (1989).

Jalal, I., E. Zmaily, and N. Najib, *Int. J. Pharm.*, *52*, 63, (1989).

Kaniwa, N., H. Ogata, N. Aoyagi et al., *J. Pharm. Sci.*, *78*, 1020 (1989).
Keseru, P., T. L. Paal, and E. Varsanyi, *Pharm. Ind.*, *51*, 532 (1989).
Khoury, N., J. W. Mauger, and S. Howard, *Pharm. Res.*, *5*, 495 (1988).
Lin, S. Y. and J. C. Yang, *Drug Dev. Ind. Pharm.*, *14*, 805 (1988).
Sande, S. A. and J. Karlsen, *Int. J. Pharm.*, *55*, 193 (1989).
Shah, V. P., N. W. Tymes, and J. P. Skelly, *Pharm. Res.*, *6*, 346, (1989).
Qiu, J. X., *J. China Pharm. Univ.*, *19*, 17 (1988).

SEVEN

Dissolution of Dosage Forms

INTRODUCTION

Dissolution testing of dosage forms (wherever applicable) is considered one of the most important quality control tools while assessing the efficacy of a product in vitro. The process of dissolution of an active ingredient from solid pharmaceutical dosage forms involves several intermediate physicochemical steps, such as wetting, swelling, capillarity, solubility, and diffusion. Among the most significant factors that control the process of dissolution are the type and nature of the dosage form within which the active ingredient is contained. Consequently, it is crucial for a pharmaceutical scientist to understand and appreciate the various intricacies associated with the dissolution of dosage forms, solid pharmaceuticals in particular. The various theories of dissolution discussed in Chapter 2 address primarily the process of dissolution employing ideal, uninterrupted conditions as well as mechanistic approaches. However, the real-life situation is often much more complicated. Additionally, these situations represent a collective picture of a multitude of factors operating concomitantly. These situations often call for a realistic approach that can satisfactorily explain the dissolution process of a solid dosage form. It is the intention in this chapter to present simplistic theories that satisfactorily explain the dissolution performance of dosage forms. To do so, we address the process(es) of dissolution of such dosage forms and identify the critical factors that not only influence, but also control, the dissolution process of the dosage form in question.

In this chapter we will focus on the dissolution of conventional solid dosage forms. However, in Chapter 8 we will address the various aspects of nonconventional solid dosage forms, particularly modified-release dosage forms, including sustained-, prolonged-, and controlled-release dosage units. Additionally, it must be noted that to avoid duplication, only aspects such as dissolution testing devices, commonly observed variables that influence the dissolution process, and so on, not covered elsewhere in the book and deemed most pertinent to the dissolution process of the dosage form in question are discussed. Readers are urged to review pertinent earlier chapters for a fuller coverage.

Dosage Form Dissolution

With the exception of nondisintegrating dosage forms, most solid dosage form(s) undergo a somewhat common sequence of events during the process of dissolution in vitro. These events can be delineated as three different types of descriptive categories (1):

1. Process parameters
2. Theoretical parameters
3. Dissolution testing device parameters

Each of these categories can be further subdivided into various classes, as shown in Table 7.1. Most of these classes are self-explanatory from the standpoint of their bearing on the process of dissolution of the solid dosage unit. However, it is crucial to further assess some of the modelistic (theoretical) parameters in light of the underlying factors common to the dissolution process of several solid dosage forms.

Wetting of Dosage Unit

The first step in the process of dissolution is the wetting of the external surface of the dosage form. The degree and the extent to which the surface is wetted are a function of the interfacial tension at the solid–liquid interface. Additionally, the process of wetting is a function of the contact angle (θ) the liquid makes with the solid surface. The value of $\theta \geqslant 90°$ is indicative of poor wetting characteristics of the solid surface. Few studies have been reported that examine the speed of wetting of the dosage form, a parameter that can potentially control the ultimate dissolution rate. However, Samyn and Jung (2) have indirectly correlated the speed of wetting with respect to the rate of penetration of liquid into a powder bed.

In a general case, dissolution of capsules containing powdered material was examined. Being hydrophilic, the gelatin shell dissolves rapidly in the dissolution medium (0.1 *N* HCl at 37°C). Consequently, the wetting associated with the dosage form is limited to the wetting and dispersion of the powder in the

Table 7.1 Descriptive Categories in the In Vitro Dissolution of Drug from Solid Dosage Forms

Process	Parameters modelistic (theoretical)	Dissolution testing device
Introduction of dosage form in dissolution medium	Wetting of dosage form	Type of device
Sampling	Penetration of dissolution medium into the dosage unit	Operating characteristics
Assay		Other controlling variables
	Deaggregation and/or deagglomeration	
	Wetting of the drug	
	Solubilization/dissolution of the drug	

Source: Ref. 1.

capsule shell. It stands to reason that the more hydrophobic the powder is, the slower the wetting and subsequent penetration of the dissolution medium across the solid surface barrier. Figure 7.1 illustrates this phenomenon, which can explain the dissolution profile that results from the presence of magnesium stearate in the formulation.

In the case of tablets, the hydrophobicity of the drug, the quantity of the drug incorporated, and the method of preparation (direct compression, slugging, etc.) can collectively and selectively cause wetting problems. It has been shown that granules prepared employing the wet granulation process can produce lower-contact angle values, a result attributed to the *hydrophilization* phenomenon associated with hydrophobic surfaces, thus promoting wetting. Additionally, the roughness of the hydrophobic surface can be instrumental in attaining high contact-angle values, thus limiting wetting (3).

Deaggregation/Deagglomeration

Most conventional solid dosage forms undergo some form of deaggregration and/or deagglomeration prior to dissolution. In most instances, deaggregation does not pose problems, if not reduce them in the process of dissolution. However, as indicated by Samyn and Jung (2), too much of hydrophobic ingredient such as talc or magnesium stearate, in a capsule formulation for example, can result in a plug formation that does not deaggregate quickly.

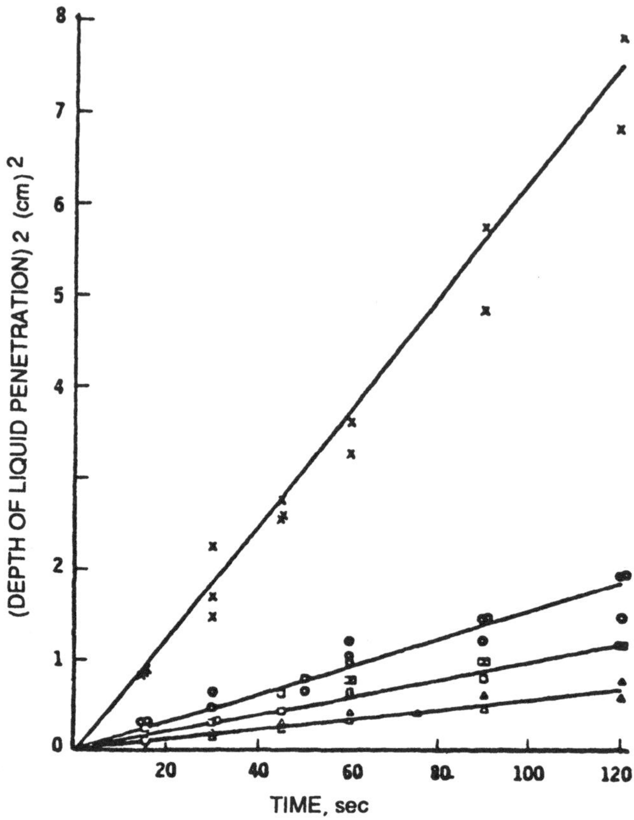

Fig. 7.1 Depth of liquid penetration in the presence of magnesium stearate. x, Lactose; ○, Lactose + 1% Mg stearate; □, Lactose + 2% Mg stearate; △, Lactose + 5% Mg stearate. (From Ref. 2.)

In such cases the *Washburn equation* can predict the time for deaggregation of a capsule:

$$D^2 = r\gamma \frac{\cos\theta}{2\eta} \tag{7.1}$$

where D is the depth of penetration, r the radius of the pore, θ the contact angle, γ the interfacial tension, and η the viscosity. This equation holds true when $\theta < 90°$. Accordingly, the time for deaggregation t' of a capsule of width w cm would then be

$$t' = \frac{(w/2)^2\eta 2}{r\gamma \cos\theta} \tag{7.2}$$

In most instances, r is a function of compaction. It implies that the greater the degree of compaction, the smaller will be the average pore radius, which results in larger time for deaggregation.

In the case of a tablet, the pore size through which the dissolution medium must penetrate to effect deaggregation is much smaller than in a capsule. To overcome this difficulty, disintegrants are employed to assure more efficient penetration and complete deaggregation. The disintegrants swell and result in physical breaking apart of the intact tablet.

It should be noted that a finite amount of time t' is necessary for penetration of dissolution medium into the pores followed by a finite time t^* to effect disintegration. Consequently, the disintegration time D_t can be given by

$$D_t = t^* + \frac{Q\eta}{r\gamma \cos\theta} \tag{7.3}$$

As t^* gets shorter, the smaller the pore radius r is. This is due to the fact that a certain swell volume of the disintegration results in a larger stress applied to a small volume of confinement (1).

The pore radius r is governed by compression force. Often the minimum is at such a low pressure that the general effect is that with an increase in the applied force of compression, there will be an increase in disintegration. Disintegrants, however, influence both r and $\cos\theta$, as illustrated in Fig. 7.2. The data on the process of disintegration imply that the weight of tablet remaining to be disintegrated is an exponential function of time (4,5):

$$M = M_0 e^{-qt} \tag{7.4}$$

where M_0 and M represent the mass of the intact tablet and mass of the tablet remaining to be disintegrated, respectively. This phenomenon is illustrated in Fig. 7.3. Other details associated with the dissolution of tablets and capsules are discussed in the following sections.

DISSOLUTION OF POWDERS

Powders are probably the only pharmaceutical dosage forms that closely approximate ideal conditions in the characterization of their dissolution. This is particularly true if they are processed in specific ways in order to obtain reasonably identical particles of known dimensions. In so doing, one can approximate, within limits, the characteristics of the powder as a whole, as well as evaluate the behavior of the particles undergoing dissolution. The process of dissolution of powders is a function not only of the particulate dimensions (size, shape, effective surface area, etc.), but also of the micromeritic proper-

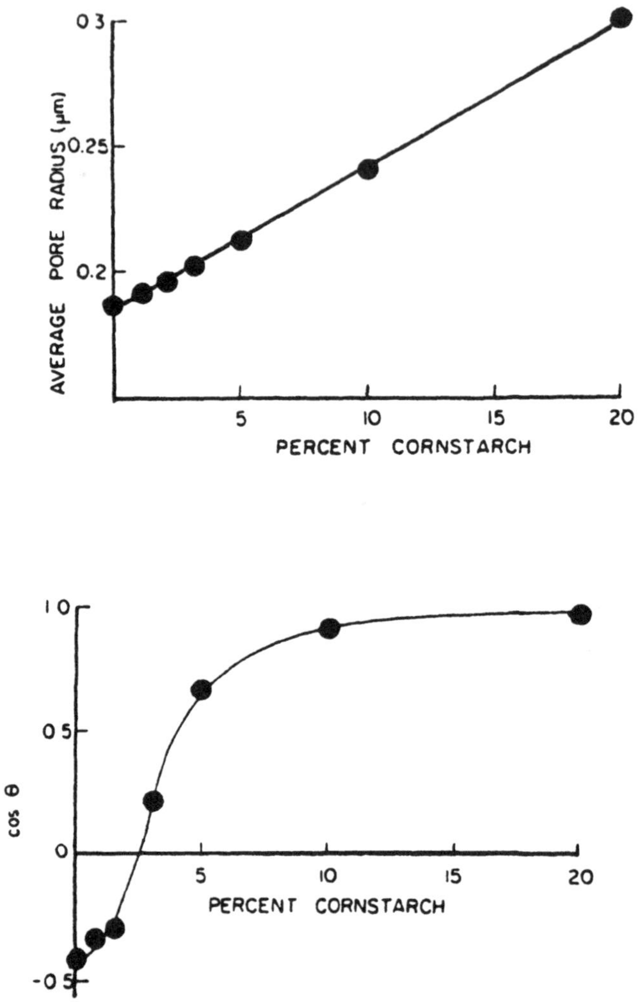

Fig. 7.2 Pore radius and contact angle as a function of percent cornstarch in the formulation (From Ref. 1.)

ties, such as particle-size distribution. Additionally, factors such as contact angle, wettability, and physicochemical properties of the drug particles have a significant bearing on the dissolution performance of the powder (6–21).

The rates and mechanisms involved in the dissolution of powders have been primarily based on monodispersed powders (6–9). For a drug consisting of uniformly sized particles, Hixson and Crowell (22) derived and expressed the

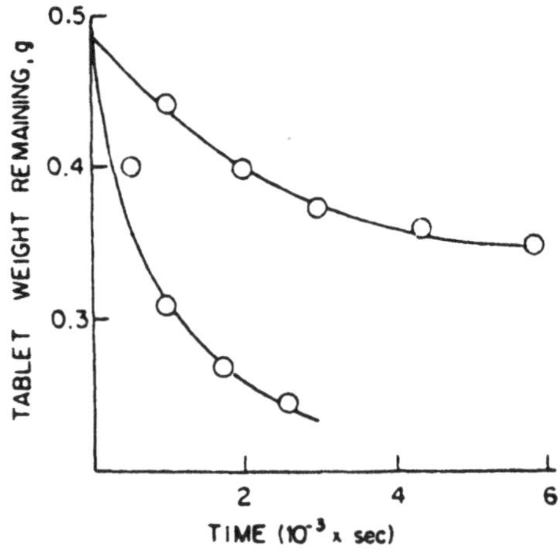

Fig. 7.3 Change in nondisintegrated tablet weight as a function of time. (From Ref. 4.)

rate of dissolution based on the cube root of the weight of the particle. The radius is not assumed to be constant (refer to Chapter 2 for details).

$$M_0^{1/3} - M^{1/3} = kt \qquad (7.5)$$

This expression is the *Hixson–Crowell cube-root law*.

Evaluation of models for single-particle dissolution based on multiparticulate dissolution data is often complicated by the distribution effect present when the particles are not truly monodispersed. In actuality, most powders exhibit a range of particle sizes. In such instances the particle-size distribution and the size and shape of the particles control the dissolution process.

A theoretical consideration of drug dissolution in relation to particle-size distribution was undertaken by Higuchi and Hiestand (19,23). Later, Brooke (16,24), and Pedersen and Brown (15) developed more exact expressions that permit calculation of spherical particles obeying log-normal distribution law. The equations derived for the amount of the substance (powder) to be dissolved as a function of time are based on the underlying assumptions: (a) particles in a multiparticulate system dissolve independently of each other, which can be approximated well under sink conditions, and (b) they dissolve in accordance with the same single-particle dissolution model having fixed parameters. Under these conditions, the ***intrinsic dissolution profile***, defined as dissolution curves having the same intrinsic dissolution rate, by a suitable scaling of time, can be brought into each other in a W/W_0 versus time plot, as shown in Fig. 7.4. W/W_0 is the ratio of the amount of powder dissolved to the initial amount of powder subjected to dissolution testing.

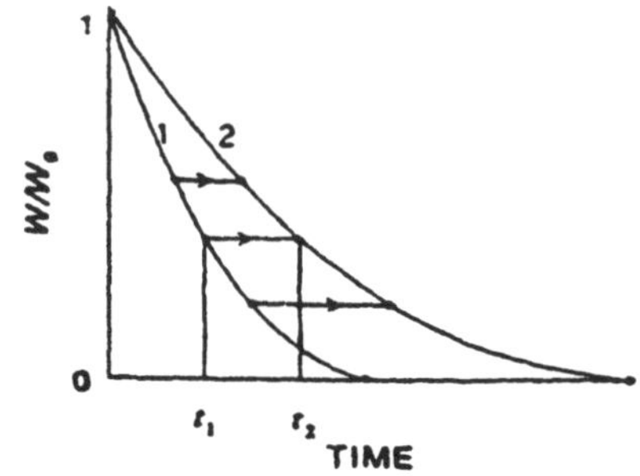

Fig. 7.4 Dissolution curves 1 and 2 that have same intrinsic dissolution profiles (refer to the text for details). (From Ref. 15.)

Pedersen and Brown (15) stated these rules as follows:

1. The intrinsic dissolution profile is independent of the rate parameter, i.e., the coefficient of time in the single-particle dissolution equation.
2. In two systems having identical particle-size distributions, the time-scaling factor that brings one dissolution curve into another is equal to the factor with which the rate parameters are proportionally related in the two systems.
3. Two powders dissolving according to the same single-particle dissolution model have the same intrinsic dissolution profile if their particle-size distributions are of the same shape on a logarithmic scale.
4. The intrinsic dissolution profile does not depend on the actual sizes of the particles but on their shape or distribution.

Dissolution patterns for powders obeying a log-normal distribution were presented by Carstensen and Musa (25), who refrained from an exact treatment of the subject since the expressions involved tended to become "analytically unmanageable." Brooke (11) derived a rigorously correct expression for dissolution profiles of log-normally distributed powders. The exact expression based on reasonable assumptions of sphericity and isotropic dissolution of particles under sink conditions requires no integration but can be evaluated by use of a calculator and readily available mathematical tables. The calculations tend to become a little tedious but can be accomplished without the use of a computer. The exact and rigorously correct expression for the weight undissolved (w) is

$$w = re^3\left(\mu + \frac{3\sigma^2}{2}\right)\left[1 - F\frac{\ln\tau - (\mu + 3\sigma^2)}{\sigma}\right]$$

$$- 3r\tau e^2(\mu + \sigma^2)\left[1 - F\frac{\ln\tau - (\mu + 2\sigma^2)}{\sigma}\right]$$

$$+ 3r\tau^2 e(\mu + \frac{\sigma^2}{2}) \left[1 - F \frac{\ln \tau - (\mu + \sigma^2)}{\sigma} \right]$$

$$- r\tau^3[1 - F \left[\frac{\ln \tau - \mu}{\sigma} \right] \tag{7.6}$$

where F is the shape factor, r the particle radius, and $\tau = 2kC_s t/\rho$, where k is the rate constant, C_s the saturation concentration (solubility), t the time interval, and ρ the density of the substance. μ and σ are the population parameters pertaining to the log-normal distribution, indicating μ to be the geometric mean diameter of the particle. A dissolution pattern resulting from this treatment along with its comparison with the earlier reported treatment (25) is shown in Fig. 7.5.

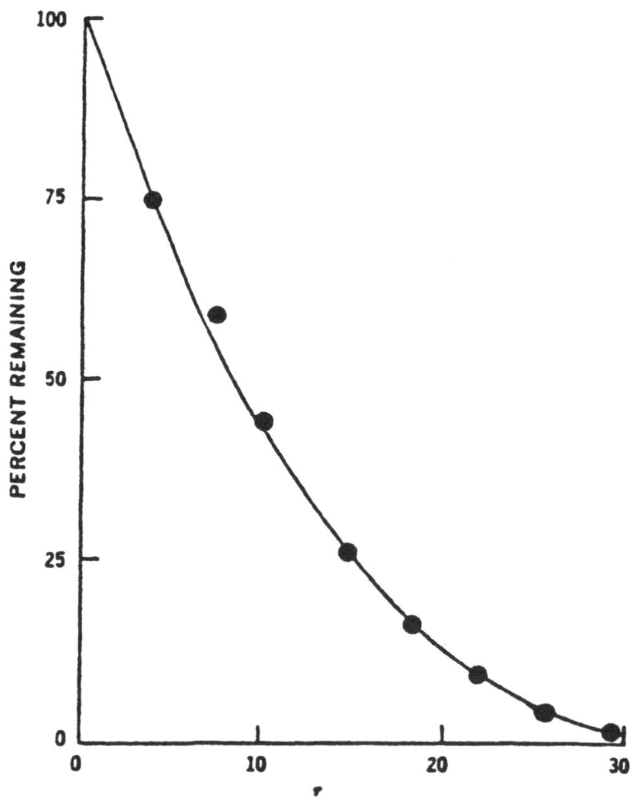

Fig. 7.5 Dissolution profile exhibited by powder with log-normal particle-size distribution with a geometric mean of 40 μm, $\mu = 3.6888$, and $\sigma = 0.03178$. (From Ref. 16.)

In most instances for simplicity, it is assumed that the particles are spherical even in a log-normally distributed sample. Relatively less attention is given in the literature to powders that contain not only finely divided multisized drug particles, but also nonspherical powders. Conventional theories assuming sphericity have limited practical value because pure drug particles are not spherical. Consequently, application of such theories to real particle systems is complicated as well as intricate. The visual approach has been to treat real particles as hypothetical spherical particles having the same surface area or volume. However, such approximations may introduce substantial errors.

Pedersen and Brown (14) derived equations for the isotropic dissolution of single particles, considering simple forms of six crystal systems as shown in Fig. 7.6. These can be summarized by three basic equations, which are approximated well, and in some cases exactly, by the dissolution equation for

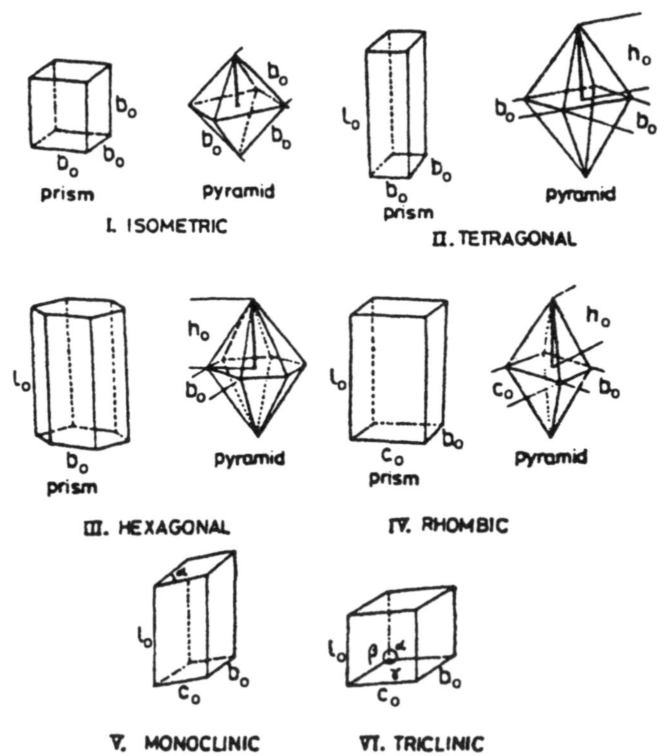

Fig. 7.6 Possible shapes of nonspherical particles. (From Ref. 14.)

a hypothetical spherical particle of specified diameter. These formulae, given in Table 7.2, enable calculation of the specified diameter and minimize weighted errors in the approximations. Table 7.2 also includes expressions for calculating the equivalent spherical diameter.

Later, Kitamori and Iga (13) further elucidated the effect of particle shape on the dissolution profile of a powder. They also discussed nonisotropic dissolution in the same report. An equation was derived for the dissolution of powders containing particles that were rectangular parallelepiped and log-normally distributed by introducing three-dimensional parameters instead of the diameter in the Brooke equation (11) for the spherical powder dissolution. By employing hypothetical values for constants in the equation, it can be shown that the smallest side length a of a particle greatly affects its dissolution profile. However, the other two side lengths, α_a and β_a, do not, even with rather large values of α and β. The Kitamori–Iga equation for the weight fraction dissolved, w, is given by

$$
\begin{aligned}
W = {} & F\frac{\ln(\tau/\mu) - 3\sigma^2}{\sigma} \\
& + \left(1+\frac{1}{\alpha}+\frac{1}{\beta}\right)(\tau/\mu)\exp(-5\sigma^2/2)\left[1-F\frac{\ln(\tau/\mu)-2\sigma^2}{\sigma}\right] \\
& - \left(\frac{1}{\alpha}+\frac{1}{\beta}+\frac{1}{\alpha\cdot\beta}\right)(\tau/\mu)^2\exp(-4\sigma^2)\left[1-F\frac{\ln(\tau/\mu)-\sigma^2}{\sigma}\right] \\
& + \left(\frac{1}{\alpha\beta}\right)(\tau/\mu)^3\exp(-9\sigma^2/2\left[1-F\frac{\ln(\tau/\mu)}{\sigma}\right]
\end{aligned}
\tag{7.7}
$$

The meaning of the various notations is explained for Eq. (7.6). The basic assumptions behind this theory are that the constituent particles are rectangular parallelepipeds that undergo isotropic dissolution under sink conditions.

It should be noted that particles undergoing dissolution lose their original physical dimensions. In doing so, they can result in changing particle-size distribution during the dissolution process. This dissolution rate can be expressed as the loss in diameter per unit time as given by

$$d_t = d_0 - kt \tag{7.8}$$

where d_t is the diameter at time t, d_0 is the initial diameter, and k is the dissolution rate constant. It is apparent from the equation that the dissolution rate is a linear function of the diameter loss of the particle. This aspect also needs to be addressed in conjunction with the other theories.

Table 7.2 Dissolution of Particle Forms, Including Expressions for Calculation of Equivalent Spherical Diameter

Crystal system	Exact dissolution expression (W/W_0 =)	Spherical approximation	Time length, t^*	Shape ratio,[a] F	Equivalent spherical diameter,[b] [a]
Prismatic particles[c]					
n-Gonal	$(1-Ft^*)(1-t^*)^2$	$\{1-[2-(2-F)^{1/3}]t^*\}^3$	$\left(\frac{2J}{b_0\rho}\tan\frac{\pi}{n}\right)t$	$\frac{b_0}{l_0}\cot\frac{\pi}{n}$	$\frac{b_0\cot(\pi/n)}{2-[2-b_0/l_0\cot\pi/n]^{1/3}}$
Tetragonal ($n=4$)	$(1-Ft^*)(1-t^*)^2$	$\{1-[2-(2-F)^{1/3}]t^*\}^3$	$\frac{2J}{b_0\rho}t$	$\frac{b_0}{l_0}$	$\frac{b_0}{2-(2-b_0/l_0)^{1/3}}$
Isometric ($n=4$, $b_0=l_0$)	$(1-Ft^*)(1-t^*)^2$	$\{1-[2-(2-F)^{1/3}]t^*\}^3$	$\frac{2J}{b_0\rho}t$	1	b_0
Hexagonal	$(1-Ft^*)(1-t^*)^2$	$\{1-[2-(2-F)^{1/3}]t^*\}^3$	$\frac{2\sqrt{3}J}{3b_0\rho}t$	$\sqrt{3}\frac{b_0}{l_0}$	$\frac{\sqrt{3}b_0}{2-[2-3(b_0/l_0)]^{1/3}}$

Rhombic	$(1-F_1t^*)(1-F_2t^*)(1-t^*)$	$\{1-[2-(2-F_1)^{1/3}(2-F_2)^{1/3}]t^*\}^3$	$\frac{2J}{b_0\rho}t$	$\frac{b_0}{c_0}, \frac{b_0}{l_0}$	$\frac{b_0}{2-(2-b_0/c_0)^{1/3}(2-b_0/l_0)^{1/3}}$
Monoclinic	$(1-F_1t^*)(1-F_2t^*)(1-t^*)$	$\{1-[2-(2-F_1)^{1/3}(2-F_2)^{1/3}]t^*\}^3$	$\frac{2J}{b_0\rho\sin\alpha}t$	$\frac{b_0}{c_0}, \frac{b_0}{l_0}\sin\alpha$	$\frac{b_0\sin\alpha}{2-(2-b_0/c_0)^{1/3}[2-b_0/l_0\sin\alpha]^{1/3}}$
Pyramidal particles					
n-Gonal (isometric, tetragonal, hexagonal)	$(1-t^*)^3$	—	$2J\frac{\sqrt{h_0^2+b_0^2/4}}{\rho}t$	—	$\frac{h_0b_0}{\sqrt{h_0^2+b_0^2/4}}$
Rhombic	$(1-Ft^*)(1-t^*)^2$	$\{1-[2-(2-F)^{1/3}]t^*\}^3$	$2J\frac{\sqrt{h_0^2+b_0^2/4}}{\rho}t$	$\frac{1}{4}+\frac{3}{4}\sqrt{\frac{h_0^2+c_0^2/4}{h_0^2+b_0^2/4}}$	$\frac{1}{[2-(2-F)^{1/3}]\sqrt{h_0^2+b_0^2/4}}$

Source: Ref. 4.

[a] When $f = 1$ [i.e., $b_0/l_0 = \tan(\pi/n)$].

[b] The diameter is equal to the biggest sphere the pyramid can contain. For n-gonal prismatic particles, $[a] = 2Jt/\{[2-(2-F)^{1/3}]\rho t^*\}$, for rhombic and monoclinic particles, $[a] = 2Jt/\{[2-(2-F_1)^{1/3}(2-F_2)^{1/3}]\rho t^*\}$.

[c] Structures I to VI in Fig. 7.6 illustrate the quantities b_0, c_0, l_0, and α used.

Wettability and Dissolution Rate of Powders

The first step in the process of dissolution is wetting of the dissolving surface, which is in contact with the dissolution medium. In order for wetting to occur, the dissolution medium should spread evenly and with relative ease over the dissolving surface. The surface tension of the solid, $\gamma_{S/A}$, will favor spreading of the liquid but is opposed by the solid–liquid interfacial tension, $\gamma_{S/L}$, the horizontal component of the surface tension of the liquid, $\gamma_{L/A}$, in the plane of the solid surface (i.e., $\gamma_{L/A} \cos\theta$, where θ is the contact angle made between the solid and the liquid). Equating these forces yields *Young's equation*:

$$\gamma_{S/A} = \gamma_{S/L} + \gamma_{L/A} \cos\theta \tag{7.9}$$

The condition for complete wetting of a solid surface is that the contact angle should be zero. This condition is fulfilled only when the forces of attraction between the liquid and solid are equal to or greater than those between liquid and liquid.

There is clearly a relationship between the ability of liquids to wet solid substances, as indicated by the magnitude of θ and the surface tension of the liquid. Various contact angles exhibited between liquid and solid surfaces are illustrated in Fig. 7.7. Extrapolation of plots of changes in contact angle as a function of surface tension to $\cos\theta = 1$ yields values for critical surface tension for spreading, γ_c. This value is a characteristic property of a solid and depends on polarity.

One frequent problem encountered when attempting to dissolve a powder in an aqueous medium (dissolution fluid) is the nonwetting of the powder. Some particles tend to float on the surface in clumps. Layers of air may adhere to the clumps, making the process of wetting even more difficult.

When a solid is immersed in a liquid, the initial wetting process that results is termed *immersional wetting*. The total decrease in surface free energy per unit area during immersional wetting can be quantified by $(\gamma_{S/A} - \gamma_{S/L})$. Substituting this expression in Eq. (7.9), which now can be written as

$$\frac{\Delta G}{a} = \gamma_{S/A} - \gamma_{S/L} = \gamma_{L/A} \cos\theta \tag{7.10}$$

where $\Delta G/a$ is the surface free energy per unit area.

It is apparent that the effectiveness of immersional wetting can be related to the contact angle that the solid makes with the liquid–air interface. The condition for complete immersion of the solid in the liquid is that there should be a decrease in surface free energy as a result of the immersion process. Only when $\theta < 90°$ is the term $(\gamma_{L/A} \cos\theta)$ positive, and the condition of complete immersion is fulfilled. Once the solid is submerged in the liquid, the process of spreading and subsequent wetting becomes important.

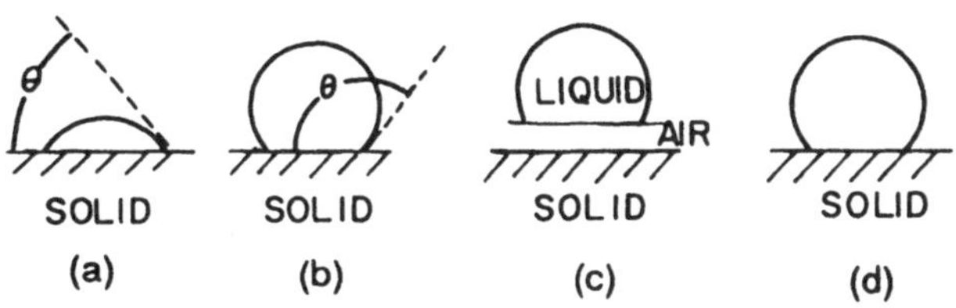

Fig. 7.7 Contact angles θ exhibited between liquid and solid surfaces: (a) good wettability; (b–d) poor wettability.

Wetting clearly plays a role in the dissolution of powders as well as other solid dosage forms (21,26–28). It is well known that improving the wettability of drug leads to less agglomeration of drug particles in contact with the liquid. Thus, the dissolution rate of the drug powder is increased because the surface area that is definitely wetted by the solvent is greater. Increasing wettability results in an evident increase of the effective surface area, which in turn leads to a higher dissolution rate.

Drugs possessing fairly good wettability, such as theophylline, amidopyrine, and phenazone, dissolve so fast in water that their concentration–time graphs increase as quickly as if drugs that are already dissolved are poured in the dissolution medium. Consequently, an evaluation of dissolution-rate constant is impossible for hydrophilic drugs. In most instances, for hydrophilic drugs it is assumed that dissolution rates follow zero-order kinetics until 20% of the used dose is dissolved.

Additionally, when the contact angle of a pharmaceutical powder is 40° or less, the resultant dissolution rates are not influenced by a decrease in the effective surface area caused by the agglomeration of the drug particles. Hence, it is assumed that in case of contact angles below 40°, the velocity of the solvent penetration into the powder agglomerates suffices to disperse the agglomerates almost instantaneously. Consequently, the powders then possess an effective surface area of 100%. Several other reports have been published addressing the various aspects of wetting and its importance in dissolution testing (29,30).

DISSOLUTION OF CAPSULES

Capsules are still considered to be the second most popular form of presentation of medicaments orally. Where all the ingredients are powders, a hard-gelatin capsule is used, but where the materials form a liquid, they are contained in a soft-gelatin shell. The use of hard gelatin capsules is almost axiomatic in the preliminary pharmacologic study of a new drug before any technological study is even contemplated. A schematic representation via which a capsule undergoes dissolution and presents its contents to the gastrointestinal medium is given in Fig. 7.8.

It is apparent from the figure that capsules must have the capsule shell dissolved before the contents are available to the gastrointestinal fluids for dissolution irrespective of it being a hard- or a soft-gelatin capsule. While capsule mass might behave as a tablet, if it is very compact it is more likely that the capsule contents will behave like a suspension and distribute quickly into the gastrointestinal fluids. Additionally, since capsules must allow the drug to go into solution for absorption to occur, the kinetics of drug release from this dosage form can be critical to its therapeutic success. Capsules contain not only the drug in solid form, but also other inert ingredients that are necessary for the manufacture, as well as the physical and chemical stability, of the dosage form. Both the manufacturing process itself and the inert ingredients in the final product can affect the dissolution rate of the drug from the dosage form. Even for a given drug in the same dosage form, it is possible to have a wide range in both the rate and the amount dissolved from capsules prepared by different manufacturers.

The fine particles placed in a capsule are usually not subjected to high compressional forces and possible fusion, which would reduce the specific surface area. A large effective surface area will be available for dissolution pro-

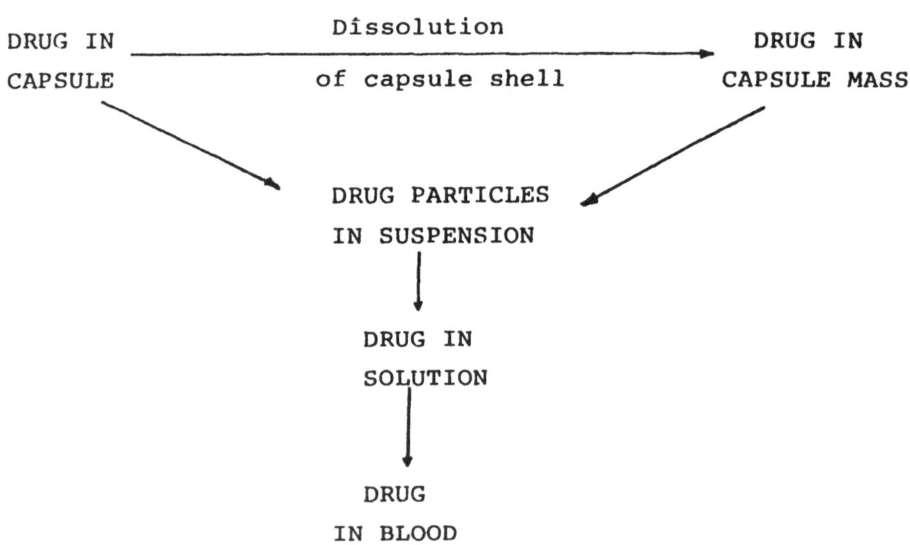

Fig. 7.8 Scheme for dissolution of capsule dosage form.

vided that the particles in a capsule are intimately wetted by the biological fluids.

The gelatin shell surrounding the drug in a capsule dosage form is usually of negligible importance as a barrier to the dissolution process. Recent studies suggest that a lag time of 10 to 20 min will be observed before measurable absorption occurs after the administration of a hard-gelatin capsule. The time-lag phenomenon is of little importance for most drugs. However, hard-gelatin capsules of the rapidly absorbed drug aspirin have been shown to be more variable in release rate in vivo than are tablets (31). Recently, El-Yazigi (32) reported a method describing the characterization of the dissolution of the capsule shell together with the dissolution rate of tetracycline–HCl from four capsule products under various conditions. The dissolution rate of the gelatin shell was determined by measuring the shell-rupture time, employing a modified version of a twin-blade-stirrer dissolution apparatus (33).

Depending on the physicochemical characteristics of the drug to be placed in the capsule shell, various other ingredients are incorporated in the formulation. These inert excipients can influence the dissolution behavior, both rate and extent, of the drug. For instance, it is important to have a suitable diluent in a capsule dosage form of a poorly soluble drug. An inert hydrophilic diluent serves to disperse the hydrophobic drug particles, increase the permeation rate of aqueous fluid to the contents of the gelatin capsule, minimize clumping of the drug particles in contact with the dissolution media, and optimize the effective surface area. The presence of a wetting agent in addition to a hydrophilic diluent is often advantageous, provided that the drug is stable in the stomach. Figure 7.9 depicts the change in dissolution rate that can be affected by the incorporation of a diluent.

It must be noted that the diluent must be truly inert and have no tendency to adsorb or interact with the drug. For example, a possible effect of diluent–drug interaction is observed when dicalcium phosphate is employed as a vehicle for tetracycline. As dissolution occurs, a poorly soluble and poorly absorbable calcium–tetracycline complex forms at the interface and the physiological availability of the antibiotic is markedly reduced (34). It is imperative that extensive studies addressing drug–diluent interaction(s) be undertaken before a suitable diluent is selected for use in a capsule formulation. Other factors that may influence bioavailability from capsule dosage forms include particle size, selection of diluents and fillers, adsorption, and other interactions of drug and fillers and crystal form of drug.

Capsule formulations have received considerably less attention in their critical evaluation of dissolution performance than tablets, presumably because of their apparent simplicity and consideration as loose powders. It has been repeatedly eluded that although the hard gelatin capsule is widely used in pre-

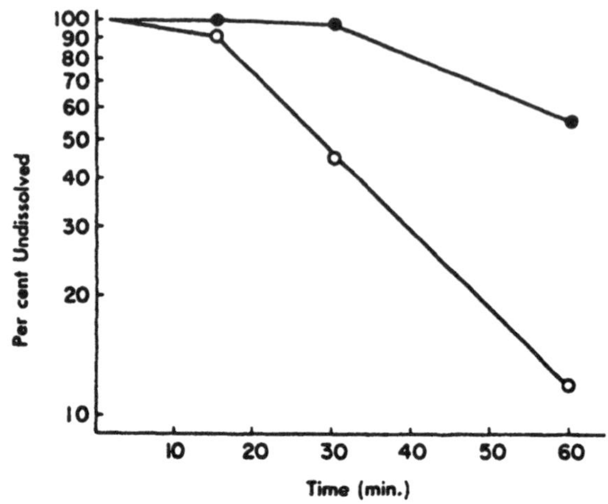

Fig. 7.9 Dissolution performance of capsules containing drug alone (●) and drug along with excipients (○). (From. Ref. 31.)

liminary studies of a new drug, very little literature on drug availability, even in vitro, exists for this type of dosage form. Only as recently as 1985, the USPXX/NFXV included an official disintegration test procedure for capsules. It is not surprising, therefore, that a review of the literature reveals a paucity of information in this area.

Formulation and process variables play a determining role in drug release from capsules and its subsequent availability for absorption. The solubility of the major component, drug or excipient, affects the rate and mechanism of drug release (35), whereas lubricants introduce hydrophobicity (36,37) and/or slug softening (38), which influence disintegration and dissolution. With fully automatic capsule-filling machines in which capsule contents are actually compressed, often to form tabletlike slugs, machine variables such as compression force and its effect on slug hardness may also affect disintegration and dissolution (39).

Even though investigators have often pointed out the importance of the rate of deaggregation of the powder mass before dissolution (40,41), few reports can be found dealing with the role of disintegrants in capsule formulations, particularly on the dissolution characteristics (36,37,42). Recently, Botzolakis et al. (43) compared super-disintegrants with starch in capsules filled on an automatic capsule-filling machine and found that in vitro drug release was improved by as much as tenfold. Botzolakis and Augsburger (44) investigated the efficacy of various disintegrants on hydrochlorothiazide dissolution from soluble (lactose) and insoluble (dicalcium phosphate) fillers at various concentrations and compression forces. Analysis of dissolution data by a three-way analysis of variance revealed that all the major factors such as disintegrant, compression force, lubricant and/or diluent, and their interactions were significant. Figures 7.10 and 7.11 depict the influence of compression force and various disintegrants on hydrochlorothiazide dissolution from capsule formulations, respectively.

Attention has also been focused on the penetration of dissolution medium into the powder bed of the capsule in predicting the dissolution characteristics

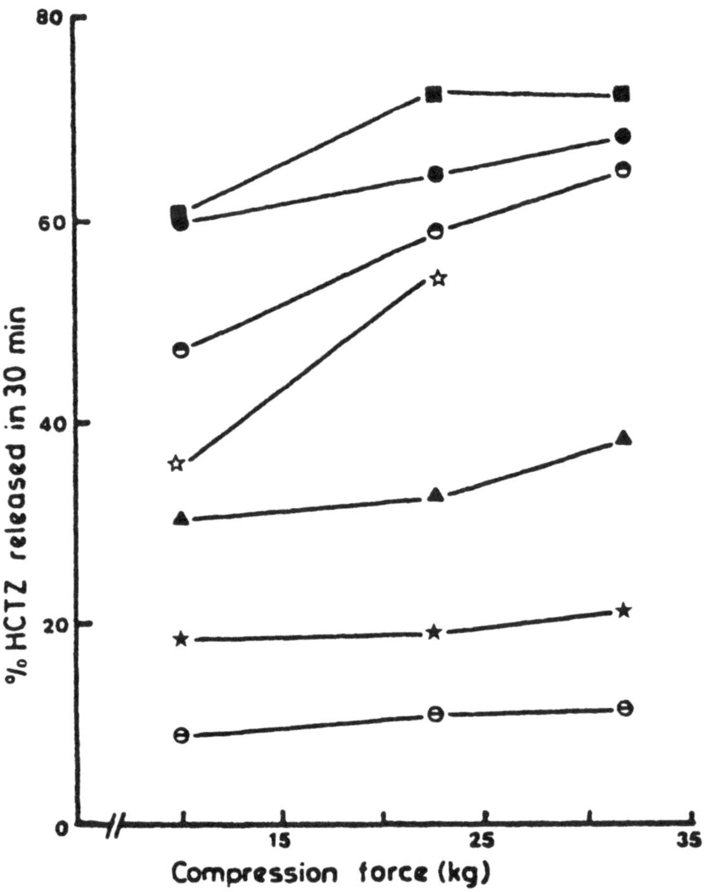

Fig. 7.10 Effect of compression force on the dissolution of hydrochlorothiazide (HCTZ) from dicalcium phosphate (CDL-2)-based capsules containing 1% magnesium stearate. Ac-Di-Sol: 4%, ◓; 6%, ●. CDL-2: 4%, ▲; 6%, ■. Primojel: 4%, ★; 6%, ☆; control, ⊖. (From Ref. 44.)

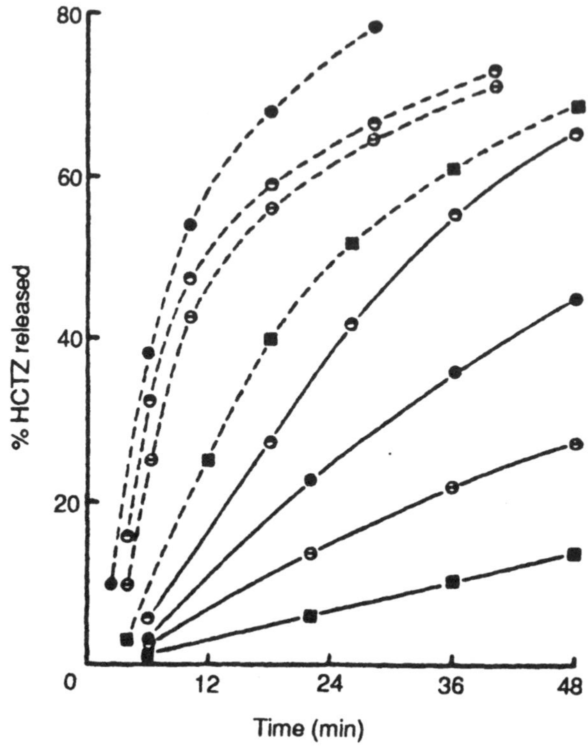

Fig. 7.11 Influence of 4% disintegrant on HCTZ dissolution form anhydrous lactose (----)- or CDL-2 (—)-based capsules containing 1% magnesium stearate. Ac-Di-Sol, ⊖; CDL-2, ●; Primojel, ⊖; control, ■. (From Ref. 44.)

and thereby the release rate of drugs from hard-gelatin capsules. In such an attempt, Samyn and Jung (2) concluded that extended dissolution rates are obtained with powder blends that exhibit reduced liquid penetration. However, this may not always be the case. Poor liquid penetration does not necessarily ensure poor dissolution of the drug from the capsule. The blend that allows no liquid penetration does, however, have the lowest dissolution. According to Rowley and Newton (45), rapid liquid penetration does not ensure good dissolution characteristics, where the presence of wetting agent readily promotes liquid penetration but does not assist dissolution. It should be noted that the liquid penetration test can only assist in the screening of wetting agents, but its extension to the prediction of drug release from capsules may not be possible.

More recently, attention has been oriented toward a dissolution test for both hard- and soft-gelatin capsules containing oily formulations. Neisingh et al., (46) have described a convenient and reproducible dissolution method for soft-

and hard-gelatin capsules containing testosterone undecanoate in oleic acid. The method employs a flow-through dissolution cell and a dissolution medium, the composition of which was optimized for both its capacity to dissolve the gelatin capsule wall completely and to give homogeneous filtrates of drug and oily excipient for convenient analysis of the fractions collected. The discriminating power of the dissolution method for oily formulations was tested with three batches of the commercial formulation Andriol and with two experimental formulations. The commercial products exhibited essentially biphasic dissolution patterns with complete dissolution within 45 min. The remaining formulations yielded dissolution over a much prolonged period of time.

In the case of soft-gelatin capsules, the rotating-bottle method is employed widely to evaluate the dissolution behavior. A rationale for using this method, along with examples, are given by Withey and Manville (47). Their dissolution studies on 13 brands of commercial chloramphenicol capsules, using modified USP dissolution apparatus, showed the soft-gelatin capsule brand to release approximately 25% of its drug content in 30 min, while hard-gelatin capsule brands B2 and D released 100.7% and 87.2%, respectively. Upon change to a rotating bottle method, the 30-minute recoveries were 100% from soft-gelatin capsules brand, 82% from brand B2, and 70% from brand D. Unfortunately, none of these studies have been correlated with bioavailability data, and thus the significance of the difference in results between the two dissolution methods is yet unclear. The difference could be attributed to greater agitation by the bottle method and less opportunity for the capsule to adhere to the sides or the bottom of the apparatus. The effect of several variables on soft gelatin capsule dissolution is discussed by Hom et al. (48), who indicate that the degree of agitation, the pH of the dissolution medium, and the presence or absence of pepsin in the medium are important to the dissolution of soft-gelatin capsules.

The overall process of dissolution testing of capsule dosage form appears to be relatively simple and straightforward. However, there are some major drawbacks and problems associated with the dissolution testing of capsules that can significantly alter their dissolution process. One of the more significant problems is floating of the dosage form during the dissolution test. This problem is usually circumvented by localizing the dosage unit (capsule) at a convenient position in the dissolution medium. This is achieved by either restraining the capsule in a stainless-steel gauge or by allowing the capsule to move in a very restricted volume (e.g., a dissolution basket). Most often, this results in uneven, nonuniform dissolution of the gelatin capsule shell, which does not permit uniform access of the medium within the contents of the capsule. Consequently, the apparent dissolution performance is under less than ideal conditions. Additionally, the dissolving gelatin shell sometimes tends to clog the pores of the basket or form barrier film along the outer surface of the restrainer. This results in an apparent increase in lag time before the shell gets ruptured and the contents are made available for absorption. In many instances, poor in vitro–in vivo correlations as well as uncomparable rank-order correlations can be attributed to the prevalance of a sum total of the multitude of such effects during the dissolution process of capsules. Currently, there is an upsurge of research activity looking closely at the various factors, including their intensity, that influence the dissolution testing of capsules, especially now that official compendia have set guidelines for the capsule dissolution test.

DISSOLUTION OF TABLETS

Compressed tablets still enjoy the status of being the most widely used dosage form. Tablets are solid dosage forms of medicinal substances usually prepared with the aid of suitable pharmaceutical adjuncts. Due to their very nature, the active ingredient is uniformly dispersed within the contents of the formulation. Consequently, it stands to reason that all factors that influence the physicochemical properties of the dosage form will influence the dissolution performance of the drug from tablets.

There are primarily two pathways via which the drug entity is made available to the dissolution medium. Either the tablet disintegrates thereby exposing the drug contents to the medium or the dissolution process continues without the disintegration of the tablet. Hence for the purpose of understanding the dissolution of tablets, they can be classified as either disintegrating or nondisintegrating solids. A schematic representation of both pathways is combined and presented in Fig. 7.12.

The rate of dissolution of a drug substance in solid form from a granule or a tablet depends to a large extent on its solubility in the solvent phase and its concentration in that phase. The rationale for testing solid dosage forms in vitro is considered in Chapter 1. Suffice it to say that the test conditions should provide a reasonable challenge to the dosage form in terms of degree of agitation, temperature, volume and pH of the dissolution medium. Additionally, factors such as wetting characteristics of the solid dosage forms, the penetration ability of the dissolution medium into the dosage forms, the swelling process, disintegration and deaggregation are critical during the dissolution testing of such dosage forms, tablets in particular.

It is apparent from Fig. 7.13 that the surface area of the solid dosage form (tablet) will change during the dissolution process. The change in surface area will alter the fluid flow dynamics involved in the dissolution rate constant. Such an effect is more pronounced in disintegrating dosage forms than in non-

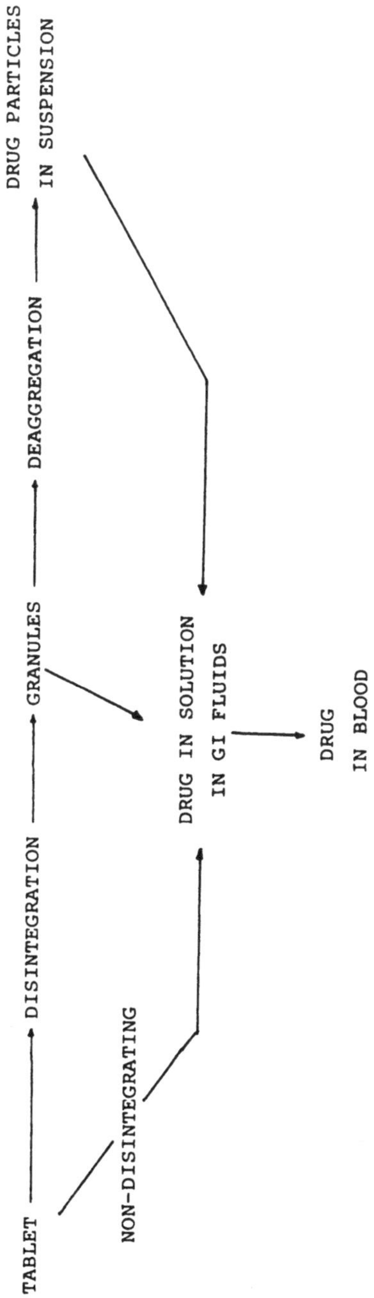

Fig. 7.12 Scheme for dissolution of tablet dosage form.

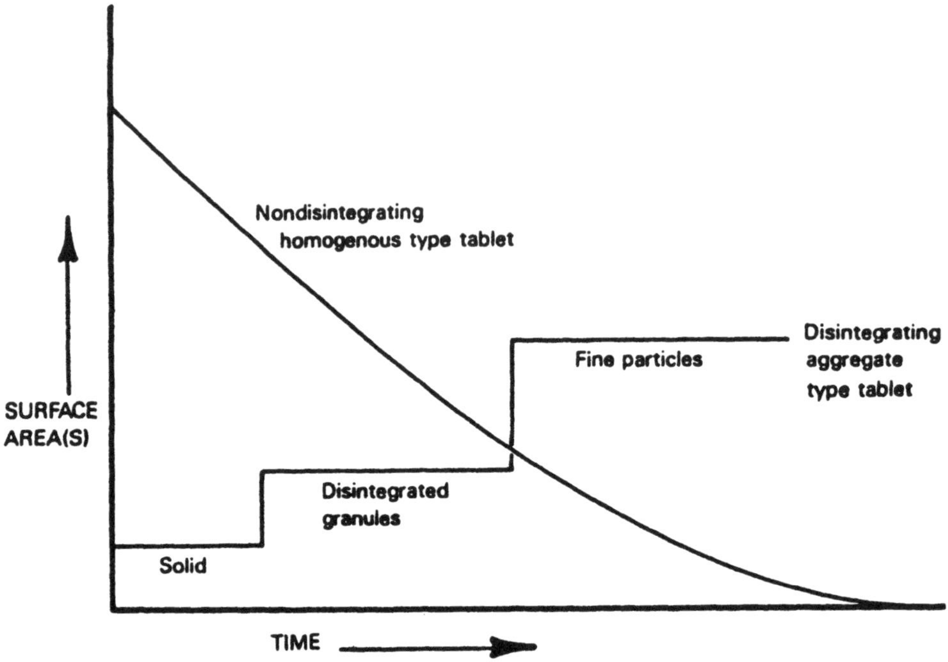

Fig. 7.13 Change in surface area with time for solids of nondisintegrating and disintegrating types.

disintegrating types. Nondisintegrating dosage forms gradually reduce their surface area during the dissolution process. Disintegrating forms, however, are subject to complicated disintegration and deaggregation as they release particles of various sizes and specific gravities into the solvent stream. The general dissolution process focusing on the change in surface area as a function of time for both disintegrating and nondisintegrating tablets is shown in Fig. 7.14. It shows particularly how surface area may vary during dissolution testing of homogeneous nondisintegration compared to nonhomogeneous disintegrating dosage forms.

The dissolution curve of a disintegrating solid does not change as abruptly, as depicted in Fig. 7.14. However, as the processes of disintegration into granules and deaggregation into fine particles take place, significant changes in the slope of the dissolution curve do occur. Any one of the three processes—disintegration, deaggregation, and dissolution—may vary in time. In some instances, one or the other may be rate limiting. When the disintegration time is rate limiting, the standard USP/NF disintegration test may correlate well with bioavailability data (49). Turbulent agitation is unsatisfactory for dosage

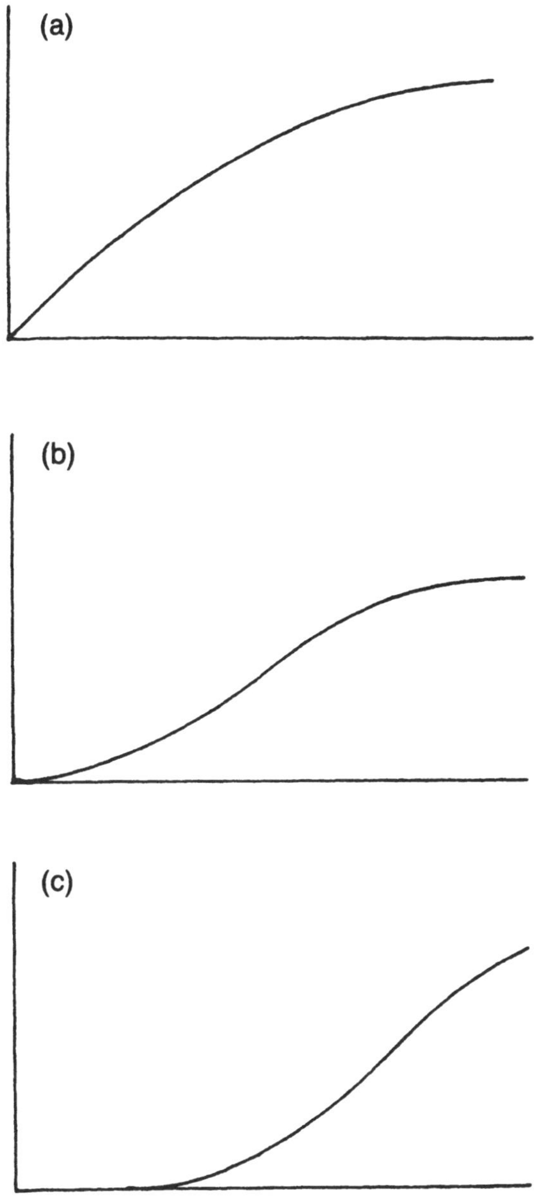

Fig. 7.14 Paths of the general dissolution process for tablets. Ordinates, concentration of ingredient dissolved; abscissas, time. (a) Nondisintegrating tablet; (b) rapidly disintegrating tablet; (c) slowly disintegrating tablet.

forms in which the process of dissolution is rate limiting. Since disintegration time is included in the total dissolution time, the Pharmacopoeial Forum in 1981 proposed elimination of the standard disintegration test.

The rate of shear of fresh dissolution medium in contact with the surface area of the solid varies with particle size, shape and density. Therefore, the flow dynamics and the surface area are indirectly related. Usually, the dissolution rate increases with decrease in particle size. However, in certain instances there may be mutual interference in the particulate motion, changes in electrical potential between particles, molecular layers of solvent tightly bound around particles, and other retarding influences, including greater influence of hydrophobic properties imparted to the liquid–solid interface by various means. In such cases, smaller particles may exhibit slower dissolution rates in actuality (50). It is thus evident that the flow dynamics of a multiparticulate mixture will be highly complex. Figure 7.15 represents typical dissolution profiles exhibited by various solids of nondisintegrating and disintegrating aggregate types.

The solid–liquid shear will change as the particle drifts in the fluid stream and the mass of the individual particle decreases. Hence repeatability of disso-

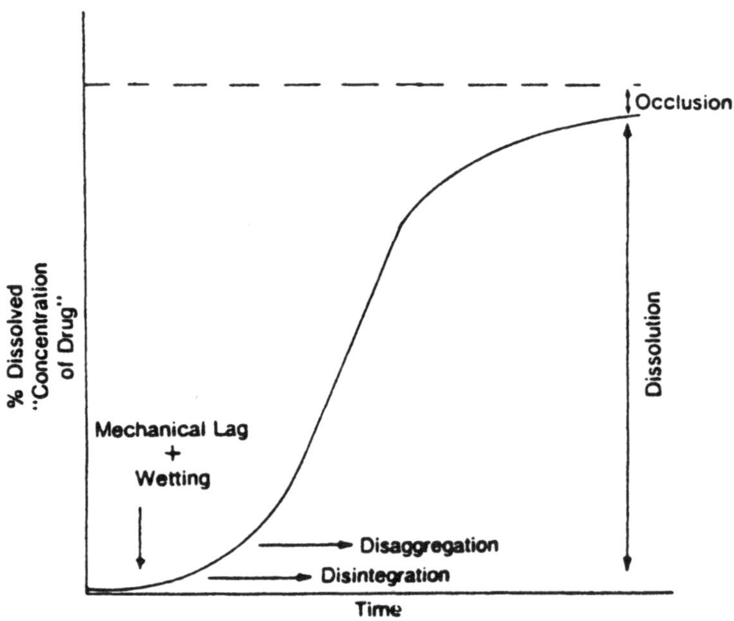

Fig. 7.15 Typical S-shaped dissolution profile of solid dosage form. (From Ref. 1.)

lution test data will not be acceptable, if the size of the particles released from aggregates varies substantially from sample to sample. A choice of the compendial methods will be crucial to minimize the intensity of this variable. Entirely different dissolution data might be expected with the basket, for example, between a solid that remains in the basket and a disintegrating solid, whose particles could become small enough to pass through the standard 40-mesh screen, drop to the bottom of the flask, and remain in random, stationary positions undisturbed by the mild agitation inherent in the basket method.

When the paddle method is employed, particles of different size and shape can float in different patterns. The particles may even accumulate at the bottom of the flask if the paddle is not centered exactly. Other factors, such as aberrations resulting from the geometrically imperfect contours of the rounded bottom of the flask can also introduce flow dynamics that deter true dissolution of solid particles. Flow dynamics related to the surface are generated by the particle size of the solid, and that relationship must be considered carefully both when selecting a dissolution test procedure and in outlining its protocol.

Carstensen (51) has proposed a general model that describes the dissolution curve of solid dosage forms, as shown in Fig. 7.16. This model incorporates the intermediate steps such as wetting, disintegration, and deaggregation, observed during the dissolution process. However, it appears that this model fits better for a disintegrating type of solid dosage unit.

The wetting of the solid surface of the dosage form controls the liquid access to the solid surface. Often, wetting of the solid dosage form is the limit-

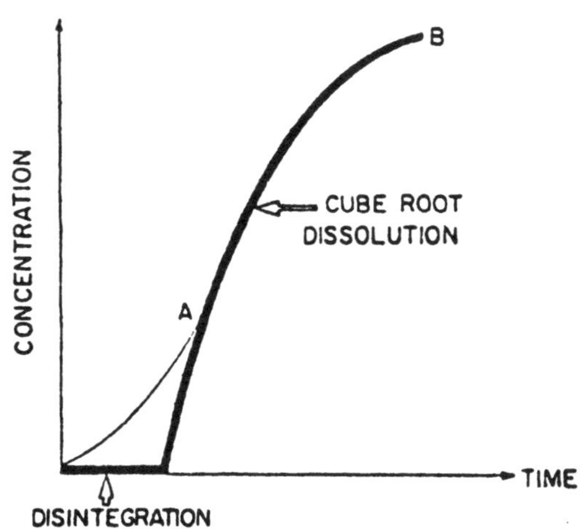

Fig. 7.16 Dissolution profile exhibited by directly compressed or slugged tablet formulation.

ing factor in the dissolution process. The speed of wetting is directly dependent on the interfacial tension and the contact angle between the solid surface and the dissolution medium. As indicated earlier, a contact angle of $>90°$ is indicative of poor wettability. Incorporation of a surfactant, either in formulation or in the dissolution medium, enhances dissolution by lowering the contact angle. Additionally, presence of air in the dissolution medium causes air bubbles to be entrapped in the tablet pores, which act as a barrier at the interface between the solid surface and the dissolution medium. Once the solid dosage form disintegrates into granules or aggregates, penetration characteristics of the dissolution medium play a prime role in the deaggregation process. Lubricants employed in tablet formulations, which are usually hydrophobic in nature, retard the rate of penetration and thereby the deaggregation process. A large pore size facilitates penetration; however, an extremely large pore size may inhibit penetration by decreasing the internal strain caused by the swelling of the disintegrant. Following deaggregation and dislodgment, the drug particles become exposed to the dissolution medium and dissolution proceeds via one or many of the different theories presented in Chapter 2.

Tablet Dissolution in Dissolution Apparatus

There is a relative abundance of literature addressing dissolution of tablets in various dissolution apparatus. However, the most pertinent tablet dissolution characterization within the scope of this book would be the elucidation of the dissolving of tablets employing the standard USP basket dissolution apparatus. Hence our discussion will focus on this aspect. This phenomenon has been studied rather extensively by Carstensen et al. (52,53) as well as by Nelson and Wang (54,55). Release of an active ingredient from a tablet involves two distinct processes: disintegration of the tablet and dissolution of the active ingredient. Although both processes commence when the tablet encounters an aqueous environment, the bulk of the active ingredient cannot dissolve until disintegration has occurred. The two processes are thus sequential and occur simultaneously until the tablet has disintegrated completely. Nelson and Wang deducted disintegration behavior from dissolution behavior, while Carstensen and co-workers did the opposite, both resulting in fairly similar conclusions, based on the above-mentioned premise.

Carstensen et al., (53) attempted to explain the basic steps involved in dissolution of a directly compressed tablet in a USP basket dissolution apparatus. They concluded that in general cases, a directly compressed tablet will disintegrate into particles from which the original blend was made. Following the disintegration time, t_1, the particles will dissolve according to a cube-root law. The amount dissolved as a function of time will therefore have an S shape if the disintegration time is not very short, as shown in Fig 7.16. The segment of

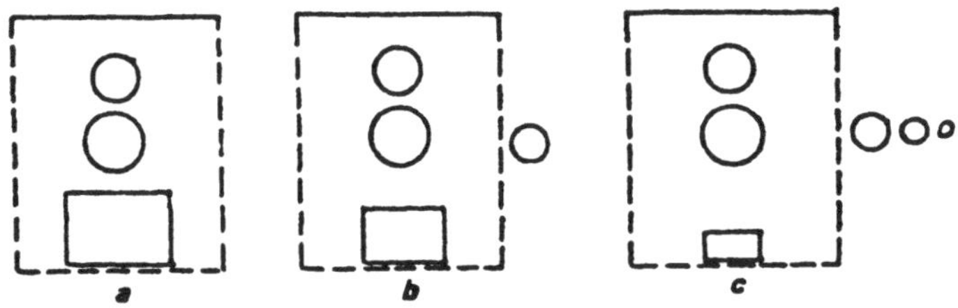

Fig. 7.17 Schematic illustration of a tablet in a basket dissolution apparatus at various stages (refer to the text for details concerning phases of dissolution). (From Ref. 53.)

the S-shaped profile corresponding to the cube-root dissolution-rate curve can be expressed as

$$M_0^{1/3} - M^{1/3} = k(t - t_1) \tag{7.11}$$

where M is the amount of drug yet to be dissolved, M_0 the initial amount of drug, and k the overall cube-root rate constant.

They attempted further to explain the entire process of dissolution of compressed tablets in USP dissolution apparatus by proposing the following model. The dissolution process can be examined in three phases as shown in Fig. 7.17. The first phase comprises the dislodging of the particles from the tablet. The resultant particles have not yet decreased sufficiently in size to pass through the basket which has an opening (Fig. 7.17, phase a). The dimensions of this opening for the USP basket will correspond to a diameter of 0.042 cm, or 40-mesh screen. The dislodged particles will then decrease in size according to the cube-root law provided that they are isometric and that sink conditions prevail.

The second phase is at time points where the earlier dislodged particles have completely dissolved as illustrated in Fig. 7.17, phase b. The third and the final phase comprises of more disintegration than in phase b and the particles formed earlier have completely dissolved (Fig. 7.17, phase c).

Expressions explaining the three phases can be generated and can elucidate further the meaning of the dissolution curves. The interested reader is advised to refer the original work (Ref. 53) for derivation and detailed explanation of the equations involved. Suffice it to say that this model explains the original shape of the dissolution curve. Furthermore, it also provides an insight into the log linearity observed for the undissolved mass as a function of time past the lag time (disintegration time).

If one assumes that after dislodgment, the drug particles are exposed to the dissolution medium and that dissolution then takes place by a cube-root law,

$$M^{1/3} - M_0^{1/3} = K^*t \tag{7.12}$$

where K^* is the cube-root dissolution-rate constant (51). K^* depends on the intrinsic dissolution rate constant k, which is primarily a function of the velocity v, of the liquid that passes by the solid surface. Therefore, it is apparent that the position of the tablet in the medium and the speed of agitation are important.

Based on this, the sequence of events wetting–penetration–disintegration–dissolution can be employed to establish the dissolution curve, as shown in Fig. 7.16. In most cases the diffusion coefficient, D, is rate determining, not the intrinsic dissolution-rate constant, k. This curve then becomes log linear, which can be expressed by

$$\ln \frac{M}{M_0} = -k^0(t - t^0) \tag{7.13}$$

where k^0 is an apparent dissolution rate constant and t^0 is the apparent lag time which is dissolution-rate-constant dependent. This phenomenon is illustrated in Fig. 7.18.

DISSOLUTION OF SUPPOSITORIES

The use of suppositories as form of medication dates back to the time of Hippocrates. Suppositories are indicated for systemic action in patients who are in a coma or who cannot tolerate oral medication due to a variety of reasons.

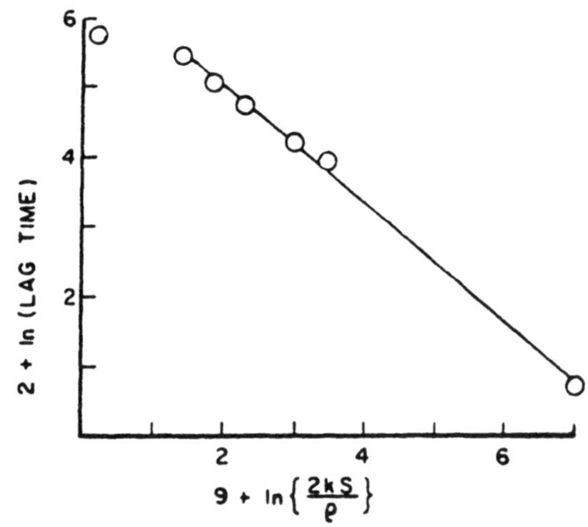

Fig. 7.18 Apparent lag time as a function of solubility and dissolution-rate constant. (From Ref. 52.)

Suppository dosage form as a method of drug delivery is not popular in the United States but is employed extensively in other countries.

Dissolution of drug from nonoral dosage forms has not been investigated to as great an extent as the oral dosage forms. Past research into drug release from suppository bases has taken a number of approaches, some of which are not very scientifically sound or reproducible. Others, however, give a good starting basis for future research.

Although most of the early work on suppositories has been concerned with their physical characteristics such as softening and liquefaction ranges, homogeneity, smoothness, and neutrality, general reports appeared in the early literature pointing to a direct correlation between their efficacy and the release characteristics of the active ingredients (56–60). Further, it has been reported that fatty bases tend to release hydrophobic drugs that are highly soluble in the oily base very slowly but that emulsification of the fatty base significantly improved the drug release rate. Additionally, incorporation of surface-active agents was found to dramatically improve the release rate of water-soluble drugs from the fatty suppository base (61). Also, in the past, drug release from suppository bases has been related to the HLB value of the surfactant used or the partition coefficient (62) as well as other parameters. However, usually no in vivo information is available.

Testing for the rate of in vitro release of drug substances from suppositories has always posed a difficult problem, owing to melting, deformation, and dispersion in the dissolution medium. Additionally, without the sound knowledge of the physical behavior of the suppository during the test often led to drawing empirical conclusions. Often, the in vivo performance failed to correlate with the in vitro data. This was one of the reasons that the suppository dosage form was looked upon unfavorably.

Suppository Dissolution Methods

The continued interest in suppositories and suppository bases has led to recognition that a dissolution test would be helpful during the initial phase of dosage form design. In addition, such a test would provide valuable information on the effect of storage time and temperature on the subsequent in vitro release profile.

General techniques have been employed in the past for the study of in vitro drug release rates from suppositories. These methods can be classified into five different types (Fig. 7.19):

1. *Beaker method.* This type consists of simple placement of the suppository in a flask or a beaker (63–67) and allowed to settle.

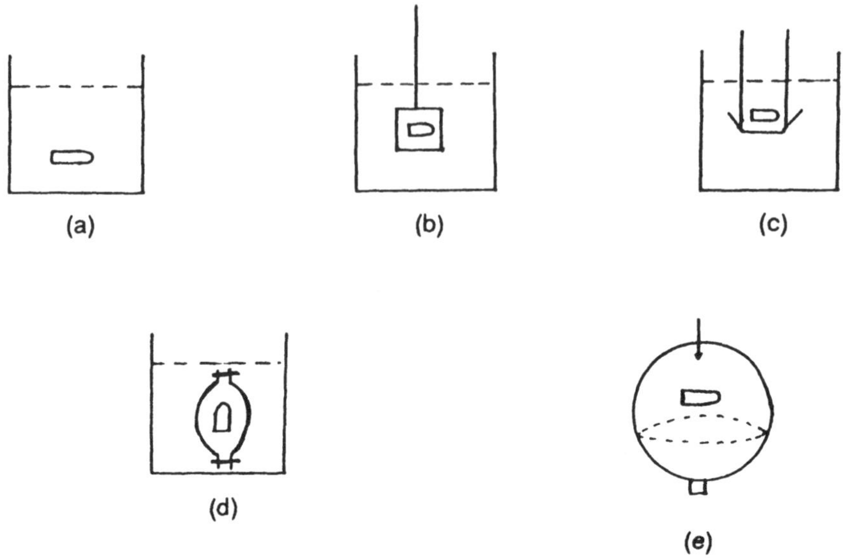

Fig. 7.19 Suppository dissolution methods: (a) beaker method; (b) basket method; (c) membrane diffusion method; (d) dialysis cell method; (e) continuous-flow method.

2. *Basket method.* This type utilizes an existing tablet dissolution apparatus that provides a wire mesh basket for holding the suppository (68–74). Also, other variations in the design that fit available tablet dissolution apparatus have also been employed (75,76).
3. *Membrane diffusion method.* This type consists of a sample chamber separated from a reservoir by a membrane (77–87). In this method, the suppository is placed inside the membrane, then in a beaker.
4. *Dialysis method.* This type employs dialysis tubing as a natural membrane (61,88–99). This apparatus has been one of the few designed where the suppository is in an upright position.
5. *Continuous-flow method.* This type involves a flow system in which the sample is placed on cotton or a wire screen (100,101). Other modifications of this basic apparatus are available. In one of the more recent ones the system entails use of a release chamber where the suppository is surrounded by glass beads or placed on a screen (101–103). The principal advantage claimed for the beaded system is that it maintains constant interfacial area while allowing direct contact between the dosage form and the dissolution medium, whereas the screen system does not. Details of the flow-through beaded system are presented in the following section.

As mentioned earlier, one basic problem in testing for drug release from a suppository is the change in the physical dimensions of the suppository (due to softening, deformation, melting, or disintegration) during the test results in exposing a variable interfacial area to the dissolution medium. The variability of this factor leads to poor test reproducibility since the release rate depends on the interfacial area.

Membranes have been employed to control the interfacial area based on the principle that when the suppository softens, it would spread over the entire membrane, restricting the area exposed to the dissolution medium (102). Bhavnagri and Speiser (78) designed a type 3 apparatus with a relatively small sample chamber. Others employed a relatively small bag in type 4 apparatus to restrict the interfacial area (92,95).

The need to control interfacial area is important, however, the introduction of an additional physical process (i.e., membrane transport) complicates matters and may mask the true release characteristics for certain drug–suppository base combinations. Consequently, a flow-through technique was developed in which a suppository is secured in a bed of glass beads. This arrangement controls the interfacial area for most suppository bases, yet permits direct contact between the suppository and the dissolution medium (102).

Flow-Through Bead-Bed Apparatus

This suppository dissolution apparatus is designed to provide reasonable control over the interfacial area for drug dissolution. A schematic representation of the apparatus along with the assembly is provided in Fig. 7.20.

A continuous eluant flow is maintained over the suppository contained in a bed of glass beads. The eluant starts in a 150-mL jacketed beaker, which is covered with an acrylic resin disk. When the pump is started, water (dissolution medium) is drawn through the polyethylene tubing from a 150-mL jacketed beaker to a 1-cm flow cell in the UV spectrophotometer. From the spectrophotometer, the water is drawn into a preheating glass coil that is submerged in the water bath to allow the water temperature to equilibrate before reaching the sample chamber, which is also submerged in the water bath. The water leaves the glass coil and enters the sample chamber from the top.

This chamber is comprised of two sections. The bottom section is a 15-mL coarse Buchner fitted disk filter modified with a 20/40 glass joint at the top and an outlet tube narrowed to 4 mm OD × 2 mm ID. The top half is a 24/40-hose connecting joint modified with an inlet tube narrowed to 4 mm OD × 2 mm ID. The dissolution medium (water) travels through the glass bead-bed and around the suppository. The dimensions of the cell containing the beads are 2.6 cm ID and 6.2 cm long. The water leaves the test chamber, is drawn into the pump and is pumped back into the 150-mL jacketed beaker, which is stirred by a magnetic stirrer.

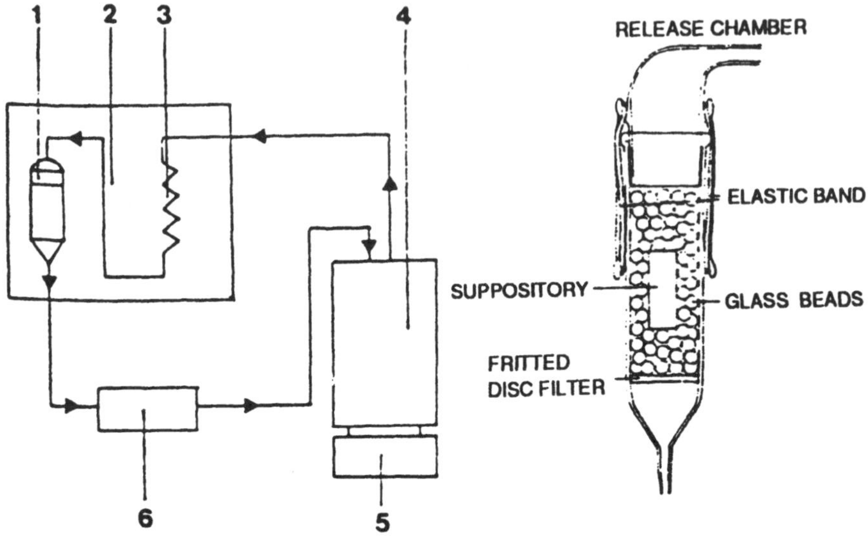

Fig. 7.20 Schematic illustration of a flow-through bead-bed dissolution method for suppositories. 1, flow-through bead-bed chamber (enlarged inset); 2, thermoregulated water bath; 3, glass heating coil; 4, insulated reservoir; 5, magnetic stirrer; 6, peristaltic pump. (From Ref. 103.)

Suppository Basket Apparatus

Palmieri (75) designed a suppository basket that adapts to the drive of the standard rotating basket apparatus of method 1. The basket is fabricated from plastic with the same external dimensions as the official basket. Employing the standard dissolution system of method 1 with the basket described, reproducible data on aspirin release from suppository were reported. The basket is commercially available, and the Palmieri method is currently under investigation in a number of laboratories.

Hanson Research Corporation markets a basket apparatus for suppository dissolution testing. Hanson's modified basket uses slots instead of mesh to provide a porosity of about 52%. Blocking and/or clogging of the mesh opening is prevented by the use of such a basket particularly when oil-based suppositories are used. Additionally, the system has the capability of testing dissolution of suppositories that float or those possessing low specific gravity such that it interferes with the flow dynamics in the paddle method.

The requirement of quality control and quality assurance of uniform, predictable drug release from suppositories clearly illustrates the need for a readily available, widely accepted dissolution testing apparatus and method. Although a number of methods have been developed, very few in vitro–in vivo correlations have been attempted, and even fewer have been successful (104). Furthermore, since most of the dissolution research has been on research lots of the drug or on extemporaneously prepared suppositories and not on commercially available suppositories, reliable comparisons of different commercial suppositories cannot yet be done. The use of pessaries will probably increase with a resultant increase in research on dissolution from suppositories. As the interest in suppository dissolution increases, standardized methods permitting meaningful comparisons will probably follow. Additionally, the procedures will be more refined and will assist in overcoming the difficulties associated with the dissolution testing as well as controlling to a better extent the variables involved in the dissolution testing of suppositories.

DISSOLUTION OF SUSPENSIONS

During the last two decades, almost all dissolution-rate research efforts have been directed toward tablets and capsules. Some studies, however, have pointed to the importance of the dissolution characteristics of drugs administered in suspensions. Suspensions share many physicochemical characteristics of tablets and capsules with respect to the process of dissolution. Since tablets and capsules disintegrate into powder suspensions, pharmaceutical suspensions share the dissolution process as a rate-limiting step for absorption and bioavailability. Several studies have shown that the bioavailability of poorly soluble drugs administered in suspension formulations is dissolution-rate limited (105,106).

In an early report, Bates et al. (107) commented that the dissolution rate of nitrofurantoin tablets and suspensions were too inconsistent to serve as a USP dissolution test without including a dissolution-rate test for suspension. They concluded that "the rationale underlying the official dissolution rate specification for nitrofurantoin tablets appears quite arbitrary and inconsistent with the dissolution profile and potential toxicity of the official suspension dosage form." This clearly substantiates the need to pursue dissolution-rate testing of suspension dosage forms.

The dissolution rate of a drug from a suspension is generally assumed to be similar to that of a postdisintegrated tablet or capsule. In the following sections we focus on the dissolution mechanisms suggested for suspensions, the methods employed for the determination of dissolution rate of suspensions, and the major factors that influence the dissolution performance of suspension dosage forms.

Dissolution Mechanisms and Factors that Influence Dissolution of Suspensions

Several models have been proposed and studied as applied to suspensions of pharmaceutical interest. Most of these models are modifications of the three primary models as summarized in Table 7.3. These models are diffusion based and represent a quasi-steady-state diffusion process. The dissolution rate is dependent on the solute diffusion coefficient, solubility and density of the suspended solid. The solubility of the drug (suspended material) may be manipulated by additives such as by addition of a surfactant or complexing agent.

The following common assumptions are employed for these models:

1. The effective particle shape approximates a sphere.
2. The diffusion coefficient is concentration independent.
3. Sink conditions exist.

The interpretation of the apparent thickness of the diffusion layer fundamentally differentiates each model, as shown in Table 7.3. In model I the diffusion layer thickness is constant over the lifetime of the particle. However, for models II and III the diffusion layer thickness is proportional to the one-half or first power of the particle diameter, respectively. It is expected that the rate of dissolution will approach infinity as the particle diameter approaches zero due to dissolution.

Several factors are included while using this convective–diffusion approach, such as viscosity of the medium and Stokes law in general. Increasing viscosity usually diminishes the rate of dissolution. This effect may be particle-size dependent, although this observation does not hold true for particles less than 10 μm in radius.

Table 7.3 Diffusion Based Dissolution Models Commonly Employed for Suspensions

Model	Equation	l characteristics
I	$\frac{da}{dt} = \frac{-2DC_s}{l}$	static
II	$\frac{da}{dt} = \frac{-2DC_s}{ka}$	a
III	$\frac{da}{dt} = \frac{4DC_s}{\alpha\rho}$	a

a = particle diameter (cm), t = time (sec.), D = diffusion coefficient (cm^2/sec.).
C_s = Solubility (g/cm^3).
l = thickness of diffusion layer (cm).
ρ = density (g/cm^3).

The models suggested in Table 7.3 are most appropriately employed for monodisperse particle systems. However, most pharmaceutical suspensions contain multisized drug particles. Particle-size-distribution effects on the dissolution rate are critical to the overall performance of the system. Employing model III to obtain dissolution data for methylprednisolone, Higuchi et al., (108) calculated the effect of particle-size distribution using a function approximating a log-normal distribution. The following expression defines the particle-size distribution:

$$W_f = a_{1t}f_1 + \cdots + a_{it}f_i \tag{7.14}$$

where W_f is the weight fraction undissolved, a_{it} is the particle diameter at time t, and f_i is the fraction of drug, by weight, having a particular size. The particle diameter, a, can be calculated from a particular dissolution model, while the sum of f_i is normalized to unity.

Later, Carstensen and Musa (109) employed computer simulation to develop two expressions describing the dissolution-rate profiles prior to the time when the smallest particle in the distribution dissolves and that subsequent to the dissolution of the smallest particle, respectively. The weight fraction undissolved at any time is inversely proportional to the mean particle size, which is congruent with the principle that smaller particles will dissolve more rapidly due to increased surface area exposed to the dissolution medium. It is also possible that this increase in dissolution rate of small particles could be due to increased solubility of very fine particles in the population. Refer to Chapter 2 for details concerning the Carstensen–Musa theory.

Brooke (110), avoiding numerical integration methods, provided an exact expression defining the dissolution profiles of log-normal powders dissolving in accordance with model I. Later, Pedersen and Brown (111) evaluated the distribution effects for all models. They concluded that it is not possible to distinguish between these dissolution models from dissolution data and particle-size measurements alone. This observation directly influences experimental verification of dissolution kinetics of pharmaceutical suspensions. It has been pointed out that mixed dissolution kinetics for multisized distributions are possible which emphasizes the difficulty in validating any model.

Howard et al. (112) developed experimental methodology employing a centrifugal elutriation technique that permits the separation of native powders with reasonably wide particle-size distributions into nearly monosized fractions. These fractions are subsequently tested for dissolution and the resultant dissolution data interpreted via a particular model. Predictions from the model are reasonably consistent with the experimental data.

Most theories for dissolution of suspensions assume sphericity of the suspended particles. It has been shown that spherical approximations yield somewhat slower dissolution than the best approximations for fitting to the exact dissolution curves (113). Also, since nonspherical particles do not grow isotropically, they probably dissolve nonisotropically (114).

Many commercial suspensions of sparingly soluble drugs (e.g., steroid suspensions) commonly include wetting agents and polymers, such as HPMC. Dissolution inequivalence was reported for three steroid formulations (105). In one case, particle size was responsible, while in the other cases, where the particle-size distributions of two formulations were reasonably consistent, polymer content seemed to influence the dissolution process. One must rigorously evaluate the influence of polymer content on the dissolution of suspension prior to deciding which polymer should be incorporated.

Shah and Sheth (115) evaluated the effect of three viscosity grades of methyl cellulose on the dissolution dialysis of nitrofurantoin suspensions. Samples containing methyl cellulose exhibited lower rates of dialysis, possibly due to complexation of the drug in solution as well as microscopic regions of high viscosity surrounding the undissolved drug particles leading to a reduction in the dissolution rate.

Dissolution Apparatus for Suspensions

Several types of apparatus have been proposed and implemented in assessing the dissolution rate of suspensions. Most of these methods are geared toward dissolution of particulate system. One of the common problems associated with most methods is retention of the dissolving material within the confines of the dissolution chamber. Sampling often poses another problem, due to interference of the smaller particles, which often get through the sampling probe. Employment of filters reduces this problem to insignificant levels, however, clogging of the filter, reducing the effective number of particles for dissolution, often results in the generation of artifactual data. It is imperative to assess all these effects before one can decide on an optimal method of dissolution for a given formulation.

As early as 1965, Edmundson and Lees (116) described a direct method for determining dissolution rates via an electronic particle counting device for suspensions containing hydrocortisone acetate. This unique method takes into account the temporal aspects of particle-size distribution during the dissolution process.

Commercially available prednisolone acetate suspensions have been evaluated for their dissolution rates by employing the spin-filter device designed by Shah et al. (117), which provides a magnetically driven rotating filter system. The filter functions as a stirring unit as well as an in situ microporous, nonclogging filter. The rotating filter assembly, secured on a jacketed flask, provides for continuous sampling via a pilot tube subsequent to filtration through the rotating filter unit. This assembly has proved to be effective in discriminating formulation effects through close monitoring of the dissolution rate determinations.

Langenbucher's flow-through apparatus has also been employed frequently to determine the dissolution characteristics of suspension (118). A valuable characteristic of this device relates to the fact that the impact of external parameters such as particle size, liquid velocity, and loading mass can be determined quantitatively using a general design equation that has elements related to convective diffusion theory. This assembly was tested under a variety of experimental conditions using benzoic acid granules (118). This dissolution cell allows for fresh dissolution medium to be circulated continuously, at a known velocity, surrounding the dissolving particles. Details concerning the design of the assembly and its workings are provided in Chapter 3.

Strum and co-workers (106) reported a methodology for determining the dissolution-rate profiles of suspensions employing the FDA's two-bladed paddle method. The feasibility and reproducibility of the method were demonstrated by determining the dissolution profile of two commercial chemically equivalent sulfamethizole suspensions. The paddle method is simple, inexpensive, reproducible, and easily adjustable to the USP basket apparatus.

Dissolution Rate and Bioavailability of Suspensions

It is anticipated that the dissolution characteristics of poorly soluble drugs administered as suspension can significantly influence drug absorption. Several reports to that effect have been published in the literature (106,119–121). Various factors, such as particle-size distribution, viscosity effects, and physiological and anatomical factors, have been shown to influence the dissolution and subsequent drug absorption characteristics. Slim-to-poor in vitro–in vivo correlations have been very common to these formulations. This can be attributed, at least in part, to the lack of a simple method to obtain narrow populations of suspended material of varying sizes (in the micrometer range), which poses a major problem in establishing the optimum size requirement of a suspension product. Unless the micromeritic characterization, particle-size distribution in particular, of a system is fully understood and evaluated rigorously, more improved in vitro–in vivo correlations can be attempted that will assist in arriving at suitable dissolution techniques that can routinely be employed as quality control tools.

DISSOLUTION OF TOPICAL DOSAGE FORMS

This category of dosage forms include gels, creams, and ointments. Drug release studies from these dosage forms are an important step during the developmental stages of new formulations, as well as a routine quality control test for assuring uniformity of the finished product. Additionally, with the increased interest in developing alternative dosage forms for existing drugs, pharmacists are investigating extensively the use of dermal products in therapy. As a result, drug release studies from topical dosage forms have become a subject of extensive investigation. These studies can often provide useful information on some physicochemical parameters involved in in vivo percutaneous absorption, such as the diffusion coefficient and the solubility of the drug in the specific vehicle employed. The release of drug from such systems involves factors of both dissolution and diffusion. In this section we will focus primarily on the characterization of drug release from ointments.

Theory of Dissolution

In all of the foregoing dosage forms, the drug is homogeneously dispersed throughout the matrix of the system. Higuchi (122) developed an equation for the release of a drug from an ointment base, in which the drug entity is distributed uniformly and homogeneously. This equation is based on principles of diffusion as expressed by *Fick's first law of diffusion*:

$$\frac{dQ}{dt} = \frac{DC_s}{l} \qquad (7.15)$$

where dQ/dt is the rate of drug released per unit area of exposed surface of the system, D the diffusion coefficient, C_s the saturation concentration or solubility of the drug in the system, and l the thickness of the diffusion layer. The drug at the surface of the system, which is in close contact with the medium gels, is released first and sets up a front. As drug passes out of the homogeneous systems, the front moves inward, forming the *boundary* of the drug. In effect, it is assumed that solid drug dissolves from the surface layer of the system first and then, as this layer becomes exhausted of drug, the next layer begins to deplete. The amount of drug depleted per unit area of the system, Q, at time t, is given by the *Higuchi equation*:

$$Q = [D(2C - C_s)C_s t]^{1/2} \qquad (7.16)$$

where C is the total concentration (amount per unit volume), dissolved or undissolved, of drug in the system.

Ordinarily, $C >> C_s$, and the instantaneous rate of release of a drug at time t can be calculated from

$$Q = (2CDC_s t)^{1/2} \qquad (7.17)$$

It is apparent from Eq. (7.17) that the rate of release of drug from such systems is proportional to the square root of time.

This original Higuchi model does not provide a fit to experimental data when the drug has a significant solubility in the ointment base. This model can be extended to drug release from homogeneous semisolid vehicles, however, by employing the modification in Eq. (7.18) as reported by Bottari et al. (123,124). This modification is particularly useful for such systems because it has been recognized that the release of drugs from topical dosage forms is affected by the composition of the vehicle (125,126). Bottari and co-workers expressed that as

$$Q^2 + 2DRC'Q - 2DC'C_st = 0 \tag{7.18}$$

where $C' = C - 0.5(C_s - C_v)$, Q is the amount of drug released per unit area of the dosage form, C_v the concentration of the drug at the vehicle–barrier interface, and R the diffusional resistance afforded by the barrier between the donor vehicle and the receptor phase. Other notations are as described earlier. The relationship between C' and C is effective when C is only about three to four times greater than C_s. When $Q^2 >> 2DRD'Q$, the expression takes the form of the Higuchi equation, where the resistance to diffusion is no longer significant at the interface between the vehicle and the receptor phase.

$$A = (2C'DC_st)^{1/2} \tag{7.19}$$

On the other hand, when $C_s << C$, the vehicle-controlled model of Higuchi takes the form expressed in Eq. (7.16).

This quadratic expression permits one to determine diffusion of drugs in ointment vehicles when C_s becomes significant in relation to C. Equation (7.18) may be solved for Q by employing the quadratic approach. This equation, and hence the value of Q, will have two roots. One of the roots will be positive, which has physical significance.

$$Q = \frac{-2DRC' + [(2DRC')^2 + (2DC'C_st)]^{1/2}}{2} \tag{7.20}$$

If a lag time is involved, then t is replaced by $(t - t')$ for the steady-state period. This approach has been used successfully for the determination of release rate of drugs from ointments, suspension-type aqueous gels, and so on.

Dissolution Apparatus

Many investigators have conducted drug release-rate studies from topical dosage forms employing a variety of apparatus. However, there does not yet appear to be a single apparatus or procedure that has emerged as the most favored or widely accepted as a quasi-standard for others in the field (127). Review of the literature reveals that two general techniques have been commonly employed. In the first technique, the sample is placed in direct contact with the receptor phase (dissolution medium), which acts as an aqueous sink. In the second technique, various types of barriers to isolate the donor and the receptor phase are utilized. These barriers can be a filter membrane, a membrane from animal origin, a dialysis membrane, or a polymer membrane.

Zuber et al. (128) developed a simple technique for studying the dissolution rate of ointments through a membrane by employing a dissolution cell and membrane assembly, as illustrated in Fig. 7.21. This assembly was used along with automated sampling equipment. Refinement of this test procedure will offer a method of evaluating and controlling the quality of various ointments. Considerable work is expected to be done in this area in the near future.

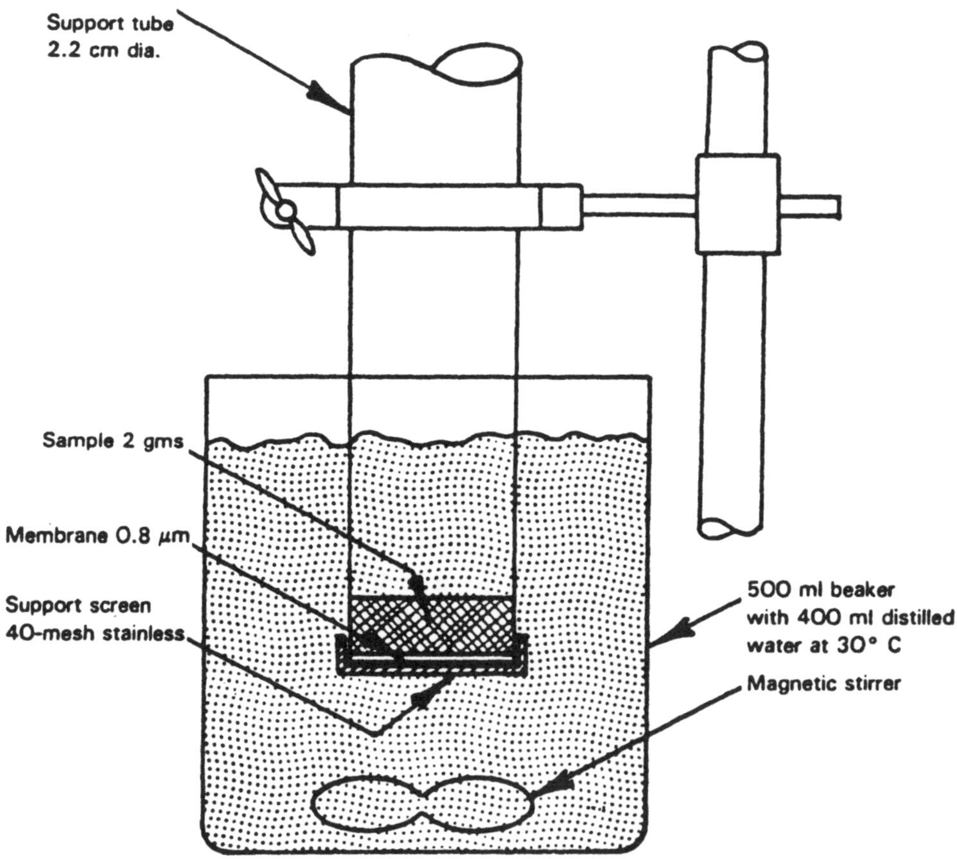

Fig. 7.21 Schematics of system proposed for dissolution of ointments. (From Ref. 129.)

CONCLUDING REMARKS

Although in vitro dissolution methodology will never replace bioavailability testing, the parameters obtained from these tests can give relative assurance that a drug in vitro will be liberated in a suitable fashion from its dosage form and afterward absorbed. The great variation observed in the dissolution characteristics of the products studied can be attributed significantly to the nature of the products themselves. The amount of research and development in improving the understanding of the dissolution process(es) of dosage forms over the last two to three decades is overwhelming. Despite this tremendous effort, the process of dissolution of various dosage forms is far from understood in its entirety. As we grow into any new technology, innovative methods will inevitably be presented that offer improvement for specific shortcomings of approaches currently in use. In this chapter, a very sincere effort has been made to present relatively simple, straightforward approaches that, possibly, explain the dissolution of conventional dosage forms from information retrieved over the last three decades. Currently, a significant effort is being oriented toward the understanding of the dissolution and/or drug release from modified-release dosage forms, sustained-, prolonged- and controlled-release dosage forms in particular. In Chapter 8 we specifically address this area, which is vast in itself, to a reasonable depth, keeping in focus the scope of this text. The reader is urged to combine the information from Chapters 2, 7, and 8 to appreciate the "flavor" of the dissolution of various types of dosage forms to the fullest extent.

REFERENCES

1. J. T. Carstensen, in *2nd Wisconsin Update Conference Proc.*, Madison, Wis. (1982), pp. 14–27.
2. J. C. Samyn and W. Y. Jung, *J. Pharm. Sci.*, *59*, 169 (1970).
3. G. Zografi and S. S. Tam, *J. Pharm. Sci.*, *65*, 1145 (1976).
4. J. T. Carstensen, J. L. Wright, K. W. Blessel, and J. Sheridan, *J. Pharm. Sci.*, *67*, 48 (1978).
5. J. T. Carstensen and K. Kothari, *J. Pharm. Sci.*, *69*, 290 (1980).
6. P. Pothisiri and J. T. Carstensen, *J. Pharm. Sci.*, *62*, 1468 (1973).
7. A. Hussain, *J. Pharm. Sci.*, *61*, 811 (1972).
8. D. Wurster and P. Taylor, *J. Pharm. Sci.*, *54*, 169 (1965).
9. J. T. Carstensen, *Pharmaceutics of Solids*, Badger-Freunc, Fon du Lac, Wis. (1974), pp. 62–67, 87, 133.
10. J. T. Carstensen and M. Patel, *J. Pharm. Sci.*, *64*, 1770 (1975).
11. D. Brooke, *J. Pharm. Sci.*, *64*, 1409 (1975).
12. I. C. Edmundson and K. A. Lees, *J. Pharm. Pharmacol.*, *17*, 193 (1965).
13. N. Kitamori and K. Iga, *J. Pharm. Sci.*, *67*, 1674 (1978).

14. V. G. Pedersen and K. F. Brown, *J. Pharm. Sci.*, *65*, 1437 (1976).
15. V. G. Pedersen and K. F. Brown, *J. Pharm. Sci.*, *64*, 1981 (1975).
16. D. Brooke, *J. Pharm. Sci.*, *62*, 795 (1973).
17. J. T. Carstensen and M. N. Musa, *J. Pharm. Sci.*, *61*, 223 (1972).
18. J. Mauger and S. Howard, *J. Pharm. Sci.*, *65*, 1042 (1976).
19. W. I. Higuchi, E. L. Rowe, and E. N. Hiestand, *J. Pharm. Sci.*, *52*, 162 (1963).
20. E. O. Parrott, *Pharm. Manuf.*, *2*(4), 31 (1985).
21. B. C. Lippold and A. Ohm, *Int. J. Pharm.*, *28*, 67 (1986).
22. A. Hixson and J. Crowell, *Ind. Eng. Chem.*, *23*, 923 (1931).
23. W. I. Higuchi and E. N. Hiestand, *J. Pharm. Sci.*, *52*, 67 (1963).
24. D. Brooke, *J. Pharm. Sci.*, *63*, 344 (1974).
25. J. T. Carstensen and M. N. Musa, *J. Pharm. Sci.*, *61*, 223 (1972).
26. S. Solvong and P. Finholt, *J. Pharm. Sci.*, *59*, 49 (1970).
27. Y. Kawashima, M. Saiko, and H. Takeraka, *J. Pharm. Pharmacol.*, *27*, 1 (1975).
28. J. G. Allen and C. A. Davies, *J. Pharm. Pharmacol.*, *27*, 50 (1975).
29. G. Buckton, A. E. Beezer, and J. M. Newton, *J. Pharm. Pharmacol.*, *38*, 713 (1986).
30. J. E. Hilton and A. E. Summers, *Int. J. Pharm.*, *31*, 157 (1986).
31. [123 of Chapter "Biopharm", Lachman 2nd Ed.].
32. A. El-Yazigi, *Drug Dev. Ind. Pharm.*, *8*, 911 (1982).
33. A. El-Yazigi, *J. Pharm. Sci.*, *70*, 535 (1981).
34. W. P. Boger and J. J. Gavin, *N. Engl. J. Med.*, *261*, 827 (1959).
35. J. M. Newton and F. N. Razzo, *J. Pharm. Pharmacol.*, *26*, 30P (1974).
36. A. Sickmüller, *Acta Pharm. Technol.*, *30*(1), 44 (1984).
37. F. W. Goodhart, R. H. McCoy, and F. C. Ninger, *J. Pharm. Sci.*, *62*, 304 (1973).
38. A. M. Mehta and L. L. Augsburger, *Int. J. Pharm.*, *11*, 327 (1981).
39. A. M. Mehta and L. L. Augsburger, *31st APhA/APS National Meeting*, Orlando, Fla. (1981).
40. A. J. Aguir, L. M. Wheeler, S. Fusari, and J. E. Zelmer, *J. Pharm. Sci.*, *57*, 1844 (1968).
41. J. M. Newton and F. N. Razzo, *J. Pharm. Pharmacol.*, *29*, 284 (1977).
42. P. T. Shah and W. E. Moore, *J. Pharm. Sci.*, *59*, 1034 (1970).
43. J. E. Botzolakis, L. E. Small, and L. L. Augsburger, *Int. J. Pharm.*, *12*, 341 (1982).
44. J. E. Botzolakis and L. L. Augsburger, *J. Pharm. Pharmacol.*, *36*, 77 (1984).
45. G. Rowley and J. M. Newton, *J. Pharm. Pharmacol.*, *22*, 967 (1970).
46. S. E. Neisingh, A. P. Sam, and H. de Nijs, *Drug Dev. Ind. Pharm.*, *12*, 651 (1986).
47. R. J. Withey and C. A. Manville, *J. Pharm. Sci.*, *58*, 1120 (1969).
48. F. S. Hom, S. A. Veresh, and J. J. Miskel, *J. Pharm. Sci.*, *62*, 1001 (1973).
49. J. G. Wagner and M. Pernarowski, *Biopharmaceutics and Relevant Biopharmaceutics*, Drug Intelligence Publications, Hamilton, Ill. (1971).
50. D. Brossard, Ph.D. Dissertation, Université René Descartes de Paris (1981).

51. J. T. Carstensen, *Proc. 2nd Wisconsin Update Conference: Dissolution—State of the Art 1982*, Madison, Wis. (1982).
52. J. T. Carstensen, T. Y. Lai, and V. K. Prasad, *J. Pharm. Sci.*, *67*, 1303 (1978).
53. J. T. Carstensen, J. L. Wright, K. W. Blessel, and J. Sheridan, *J. Pharm. Sci.*, *67*, 49 (1978).
54. K. G. Nelson and L. Y. Wang, *J. Pharm. Sci.*, *67*, 87 (1978).
55. K. G. Nelson and L. Y. Wang, *J. Pharm. Sci.*, *60*, 1758 (1977).
56. M. Gibaldi and B. Grundhofer, *J. Pharm. Sci.*, *64*, 1064 (1975).
57. W. Lowenthal, J. G. Borzeldeca, and C. D. Corder, Jr., *J. Pharm. Sci.*, *59*, 1353 (1970).
58. E. L. Parrott, *J. Pharm. Sci.*, *60*, 867 (1971).
59. M. Bornschein, R. Voigt, and K. Hoffmann, *Pharmazie*, *40*, 718 (1985).
60. F. Hackenberger, T. Gabrio, D. Grune, M. Bornschein, B. Dietzsch, and R. Voigt, *Pharmazie*, *41*, 244 (1986).
61. J. M. Playco, Jr., C. B. Free, Jr., and C. R. Rowland, *J. Pharm. Sci.*, *56*, 809 (1967).
62. G. Mezey and G. Kedressy, *Acta. Pharm. Hung.*, *40*, 200 (1970).
63. C. W. Whitworth and J. P. LaRocca, *J. Am. Pharm. Assoc. Sci. Ed.*, *48*, 353 (1959).
64. A. J. M. Schoonen, F. Moolenaar, C. Haverschmidt, and T. Huizinga, *Pharm. Weekbl.*, *111*, 585 (1976).
65. H. M. Gross and C. H. Becker, *J. Am. Pharm. Assoc. Sci. Ed.*, *4*, 96 (1953).
66. S. N. Pagay, R. I. Poust, and J. L. Colaizzi, *J. Pharm. Sci.*, *63*, 44 (1974).
67. P. Vahby and P. Vaghy, *Gyogyszereszet*, *22*, 27 (1978).
68. C. J. deBlaey and J. J. Rutten-Kingma, *Pharm. Acta Helv.*, *52*, 11 (1977).
69. I. W. Kellaway and C. Marriott, *J. Pharm. Sci.*, *64*, 1162 (1975).
70. V. E. Krogerus and M. Tolvi, *Acta Pharm. Suec.*, *2*, 327 (1965).
71. E. L. Parrott, *J. Pharm. Sci.*, *64*, 878 (1975).
72. L. Roller, *Aust. J. Hosp. Pharm.*, *7*, 97 (1977).
73. S. E. Leucuta, L. Popa, M. Ariesan, L. Popa, R. D. Pop, M. Kory, and S. Toader, *Pharm. Acta Helv.*, *52*, 261 (1977).
74. A. Pech, Y. Lasserre, and M. Jacob, *Trav. Soc. Pharm. Montpellier*, *37*, 165 (1977).
75. A. Palmieri, *Drug Dev. Ind. Pharm.*, *7*, 247 (1981).
76. A. Palmieri, *Pharm. Technol.*, *6*(6), 70 (1982).
77. L. Bardet and J. Cemeli, *Pharm. Technol.*, *16*, 200 (1956).
78. V. P. Bhavnagri and P. Speiser, *Pharm. Acta Helv.*, *51*, 10 (1976).
79. M. A. Ghafoor and C. L. Huyck, *Am. J. Pharm.*, *134*, 63 (1962).
80. A. A. Kassem, E. N. El-Din, A. A. El-Bary, and H. M. Fadel, *Pharmazie*, *30*, 472 (1975).
81. L. Krowczynski, *Acta Pol. Pharm.*, *19*, 127 (1962).
82. Z. Kubiak, *Gyogyszereszet*, *21*, 322 (1977).
83. V. H. Muhlemann and R. H. Neuenschwander, *Pharm. Acta Helv.*, *31*, 305 (1956).
84. M. Kapas, E. Regdon, and G. Regdon, *Acta Pharm. Technol.*, *25*, 109 (1979).

85. G. Regdon, A. Magyarlaki, G. Kedvessy, E. Minker, and E. Regdon, *Pharmazie, 33*, 67 (1978).
86. R. Voigt and G. Falk, *Pharmazie, 23*, 709 (1968).
87. G. B. Carp, D. Brossard, C. Chemtob, and J. C. Chaumeil, *Sci. Tech. Pharm., 7*, 159 (1978).
88. W. H. Thomas and R. McCormack, *J. Pharm. Pharmacol., 23*, 490 (1971).
89. T. Stozek, *Pol. J. Pharmacol. Pharm., 27*, 227 (1975).
90. L. Turakka and V. E. Krogerus, *Farm. Aikak., 83*, 59 (1974).
91. L. Turakka and V. E. Krogerus, *Farm. Aikak., 83*, 105 (1974).
92. J. W. Ayres, D. Lorskulsint, A. Lock, L. Kuhl, and P. A. Laskar, *Farm. Aikak., 65*, 832 (1976).
93. C. G. Hartman, *Ann. N.Y. Acad. Sci., 83*, 318 (1959).
94. H. P. M. Kerckhoffs and T. Huizinga, *Pharm. Weekbl., 102*, 1187, 1255 (1967).
95. C. F. Peterson and A. J. Guida, *J. Am. Pharm. Assoc. Sci. Ed., 42*, 537 (1953).
96. H. Piasecka and Z. Zakrzewski, *Pol. J. Pharmacol. Pharm., 28*, 199 (1976).
97. W. A. Ritschel and M. Banarer, *Arzneim.-Forsch., 23*, 1031 (1973).
98. S. Tsuchiya, M. Hiura, and H. Matsumaru, *Chem. Pharm. Bull., 25*, 667 (1977).
99. W. A. Ritschel and J. Rotmensch, *Pharm. Int., 3*, 4 (1974).
100. M. R. Baichwal and T. V. Lohit, *J. Pharm. Pharmacol., 22*, 427 (1970).
101. H. W. Puffer and W. J. Crowell, *J. Pharm. Sci., 62*, 242 (1973).
102. T. J. Roseman, G. R. Derr, K. G. Nelson, B. L. Lieberman, and S. S. Butler, *J. Pharm. Sci., 70*, 646 (1981).
103. J. C. McElnay and A. C. Nicol, *Int. J. Pharm., 19*, 89 (1984).
104. A. Palmieri III, *Proc. 2nd Wisconsin Update Conference: Dissolution—State of the Art 1982*, Madison, Wis. (1982), pp. 92–96.
105. S. A. Howard, J. W. Mauger, and L. Phusanti, *J. Pharm. Sci., 66*, 557 (1977).
106. J. D. Strum, J. L. Colaizzi, T. J. Goehl, J. M. Jaffe, W. H. Pitlick, V. P. Shah, and R. I. Poust, *J. Pharm. Sci., 67*, 1399 (1978).
107. T. Bates, H. Rosenberg, and A. Tembo, *J. Pharm. Sci., 62*, 2057 (1973).
108. W. I. Higuchi, E. L. Rowe, and E. N. Heistand, *J. Pharm. Sci., 52*, 162 (1963).
109. J. T. Carstensen and M. Musa, *J. Pharm. Sci., 61*, 223 (1972).
110. D. Brooke, *J. Pharm. Sci., 62*, 795 (1973).
111. P. V. Pedersen and K. Brown, *J. Pharm. Sci., 64*, 1981 (1975).
112. S. Howard, J. Mauger, A. Khwangsopha, and P. Lee, *J. Pharm. Sci., 67*, 673 (1978).
113. P. V. Pedersen and K. Brown, *J. Pharm. Sci., 65*, 1437 (1976).
114. N. Kitamori and K. Iga, *J. Pharm. Sci., 67*, 1674 (1978).
115. N. Shah and B. Sheth, *J. Pharm. Sci., 65*, 1618 (1976).
116. I. C. Edmundson and K. A. Lees, *J. Pharm. Pharmacol., 17*, 193 (1965).
117. A. C. Shah, C. B. Poet, and J. F. Ochs, *J. Pharm. Sci., 62*, 671 (1973).
118. F. Langenbucher, *J. Pharm. Sci., 58*, 1265 (1969).
119. J. Lima and W. Jusko, *Clin. Pharmacol. Ther., 28*, 262 (1980).
120. F. Nimmerfall and J. Rosenthal, *J. Pharm. Sci., 69*, 605 (1980).
121. M. Soci and E. Parrott, *J. Pharm. Sci., 69*, 403 (1980).

122. T. Higuchi, *J. Soc. Cosmet. Chem.*, *11*, 85 (1960).
123. F. Bottari, G. Dilolo, E. Nannipieri, M. F. Saettone, and M. F. Serafini, *J. Pharm. Sci.*, *63*, 1779 (1974).
124. F. Bottari, G. Dilolo, E. Nannipieri, M. F. Saettone, and M. F. Serafini, *J. Pharm. Sci.*, *66*, 927 (1977).
125. S. Tanaka, Y. Takashima, H. Murayama, and S. Tsuchiya, *Int. J. Phar.*, *27*, 29 (1985).
126. B. J. Poulsen, E. Young, V. Coquilla, and M. Katz, *J. Pharm. Sci.*, *57*, 928 (1968).
127. H. M. Abdou, "Dissolution", Ch. 35 in *Remington's Pharmaceutical Sciences*, 17th ed., Mack Publishing, Easton, Pa. (1985), p. 665.
128. M. Zuber, C. Chemtob, and J. Chanmeil, *Sci. Tech. Pharm.*, *8*(1), 1979.

ADDITIONAL READING

Aiache, J. M., J. C. Maublant, M. Dopogny et al., *S T P Pharma.*, *4*, 215 (1988).
Baumann, T. J., M. A. Smythe, K. Kaufmann et al., *Am. J. Hosp. Pharm.*, *45*, 1667 (1988).
Block, L. H. and U. V. Banakar, *Drug Dev. Ind. Pharm.*, *14*, 2143 (1988).
Graffner, C., *Manuf. Chem.*, *60*, 50 (1989).
Jalal, I., E. Zmaily, and N. Najib, *Int. J. Pharm.*, *52*, 63 (1989).
Kaniwa, N., H. Ogata, N. Aoyagi et al., *J. Pharm. Sci.*, *78*, 1020 (1989).
Keseru, P., T. L. Paal, and E. Varsanyi, *Pharm. Ind.*, *51*, 532 (1989).
Khoury, N., J. W. Mauger, and S. Howard, *Pharm. Res.*, *5*, 495 (1988).
Lin, S. Y. and J. C. Yang, *Drug Dev. Ind. Pharm.*, *14*, 805 (1988).
Sande, S. A. and J. Karlsen, *Int. J. Pharm.*, *55*, 193 (1989).
Shah, V. P. and N. W. Tymes, *J.P. Skelly, Pharm. Res.*, *6*, 346 (1989).
Qiu, J. X., *J. China Pharm. Univ.*, *19*, 17 (1988).

EIGHT

Dissolution of Modified-Release Dosage Forms

INTRODUCTION

The recognition of the fact that the absorption rate of drugs into the body can be decreased by reduction of the rate of release of the drug from the dosage form is one of the more interesting results of pharmaceutical research. Accordingly, some dosage forms are designed to release their medication to the body for absorption rapidly and completely, whereas other products are designed to release the drug slowly for more prolonged drug release and sustained drug action. Products formulated for the latter purpose have been described as sustained action, sustained release, prolonged action, depot, repository, delayed action, retarded release, and timed release.

The term *controlled release* or *rate-controlled release* and similar terms indicate that the release of the drug from the dosage form occurs in a planned, predictable, and slower than normal manner. Controlled-release dosage forms release the drug (in vitro) as predicted by physicochemical mechanisms believed to be operating in physiological in vitro test conditions. Apparently, the rate and extent of absorption of the drug occur in humans as predicted from the rate and extent of drug release.

Pharmaceutical preparations with controlled-release characteristics have been a part of the pharmacists' armamentarium since the 1950s, with the purpose of optimizing the bioavailability through the modulation of the time course of the drug concentration in the blood. These dosage forms add an extra dimension to the traditional functions of the dosage form, being a mere carrier for drug storage, portability, and administration. It is apparent that any dosage form other than conventional, be it prolonged-release, sustained-release, controlled-release, or others, involves some sort of modification in the release characteristics of the drug incorporated within it.

Compendia describe *modified-release dosage forms* as those forms for which the drug release characteristics as a function of time and/or conditions at the site of dissolution are chosen to accomplish therapeutic or convenience objectives not offered by conventional dosage forms such as solutions, ointments, or compressed tablets and capsules. Currently, *Pharmacopoeial Forum* proposes two modified-release dosage forms.

Delayed-release dosage forms are defined as those that release a drug (or drugs) at any time other than promptly after administration (e.g., enteric-coated products). The USP limit for enteric-coated tablets requires that the tablets survive a 1-h acid treatment in the disintegration apparatus without disks. On successful passing of this step, they must show 75% dissolution in 45 min in pH 6.8 buffer.

Extended-release dosage forms are defined as those that allow at least a twofold reduction in frequent dosing compared to the drug presented in a conventional form (e.g., a solution or fast-releasing conventional solid dosage form). These dosage forms are popularly known as *timed-release, sustained-release*, or *prolonged-release dosage forms*.

Like any other solid dosage form, the rate of drug release from modified-release solid dosage forms depends on the rate of dissolution. In the case of solutions, it depends on the rate of diffusion. Present technology utilizes either of these possibilities alone or in combination. On the basis of the Noyes–Whitney equation describing the dissolution process and Fick's law of diffusion, Huttenrauch (1) defined the principles of modified-release dosage forms depicted in Table 8.1. Depending on the dosage form, the dissolution rate can be further modified by excipients, formulation, and technology of production.

The mechanism of release of the drugs from various modified-release dosage forms is different for each form. Additionally, it has long been recognized that these dosage forms are not only drug products but also devices and therefore "no single in vitro test will completely reflect the availability of the drug" (2). The usual tests of disintegration time found in pharmacopoeias do not apply to oral modified-release dosage forms, since the release rate per unit time is the critical factor (3).

Without entering into questionable and conflicting controversies regarding the true validity of these dosage forms as to their being either, prolonged-, sustained, or controlled-release characteristics, in this chapter we focus on the

Table 8.1 Principles of Modified-Release Dosage Forms

1. Dissolution-rate modification
   a. Solubility modification
   b. Specific area modification
   c. Particle shape and surface structure modification
   d. Crystallographic modification
   e. Modification of dissolution condition
2. Diffusion-rate modification
   a. Modification of thickness of separating layer
   b. Concentration modification
   c. Partition-coefficient modification
   d. Porosity modification
   e. Diffusion-coefficient modification
      (1) Efficient modification of molecular size
      (2) Viscosity modification

various critical aspects of the dissolution characteristics of modified-release dosage forms in general. Discussions will focus on dosage forms exhibiting prolongation in drug dissolution behavior over a period of time since this characteristic is common to all modified-release dosage forms. These discussions will include theoretical concepts, dissolution testing devices, factors influencing dissolution/diffusion-rate modifications, and general graphic interpretation of dissolution test data for a modified release preparation. It is anticipated that the contents of this chapter, together with Chapters 2, 5, and 6, will provide a critical mass of information to the development scientist for a rational formulation development of a modified-release preparation.

THEORIES OF DISSOLUTION

Most of the theories describing the dissolution of modified-release solid dosage forms are based on the classical theories described in Chapter 2. Modifications are introduced to describe the dissolution characteristics of modified-release dosage forms more meaningfully. In the following sections we allude to the classical approaches as well as other modified approaches described in the literature broadly covering these modified-release dosage forms.

Film Theory

Film theory is based on the assumption that the surface of the dosage form in contact with the solvent does not change during the process of dissolution and that the dissolution medium is stagnant. Under these simplified conditions,

Noyes and Whitney (4) described the quantitative kinetics of dissolution of a substance from an even surface by the movement of molecules at the solid–liquid interface and diffusion of dissolved molecules in the liquid (dissolution medium). Equation (8.1) best describes this theory.

$$\frac{dc}{dt} = K(C_s - C) \tag{8.1}$$

where dc/dt is the change in concentration as a function of time, K the dissolution rate constant, C_s the saturation concentration (solubility), and C the solution concentration at time t.

Due to the motionless nature of the liquid, a saturated solution is formed at the solid–liquid interface and the concentration decreases with growing distance from the interface reaching a finite concentration C' in the surrounding liquid. The layer of saturated solution functions as the diffusion barrier layer. Consequently, according to Fick's Law of Diffusion, the dissolution-rate constant, K, is directly proportional to the coefficient of diffusion, D. Hence $K = D/Vl$ where V is the solution volume and l is the thickness of diffusion layer.

Recognizing that the rate of dissolution is proportional to the surface area of the dissolving substance, S, and employing the assumption of Noyes and Whitney, Nernst and Brunner (5) modified Eq. (8.1) to incorporate the diffusion coefficient and the surface area of the dissolving substance:

$$\frac{dc}{dt} = \frac{DS}{Vl}(C_s - C') \tag{8.2}$$

The dissolved substance moves according to differences in the concentration gradient between the layer that is in direct contact with the solid surface and the other layers of the medium, provided that there is now accelerated movement of the liquid. It is also well known that if the liquid surrounding the dissolving substance is set in motion by either laminar or turbulent flow, the dissolved molecules will move more quickly into the ambient liquid. In such instances the resultant solution is homogeneously mixed at all times. In case of sparingly soluble substances, C' is very low in the surrounding medium and Eq. (8.2) simplifies to

$$\frac{dc}{dt} = KSC_s \tag{8.3}$$

In addition to the diffusion model described, Nelson (6) proposed a convection–diffusion model based on the hanging pellet method. This model was based on the assumption that dissolution is comprised of two parallel processes: diffusion and free convection. Molecular movement is perpendicular to the solute surface in diffusion and parallel in convection. Dissolution characteristics based on film theory have been discussed in detail in Chapter 2.

Dissolution from Particle Mixture

Early theories of dissolution were based on the assumption that dissolution occurs on and from a flat surface with minimal to no change in its area, or from a spherical surface. However, multiparticulate systems exist in which dissolution occurs simultaneously on the surface of many particles.

A cube-root law deduced by Hixon and Crowell (7) describes the dissolution of a multiparticulate system. In addition to the foregoing assumptions, it is assumed that each dissolving particle dissolves isotropically, decreasing its volume and mass and hence its surface area, and that in laminar liquid flow, the value of l remains constant. If W_0 and W_t represent the weight of the particle at the start of dissolution process ($t = 0$) and the weight of the particle at time t, respectively, then

$$W_0^{1/3} - W_t^{1/3} = -\left[\frac{DC_s}{l\rho}\frac{(N\pi d)^{1/3}}{3}\right]t \tag{8.4}$$

where N and ρ, respectively, denote the number and density of the particles undergoing dissolution. The value in parentheses is simply a representation of the dissolution rate constant, K. This cube-root law makes it possible to exclude any definite geometrical shape of particle undergoing dissolution, thus decreasing the necessity for any other measurements beyond weight.

Dissolution of a drug from modified-release dosage forms, extended-release dosage forms in particular, was described by Wagner (8,9). According to Wagner, the kinetic equation describing the drug release mechanism essentially follows a pseudo-first-order path:

$$\ln W = \ln W_0 - Kt \tag{8.5}$$

where W represents the amount of drug remaining in the dosage form awaiting dissolution at any given time t, and W_0 is the initial amount of drug in the dosage form. W will equal W_0 when $t = 0$, indicating that the dissolution rate is dependent on the amount of drug present in the dosage form to begin with.

Dissolution from Matrix

Modified-release dosage forms can be characterized for the most part by solid drugs randomly dispersed in some sort of solid matrices. The simplified treatment of dissolution kinetics based on several assumptions, as described earlier, cannot be applied in these cases. When the drug is mixed with an excipient forming homogeneous solid matrices, the dissolution characteristics change, resulting in different theoretical considerations. Two major classes can result; one where the matrix does not dissolve, and the other where the matrix is soluble along with the drug. Systems of this type or types have been studied widely and utilized recently as bases for dosage forms that provide more or less continuous release of medicaments over relatively long periods. The deduction of the rate of release of drugs from such systems to the pertinent physical constants based on simple laws of diffusion will be presented.

Two geometric systems can be considered, one involving unidirectional leaching or extraction from a simple planar surface and a second involving three-dimensional leaching or extraction from a spherical dosage form, such as a pellet. This corresponds most closely to the release process from an insoluble matrix (tablet) or certain sustained- or controlled-release pellets. The mechanisms of release from these systems can be treated in two ways (10):

1. Extraction of the medicament by a simple diffusional process through enveloping homogeneous matrix.
2. Leaching of the medicament by the bathing fluid, which is able to enter the drug–matrix phase through pores, cracks, and intergranular spaces.

In the former case, the drug is presumed to go successively from the crystal surfaces into the uniform matrix and out into the bathing solvent, which in turn acts as a perfect sink. In the latter case, however, the drug is presumed to dissolve slowly into the permeating fluid phase and to diffuse from the system along the cracks and capillary channels filled with the extracting solvents (dissolution medium). In most instances it is assumed that intergranular diffusion is minimal. Schematics of both these mechanisms are shown in Fig. 8.1.

Treatment of data by Weigand and Taylor (11) and Wagner (8) relate to release data derived from formulated modified-release (sustained or prolonged) preparations. However, the following treatment relates to model systems. Modified-release dosage systems may actually be complicated, due to one or a combination of the following factors:

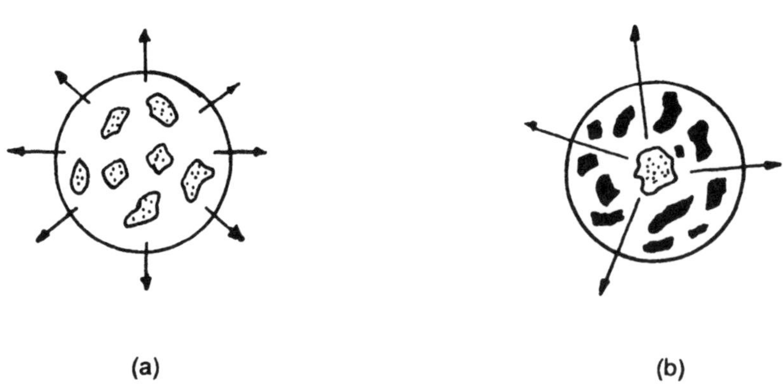

Fig. 8.1 Mechanisms of drug release from homogeneous matrix (a) and from granular matrix with connecting capillaries (b). (From Ref. 10.)

1. Partial dissolution of matrix substances
2. Simultaneous breakup of matrix
3. Drug on the surface of the matrix being released more rapidly than the drug in the matrix
4. One fraction of the dose being in a different, nonmatrix, readily available form

These complicated combinations or individual situations have to be addressed on a case-by-case basis.

Homogeneous Matrix: Planar Geometry

Assuming that the matrix does not dissolve and that the drug is uniformly distributed in it, drug release from this matrix surface under perfect sink conditions is described by

$$Q = [DtC_s(2W - C_s)]^{1/2} \tag{8.6}$$

where Q is the amount of drug released after time t per unit exposed area, D the coefficient of diffusion of the drug in the homogeneous matrix media, W the total amount of drug present in the matrix per unit volume, and C_s the solubility of the drug in the matrix substance. Initially, this expression was derived for release of drug substance from an ointment base containing finely divided drugs. However, it is evident that this expression is equally applicable for release from sustained-release matrix of this type. Equation (8.6) can be reduced and rewritten as

$$Q = f\sqrt{t} \tag{8.7}$$

indicating that the release of drug is dependent on the square root of time. This equation is more popularly known as the $\sqrt{t}$ equation.

Homogeneous Matrix: Spherical Geometry (Pellet)

An exact coordinate description of the distribution pattern of the dispersed particles is extremely difficult to acquire. Hence any attempt to derive an exact solution for a system of this type is impossible. However, a reasonably accurate and useful mathematical solution can be based on a similar assumption that permits solution of the two-dimensional system.

Assuming that $W >> C_s$, a pseudo-steady-state condition exists during the leaching or extraction process. Additionally, as a result, a sharp front will be formed between the partly leached or extracted part of the sphere and the untapped portion. If r_0, r', and r represent the radii of the whole pellet, of that part to be extracted, and of the polar radius of any region under consideration, it is apparent that the total amount of drug contained by the pellet at time t is the sum of the unleached portion ($r < r'$) and that in the region no longer saturated with the drug ($r' < r < r_0$). Equation (8.8) presents a general solution to the proposed problem since it permits determination of r' as a function of time provided that r_0, W, C_s, and D are known for any given system.

$$W[r_0^3 + 2(r')^3 - 3r_0(r')^2] + C_s[4(r')^2 r_0 + r_0^3 \ln \frac{r_0}{r'} - r_0^3 - r_0^2 r' - 2(r')^3] = 6DC_s r_0 t \tag{8.8}$$

In the event of $C_s << W$, the above expression simplifies to

$$r_0^3 + 3(r')^2 r_0 + 2(r')^3 = \frac{6r_0}{W} DC_s t \tag{8.9}$$

An explicit solution for r' as a function of time is relatively difficult. It is more feasible to obtain t as a function of r' and the amount of release as a function of r' and correlate the dependent variables. Transferring Eq. (8.9) into a dimensionless relationship, the factor B can readily be calculated from the constants of the system.

$$1 + 3\left(\frac{r'}{r_0}\right)^2 + 2\left(\frac{r'}{r_0}\right)^3 = \frac{6DC_s t}{Wr_0^2} = BT \tag{8.10}$$

The fraction of the drug remaining, $(r'/r_0)^3$, in the pellet to be dissolved, where $W >> C_s$ can readily be calculated. For real systems, actual time units can be substituted where the constants comprising B are determinable. It should be noted that the physical significance of B is that the reciprocal of $W >> C_s$ corresponds to that time when the last trace of the solid drug dissolves into the matrix.

By and large, the fraction of drug released per unit time [i.e., the relative release rate(s)] from spherical pellets is inversely proportional to the square of the radius of the pellet and the drug concentration. However, the release rate per unit time is directly proportional to the solubility and the diffusivity of the drug. Actually, the $C_s : W$ ratio should be considerably smaller for the spherical three-dimensional system for a steady-state condition to occur and exist than for a planar system.

Granular Matrix: Planar Geometry

The dissolution and ensuing release of drug from a granular matrix system under perfect sink conditions for the leaching type of release mechanism occurring through diffusion movement utilizing intergranular openings can be expressed as

$$Q = \left[\frac{D\epsilon}{\tau}(2W - C_s)C_s t\right]^{1/2} \tag{8.11}$$

where τ is the tortuosity factor of the capillary system and ϵ is the porosity of the matrix. All other notations are as defined earlier. This expression is based on the existence of a pseudo-steady-state condition during the release process and on the assumption that the drug particles are quite small relative to the average distance of diffusion and are uniformly distributed in the matrix. As long as $W > C_s$ or ϵC_s by a factor of 3 or 4, this equation can satisfactorily define the release of drug from such a system. A different expression would apply if $W < C_s$ or ϵC_s because the drug would no longer be present as a solid.

The porosity of the matrix increases as the drug is released, in a degree depending on the volume of the drug. This difference in porosity would correspond directly to the volume of free space previously occupied by the extracted component(s). Hence

$$\epsilon = \epsilon_0 + VW \tag{8.12}$$

where ϵ_0 and ϵ represent initial and final porosities, respectively, of the matrix. If W (amount of drug per unit volume of matrix) is expressed in g/mL, then V (specific volume of the drug) will be inversely proportional to density of the drug ($V = 1/\text{density}$). When the initial porosity ϵ_0 is very small or when the drug has a large volume compared to the volume of matrix, the porosity at any later time, ϵ, approximates the product of V and A. Accordingly, Eq. (8.11) gets modified to

$$Q = W\left[\frac{DK}{\tau}(2 - VC_s)C_s t\right]^{1/2} \tag{8.13}$$

Equation (8.13) implies that the fraction of the drug released at any time is essentially independent of the total amount of the drug in the matrix, W.

Granular Matrix: Spherical Geometry

One of the most common mechanisms by which a drug is uniformly mixed in a granular spherical pellet is released is through leaching. A mathematical expression defining the rate of leaching by external solvent, such as gastric medium, for spherical geometry can be developed employing a pathway similar to that described in the section "Homogeneous Matrix: Spherical Geometry (Pellet)." A dimensionless expression corresponding to Eq. (8.10) will take the form

$$(1-\alpha)+2\left[\frac{r'}{r_0^3}\right](1-\alpha)-\left[\frac{r'}{r_0}\right]^2(3-4\alpha)-\left[\frac{r'}{r_0}\right]+\ln\frac{r_0}{r'}=\frac{6D\epsilon C_s t}{\tau W r_0^2} \tag{8.14}$$

where $\alpha = \epsilon C_s/W$, $\epsilon = \epsilon_0 + VA$, and D = diffusivity in the medium. All other notations are as described earlier. It can be shown that when $\epsilon_0 \sim 0$ (initial porosity) and $\alpha << 1$, the expression reduces to

$$1 + 2\left[\frac{r'}{r_0}\right]^3 - 3\left[\frac{r'}{r_0}\right]^2 = \frac{6DVC_s t}{\tau r_0^2} \tag{8.15}$$

where $(r'/r_0)^3$ represents the residual fraction of the drug remaining to be dissolved at time t.

The basic assumption underlying this theory is that the time of extraction begins with the slightly porous pellet already permeated by the extracting solution. This closely represents true conditions since such pellets will be consumed dry and a short lag time will be involved, corresponding to that required to wet the interior of the matrix. In practice this time period is usually very short compared to the duration of action of such dosage forms.

Other Models

A relatively new model based on Michaelis considerations was proposed for plastic matrix tablets by Rowe et al. (12). This model is comprised of two cylindrical capillary tubes that have different inner radii, r_1 and r_2, and are of different lengths, l_1 and l_2. These capillary tubes are joined in one system. The capillary tubes with smaller diameter correspond to the free pores remaining between aggregates of plastic, and the larger-diameter capillary tubes represent the free space that remains following removal of the dissolved drug. They expressed the following equation, which determines the ratio of apparent diffusion coefficient, D, to actual diffusion ability, D_0, which is an indirect measure for the dissolution/diffusion characteristic of the drug contained within such a matrix.

$$\frac{D}{D_0} = \frac{r_0}{l_1 + l_2}\left(\frac{l_1}{r_1} + \frac{l_2}{r_2}\right) \tag{8.16}$$

where r_0 is the radius equivalent of the cylindrical capillary in terms of mean volume per unit length. The drug-release rate for plastic matrix tablets can be calculated by determining D_0 from Eq. (8.16) and substituting this value in Eq. (8.13)(Higuchi equation).

Roseman and Yalkowski (13) described drug release from silicone rubber employing the following expression:

$$Q = \left[\left(\frac{D_s l_a K W \epsilon}{D_a \tau}\right)^2 + \left(\frac{2WD_a C_s \epsilon}{\tau}\right) t\right]^{0.5} - \frac{D_s l_a K W \epsilon}{D_a \tau} \tag{8.17}$$

where Q is the amount of drug released from the unit of area at time t; D_a and D_s represent the diffusion coefficients of drug in aqueous and matrix phases, respectively; C_s is the drug solubility in the matrix; and l_a is the thickness of the boundary diffusion layer. All other notations are as described earlier.

Differentiation of Eq. (8.17) yields

$$\frac{dQ}{dt} = \frac{\alpha C_s}{2(\beta^2 K^2 + \alpha C_s t)^{1/2}} \tag{8.18}$$

where $\alpha = 2AD_a\epsilon/\tau$ and $\beta = D_s l_a W\epsilon/D_a\tau$. These considerations relate to drug release from a flat surface. However, in reality a three-dimensional dosage form needs to be considered. On the basis of Fick's law, it can be shown that

$$\frac{AdQ}{dt} = \frac{4DC_s}{(1/r' - 1/r_0)} \tag{8.19}$$

where $A\,dQ$ represents the amount of drug released in the period dt, from a diffusing surface A, and r' and r_0 represent the radius of the bead that contains drug in time t and the radius of the initial bead, respectively.

Over the last decade, several other models have also been proposed. They are either modifications of these basic principles or extensions of these concepts (14–17). Christensen and co-workers (18) rigorously evaluated the in vitro release of drugs from modified-release dosage forms for propoxyphene hydrochloride pellets in terms of a diffusion model. They described a model that may be used to predict the drug release profile adequately when the pellet size is changed and when the thickness of the coating is varied as well. The size distribution of pellets in an experiment may be too broad to justify a simulation with just one average pellet size. Consequently, the results for pellets of the same size are generalized to any size distribution of pellets in an experiment. This is trivial only if sink conditions exist in the dissolution medium, because under such conditions, drug release from each pellet type is independent of releases from other pellet types. The total drug release in such an instance may therefore be determined as a sum of the individual releases.

Membrane-Modified Dissolution

A significant number of modified-release dosage forms involve modification of membrane that ultimately controls the drug release characteristics of the final dosage form. Most drug release mechanisms from membrane-modified drug delivery systems are essentially based on diffusion principles. An analogy can be made to multiple emulsions containing drugs that are uniformly dispersed (in analyzing drug release from dosage forms covered by a membrane, such as coated pellets or tablets). In such instances the conditions in the delivery compartment when drug is permeating through the membrane are crucial. Three such cases are illustrated in Fig. 8.2.

Nakano and co-workers (19), employing Fickian diffusion principles, analyzed controlled drug permeation through silicone membrane in relation to the form in which the drug appears in the donor compartment (see Fig. 8.2 for details). The drug release rate dQ/dt at steady state via Fickian interpretation is given by

$$\frac{dQ}{dt} = DA\frac{C_d - C_m}{l} = DA\frac{K_d C_d - K_r C_r}{l} \tag{8.20}$$

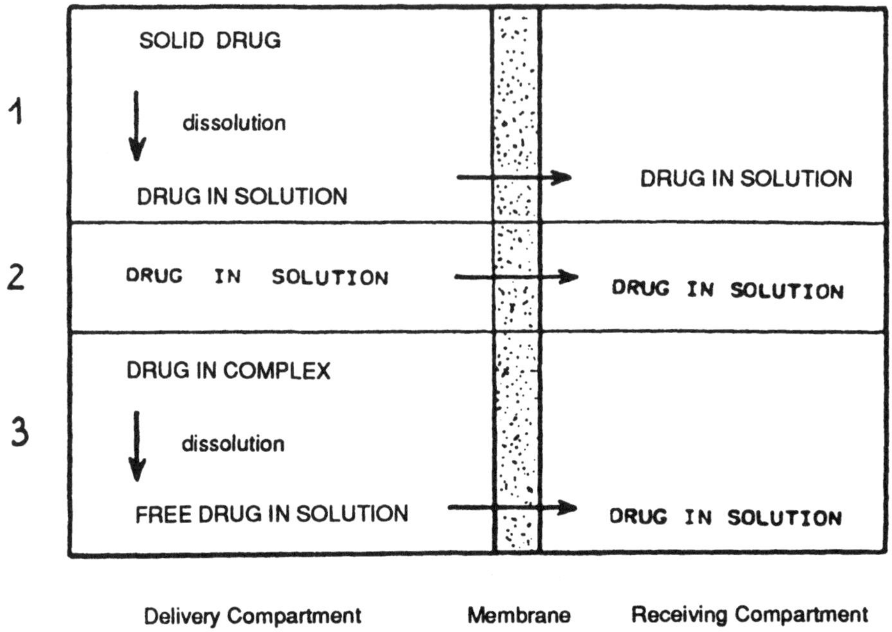

Fig. 8.2 Permeation of a drug under different conditions. (From Ref. 19.)

where D is the coefficient of diffusion through the membrane, A the membrane area, C_d the drug concentration in the delivery compartment, C_r the drug concentration in the receptor compartment, and K_d and K_r represent the partition coefficients between the membrane of drug in delivery and receptor solutions, respectively.

Under sink conditions $C_r << C_d$ in the delivery compartment. Consequently, Eq. (8.20) transforms to

$$\frac{dQ}{dt} = \frac{DAK_d}{l} C_d = \frac{PAC_d}{l} \tag{8.21}$$

where $P = K_dD$, which represents the permeability behavior of the drug from such a system.

The drug in the delivery compartment is in the form of a suspension, as shown in Fig. 8.2, case 1. Therefore, the concentration of the resulting solution has a constant value, since the amount of drug lost due to permeation into the receiving compartment is replaced by drug from the depot in solid form, thus yielding drug release that can be described by zero-order kinetics. Equation (8.22) describes such dissolution behavior, in which the right-hand side is a constant.

$$\frac{dQ}{dt} = \frac{PAC_s}{l} \tag{8.22}$$

where C_s represents drug solubility in the delivery compartment solution. On the other hand, if a saturated aqueous drug solution is in the delivery compartment, the concentration of drug diminishes due to permeation into the receptor compartment, as shown in Fig. 8.2, case 2. This dissolution characteristic can be described by an exponential function:

$$\frac{dQ}{dt} = \frac{PAC_s}{l} e^{-(PA/v)t} \tag{8.23}$$

where V represents the volume of solution in the delivery compartment. The drug release in this case is similar to a first-order reaction. If, however, the donor compartment contains a saturated solution with the addition of a drug-complex binding substance, similar release to a zero-order process can be observed. This dissolution characteristic is shown by the preparation represented in Fig. 8.2, case 3. The complex-bound form is a drug depot that releases by diffusion and substitutes partially for the drug permeating through the membrane. If the concentration of complex-bound drug in the donor compartment is high enough, the concentration of the free drug form available for permeation can be maintained at an almost constant rate and level.

Starting with the theoretical assumptions of the diffusion process, Brodin, et al. (20) calculated the actual coefficient of diffusion for the multiple emulsion system from the slope of the straight line derived from the graph of the dependence of the percentage of drug released as a function of the square root of time, as exemplified by

$$Q(\%) = \frac{200A}{V} \frac{Dt^{1/2}}{\pi} \tag{8.24}$$

The control of drug release from matrix tablets occurs according to the law $Q = f(t)^{1/2}$, while control of the drug release rate by tablet coating provides for release by zero- or first-order kinetics.

According to Fick's law, the rate of release, dQ/dt, depends on the coefficient of diffusion of drug through the coating D_m, coating area A, and thickness of coat l; partition coefficient of the coating/water VK; and concentration of the saturated solution C_s. All these parameters can be expressed collectively as

$$\frac{dQ}{dt} = \frac{D_m AVK(C_s - C)}{l} \tag{8.25}$$

Under sink conditions and integrating Eq. (8.25) yields

$$Q = KAC_s t = \frac{PAC_s}{l} t \tag{8.26}$$

where K and P represent the diffusion rate and penetration rate constants, respectively.

Lippold (21) reports, however, that the drug release from coated tablets is more complex than indicated by the foregoing equations. Lipid coating is practically impermeable to hydrophilic molecules and weakly permeable to water but permeable only to undissociated lipophilic molecules. This inhibits the formation of a saturated drug solution within the tablet. Consequently, these coatings act more like filters. These are porous membranes permeable to both hydrophilic/lipophilic molecules and water.

DISSOLUTION TESTING DEVICES

The pharmaceuticals designed to permit longer dosage intervals for short-acting drugs, such as that provided by extended-release dosage forms, must meet the same requirements as other dosage forms from the standpoint of quality control. The important factors, in addition to specification of the drug content in the dosage form, include the timed-release pattern and the time course of the drug plasma concentration level after the dosage form is administered. Disintegration tests are usually not required for extended-release dosage forms (e.g., for inert-matrix tablets they are of no use). A carefully monitored and devised dissolution test can successfully evaluate in vitro drug release behavior from such modified-release dosage forms. Advantages of the dissolution test are the simplicity and good reproducibility of results when the parameters are constant. For these reasons, the dissolution test was introduced as a method of quality evaluation for modified-release dosage forms. However, the value of this test depends on correlation with the in vivo performance of the same dosage form.

All factors that affect the dissolution performance of any conventional dosage form affect the in vitro dissolution characteristics of these dosage forms. Additionally, factors such as prolonged residence time in the biological space can contribute to the dissolution behavior of such dosage forms. The resultant physiological changes that are encountered during passage of these dosage forms need to be understood and evaluated carefully, which can decide the absorption characteristics of modified release drug products. This imparts additional responsibilities on the research personnel to devise not only a method or device for the dissolution testing of such products but also to ensure that this method/device closely mimics the in vivo microenvironment so that the results will be more meaningful and credible.

Drug properties usually determine the optimal dissolution profile. It is important that within the initial release period the amount of drug delivered provides for minimal effective concentration in the body for drugs with a relatively long half-life. Then amounts of drug released as maintenance doses can be smaller. On the other hand, in drugs characterized by short biological half-lives, it is necessary that in addition to the attainment of minimum effective concentration, the delivered maintenance dose equals amount of drug excreted from the biological system relatively quickly. Consequently, the drug release in the second stage must be considerable. It can be appreciated that it is impossible to assume, a priori, the same drug release profiles for either various types of extended-release dosage forms or for drugs with different biological half-lives. These difficulties were the reasons why the official pharmacopoeial requirements for an in vitro dissolution test have been introduced only and not for in vivo tests.

Many types of apparatus for dissolution testing of these dosage forms have been reported (21–28). The reproduction of gastrointestinal conditions in vitro has always been a problem despite the construction of the apparatus. The factors that can be reproduced to a reasonable degree of similarity are an approximation of sink condition, constant temperature at 37°C, and to some extent, pH changes in the various parts of the gastrointestinal tract and the action of gastrointestinal enzymes. However, these are only some of the factors that contribute to the release of drug from dosage forms. In the following sections we briefly review the history of various noteworthy attempts to characterize the dissolution of modified-release dosage forms. This is followed by brief description(s) of dissolution device(s) currently employed for the dissolution testing of such dosage forms.

As early as 1958, Campbell and Theiragt (30) employed the USP XV tablet disintegration apparatus with certain procedural as well as apparatus changes for determination of drug release from gradual-release preparations. They reported that in vitro tests correlate with clinical in vivo results. Later in the same year, Souder and Ellenbogen (31) devised a rotating-bottle apparatus for tests with sustained-release tablets containing dextroamphetamine sulfate as the active ingredient. The bottles are rotated at 40 rpm in a water bath maintained at 37°C. Each bottle of 90 mL capacity contains 60 mL of simulated gastric fluid. After 0.5 and 1.5 h one bottle is removed and microcapsules are filtered and washed with water to remove excess gastric fluid from the surface. The amount of drug remaining in the microcapsules is assayed. From the remaining three bottles, the microcapsules are separated from liquid by filtration and then placed in the bottles containing simulated intestinal fluid. The drug remaining in the microcapsules is assayed after 2, 4, 5, and 7 h. From the standpoint of changes in the environmental medium and the time protocol, this test setup has become a prototype for several dissolution testing apparatus that followed later.

Chiaramonti et al. (32) described the Diffutest apparatus, based on the same principle. A 16-place wheel holder rotates at a speed of 30 rpm inside a thermostatic chamber maintained at 37°C, as shown in Fig. 8.3. In 40-mL bottles,

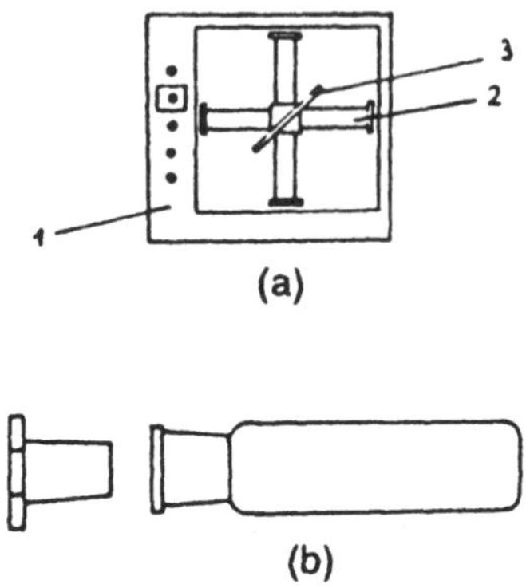

Fig. 8.3 Diagrammatic representation of a Diffutest apparatus. (a) Frontal view: 1, thermostatic chamber; 2, sample holder bottles; 3, thermometer. (b) Sample bottle and stopper.

a weighted pellet sample is placed in exactly 25 mL of elution fluid. The tightly stoppered bottle containing the sample is rotated at 30 rpm. Initially, the sample bottles are filled with simulated gastric fluid. After 1 h, the bottles are removed and the contents are filtered through a 30-mesh nylon screen. The pellets and the insides of the container are washed with 5-mL portions of distilled water. The element is assayed for drug content. Now, in addition to the pellets in the sample bottle, exactly 25 mL of simulated intestinal fluid at pH 4.5 is added. Dissolution is continued as before for 1 h. Subsequent changes of the elution fluid take place every 2 h, using twice the simulated intestinal fluid at pH 6.9 and after 6 h simulated intestinal fluid at pH 7.2. The experiment lasts 8 h. The authors claim that this procedure closely reproduces in vivo conditions.

Souder and Ellenbogen's apparatus was modified by Kreuger and Vliet (33) from a procedural standpoint and adjusted for extended-release dosage forms (tablets). They also applied a mixture of simulated intestinal and gastric fluids, so that after 1 h the pH would be 2.5; after 2 h, 4.5; and after 3.5 h, 7. After 5 h, simulated intestinal fluid at pH 7.5 was used. Based on these experiments. the second supplement of National Formulary (NF XII 1965), for the first time, described an in vitro test procedure for timed-release tablets and capsules.

In many publications, the Levy and Hayes (34) beaker method has gained popularity. This basic model, which has been modified and improved many times, resulted in a variety of dissolution apparatus for in vitro dissolution assessment of modified-release dosage forms. These modifications have been predominantly in the area of agitation/hydrodynamic conditions, flow-through cell units, composition of the dissolution media, and the structural design of the apparatus (35–40). The reader is directed to Chapter 3 for details concerning various representative dissolution devices. The apparatus were the basis on which the official method and apparatus for dissolution testing of oral solid dosage forms, also employed in testing modified-release dosage forms, were introduced to the National Formulary XII (NF XII) and later to the United States Pharmacopoeia XVIII. In the following sections we describe and discuss official and unofficial method(s) currently used to assess the in vitro dissolution of modified-release dosage forms.

National Formulary Apparatus

This NF XII device consists of round, screw-capped bottles held by clamps which are attached to a horizontal rotating shaft. The long axis of the bottle is at a right angle to the axis of the shaft. The distance between the axes is about 47.5 mm. The rotating shaft with the attached bottles is mounted in a constant temperature bath and connected by a chain drive to an electric motor equipped with a speed-regulating device capable of altering the rotational speed from 6 to 50 rpm.

Sixty milliliters of simulated gastric fluid at 37°C is used as an elution fluid in the first hour. It is then replaced by a mixture of simulated gastric and simulated intestinal fluid at different ratios with gradually increasing pH, as shown in Table 8.2.

At the end of each interval, the liquid is filtered through a 40-mesh sieve. Care is taken to retain as much residue as possible in the bottles. The content of the first bottle is passed through the sieve using 25–30 mL of distilled water and the amount of drug in the undissolved particles of the dosage form is

Table 8.2 Procedure for Extended-Release Testing of Tablets and Capsules and Composition of Dissolution Medium (Elution Fluid)

	Proportion of:			
pH	Simulated gastric fluid (mL)	Simulated intestinal fluid (mL)	Bottle number	Time of elution (h)
1.2	100	0	1,2,3,4,5	0–1
2.5	46	54	2,3,4,5	1–2
4.5	39	61	3,4,5	2–3.5
7.0	17.5	82.5	4,5	3.5–5
7.5	0	100	5	5–7

assayed. Sixty milliliters of dissolution fluid at pH 2.5 at 37°C is added to the remaining four bottles, and the procedure is repeated.

This test has been used routinely not only during the development of such products, but also to ensure quality control and quality assurance of the products.

Sustained-Release Rotating-Bottle Apparatus

A rotating-bottle apparatus for determining dissolution rates for sustained-release dosage forms appeared as a suggestion in NF XIII. Although this suggestion was repeated in subsequent compendia, it has never achieved official status. An extensive data base exists from its use, but it is probable that this apparatus will ultimately be replaced by standard dissolution methods.

The schematics of the apparatus are shown in Fig. 8.4. The individual bottles have an internal diameter of 30 mm and are approximately 150 mm in length. The distance between the right-angle axes is held at about 47.5 mm. The rotating shaft with the dosage form, along with 60 mL of extracting fluid (dissolution medium at a specific pH) in each bottle, is immersed in a 37°C water bath. The normal rotational speed is 30 rpm. However, it may change, as will the sampling intervals, as the product and drug demand. The speed may be varied from 5 to 50 rpm for specific tests.

At the end of each sampling interval, the apparatus is stopped. Each bottle is decanted through a 40-mesh screen and the residue is retained. The bottles, along with the residue, are exposed to new, fresh dissolution medium for a specified time, with the residue from one bottle being retained for analysis. The procedure is repeated five times, with recommended sampling intervals and dissolution medium pHs as shown in Table 8.3.

After a total of 7 h with five different extraction fluids (at increasing pH values), the residues from each time interval are assayed. As noted earlier, the dissolution media are prepared by mixing simulated gastric and simulated intestinal fluids, without addition of enzymes. A detailed procedure described in NF XV, although not an official method, is suggested as a suitable test that could be helpful in assuring product uniformity of timed-release tablets and capsules.

This method is rapidly losing popularity since all new sustained-, controlled-, or timed-released dosage forms are being tested by the conventional, compendial dissolution methods. Additionally, this method does not readily lend itself to automation, which seriously limits its use and adoption for routine purposes. Automation of dissolution testing is particularly important in testing sustained-release preparations.

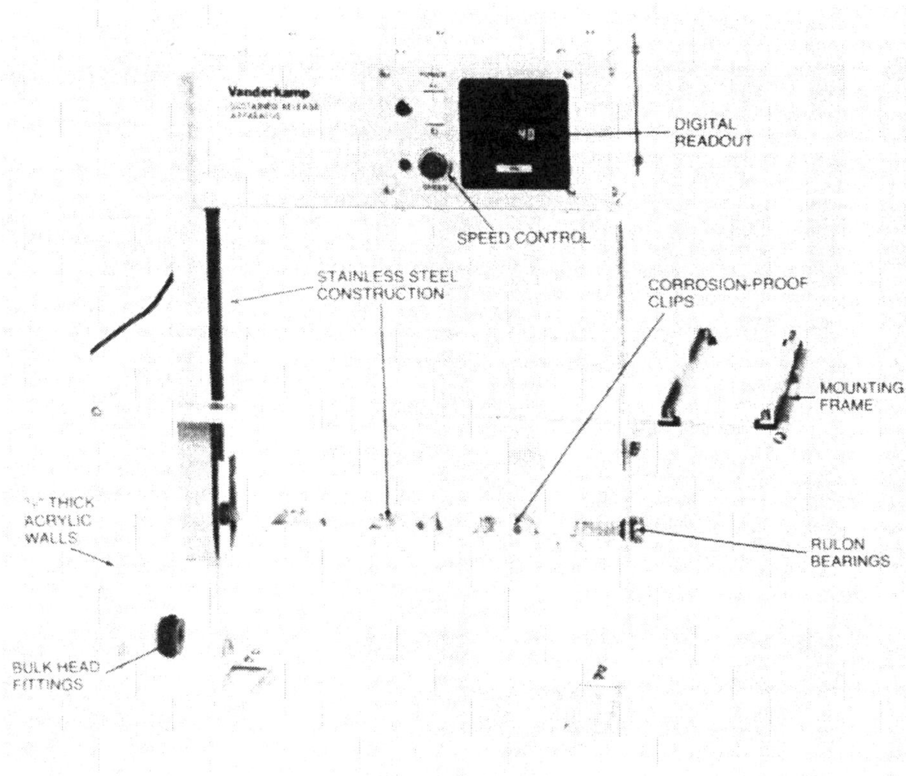

Fig. 8.4 Rotating bottle sustained-release dissolution apparatus. (Courtesy of VanKel Industries, Inc.)

Table 8.3 Sampling Interval Specifications Recommended for Sustained-Release Rotating Bottle Apparatus

Time (h)	Dissolution medium pH
0–1	1.2
1–2	2.5
2–3.5	4.5
3.5–5	7.0
5–7	7.5

Dissolution Testing Devices for Other Modified-Release Dosage Forms

These dosage forms include suspensions, emulsions, transdermal preparations, suppositories (special types), and bioadhesive preparations. In vitro dissolution tests for these dosage forms are based on principles similar to those described earlier. The construction of the apparatus described in various publications is mainly intended for separation of dosage form from the dissolution medium.

In vitro dissolution testing of drugs from extended-release suspensions has been conducted employing either a flask and stirrer assembly of some sort or dialysis membranes (42–47). Based on the stirrer–flask assembly by Poole (44), Barzegar-Jalali and Richards (43) devised a similar method for evaluating the drug release characteristic of suspensions. Approximately 1.5 L of dissolution medium was placed in a 2-L flask and placed in a water bath maintained at 37°C. An 8.1-cm-diameter stirrer, rotated at speeds varying from 20 to 50 rpm, provided the agitation required. Five milliliters of suspension is pipetted into the flask. A sample of 3 mL of dissolution medium was removed and passed through a Millipore filter (0.45 m pore diameter), following which the sample was analyzed for drug content at preset time intervals. A volume of fresh dissolution medium at the same temperature was replaced immediately after the sample was removed in order to return to original conditions as soon as possible.

Two other dissolution testing devices employed for extended-release suspension dosage forms, one employing a semipermeable membrane and the other employing a dialysis membrane, have been reported (46,47). A glass tube closed at the bottom by a semipermeable membrane is suspended in a beaker on a special holder. A sample of the suspension to be tested is poured in the tube above the membrane, and the entire assembly is immersed in the dissolution medium at a depth of 5 cm. Samples are withdrawn at set intervals and assayed for drug content. A magnetic stirrer is placed at the bottom of the beaker for better agitation of the dissolution fluid. The apparatus assembled by Shah and Sheth (46) consists of a plexiglas dissolution chamber that supports a cellulosic dialysis tubing. This assembly is placed in a 2-L resin-reaction kettle, which serves as a recipient chamber. Fifty milliliters of the dissolution fluid is placed in the chamber and agitated at 70 rpm using a stainless steel propeller. The desorbing fluid (500 mL), like the dissolution medium, is placed in the dialysis chamber and agitated at 500 rpm with a magnetic stirrer. The entire assembly is maintained at 37°C. Samples of desorbing fluid are withdrawn for analysis and replaced with fresh desorbing medium immediately. Careful monitoring of the dissolution testing of suspension is recommended because release of a drug from suspensions employing dialysis methods essentially occurs via a two-step process (48).

Parenteral water-in-oil emulsions are tested for dissolution using a similar apparatus without a membrane (49). In a water-jacketed vessel maintained at 37°C, 250 mL of buffer simulating blood is placed, and this constitutes the dissolution medium. A test sample of the emulsion (100 mL) is carefully placed on its surface. The lower portion of the aqueous fluid (simulated blood buffer) is agitated by a magnetic stirrer at 60 rpm. The aqueous phase is sampled at regular intervals and assayed for dissolved drug. Similar testing methods have also been reported for testing of viscous eyedrops (50).

FACTORS INFLUENCING DISSOLUTION OF MODIFIED-RELEASE DOSAGE FORMS

Most factors that affect the dissolution of conventional dosage forms influence the dissolution process of modified-release dosage forms. However, a few factors are critical and need to be mentioned. They are especially important since most of the modified-release dosage forms incorporate modifications in the structural components of the dosage unit such as crystallographic changes of the drug molecule, modifications in the dissolution surface, etc., as well as diffusion-rate modifications. As a result, it is crucial to elaborate on these factors pertinent to the dissolution of such drug products.

In many instances, excipients are incorporated in a formulation, which impedes the contact of drug and the dissolution medium. This is accomplished by embedding the drug particles within the excipient undergoing slower dissolution or enzymatic breakdown. In the latter case, it influences the dissolution kinetics more directly. For example, if the enzymatic hydrolysis (breakdown) follows first-order kinetics, the drug release process also follows first-order kinetics (51).

Polymorphic forms of a drug substance are indicative of different crystalline forms. With a change in the crystalline form, there is a change in the lattice-energy level associated with each form. This energy is primarily responsible for physicochemical properties such as solubilizing potential and dissolution rate. This phenomenon is particularly applicable to steroids. As a result, crystallographic modifications can significantly influence dissolution of the drug substance itself as well as the dosage unit it is contained within.

The surface area parameter (S) of the dissolving substance is directly proportional to its dissolution rate [refer to Eq. (8.2)]. In most instances, when S is diminished, retarded dissolution, and thereby retained release of the drug, is obtained. Assuming sphericity of the drug particle, the magnitude of specific surface S_w varies inversely with the particle diameter d:

$$S_w = \frac{6\rho}{d} \tag{8.27}$$

where ρ is the density of the particle. Consequently, it is apparent that the dissolution surface plays an important role in the dissolution behavior of such products. Several examples reported in the literature allude to this fact (52,53).

Several other factors of equal importance—including particle size, crystal surface anisotropy, the drug's solubility, diffusion-layer thickness, partition and diffusion coefficients, viscosity, molecule size, and concentration gradient difference—have a bearing on the dissolution performance of modified-release products.

Modified-release dosage forms, unlike conventional rapid-release dosage forms, spend more time in the dissolution medium or the biological system, whichever the case may be. Hence they are exposed to a milieu of varying pH in the gastrointestinal tract (pH approaching 1.2 in the acid-secreting stomach region to pH approaching 7.8 in the distal region of the intestinal tract). Consequently, pH becomes a major variable that must be considered in both design and evaluation of these products since it can control the dissolution process to a significant degree. Also, it becomes apparent that not only must pH dependency and dissolution characteristics be investigated, but proper attention must be paid to selection of the appropriate media for dissolution testing of modified-release dosage forms (54). Although all physiological conditions cannot be reproduced during dissolution testing, one should bear in mind that a variety of physiological parameters, in addition to those discussed here, can significantly influence the dissolution performance and thereby the bioavailability of such specialized dosage forms.

INTERPRETATION OF DISSOLUTION DATA

The in vitro dissolution data obtained for modified-release dosage forms can be expressed in different ways. However, algebraic functions have customarily been employed to define the dissolution kinetics of both conventional fast-release dosage forms and nonconventional modified-release dosage forms. In the latter case, owing to the very nature of the dissolution process, the resultant data can be interpreted employing algebraic functions more reliably and with relative ease. These functions relate the cumulative amount of drug dissolved Q as a function of time. These functions can be further transcribed into respective graphical representations. These functions fall into four basic types of $Q = f(t)$ functions, as shown in Fig. 8.5a–d.

For a dosage form in which the amount of drug permeating to the solution is constant for each time interval, $Q = kt$ can express this process. This dissolution process is said to follow zero-order kinetics (Fig. 8.5a). In many of the modified-release dosage forms, particularly controlled- or sustained-release dosage forms, this type of dissolution kinetics is expected.

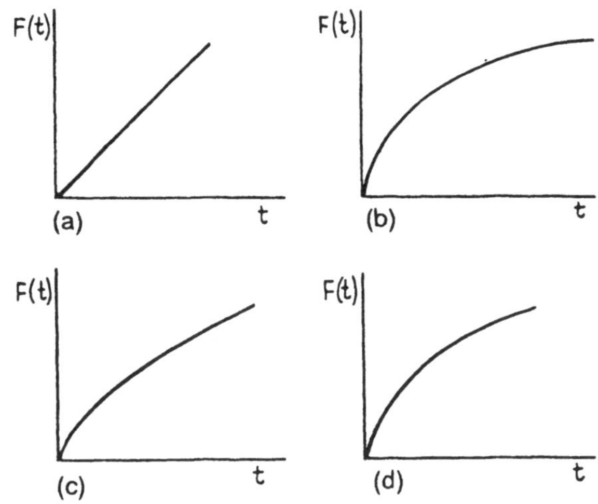

Fig. 8.5 Graphic interpretation of dissolution profiles in terms of cumulative amount dissolved, $F(t)$, as a function of time. (a) Zero-order process; (b) first-order process; (c) dissolution adhering to cube-root law; (d) dissolution adhering to square-root equation.

When the dissolution kinetics can be explained via a $Q = 1 - kt$ function, we have a first-order process (Fig. 8.5b). Most conventional dosage forms exhibit this dissolution mechanism, and some modified-release preparations, particularly prolonged-release formulations, adhere to this type of dissolution process.

Some specialized dosage forms contain many drug particles of the same size and shape or their agglomerates that dissolve evenly. In such instances the dissolution process can be expressed employing the cube-root law, where $Q = 1 - (1 - kt)^3$, as shown in Fig. 8.5c.

A large number of modified-release dosage forms contain some sort of a matrix system. In such instances, the drug dissolves from this matrix; when it is dissolved in the matrix-forming substance, the process is controlled by diffusion. The diffusion-controlled dissolution process can be expressed via the square-root equation, where $Q = k\sqrt{T}$, as shown in Fig. 8.5d.

In many cases the dissolution process cannot be delineated as outlined above. Complex dissolution profiles result and the process cannot be explained with relative ease. In such instances, a conventional method is followed wherein the entire dissolution profile, with cumulative amount dissolved as a function of time from $t = 0$ to $t = \infty$, is considered. The $t = \infty$ is characterized by total release of the drug from the dosage form where no more drug is being released into the dissolution medium. A dissolution-time profile is thus constructed from which parameters such as area-under-dissolution curve $AUC_{\text{in vitro}}|_{t=0}^{t=\infty}$, and others are determined. These parameters are then employed for subsequent in vitro–in vivo correlations. According to one school of thought, consideration and quantification of the entire dissolution profile is a truer, more meaningful indication or reflection of the dissolution process exhibited by a dosage form.

REGULATORY ASSESSMENT

Over the past two decades significant advances in biopharmaceutics and analytical techniques, including analytical chemistry, have led to the recognition that assurance of reliable drug release from solid oral dosage forms must be included in compendial standards. Significant improvements in dissolution technology, followed by an increase in obvious variations in bioavailability and bioequivalence, added impetus to adoption of dissolution testing for product development and quality control during the same period. In 1976 the USP adopted a policy favoring dissolution tests for all official tablet and capsule monographs. A comprehensive policy for dissolution standards for all capsules and tablets was developed in 1980 (54).

Modern pharmaceutical technology makes it possible to design dosage forms that modify bioavailability of a drug into the blood stream, in addition to being vehicles for storage, portability, and administration. It is well known that in vitro dissolution data alone cannot predict in vivo performance. This is particularly true for modified-release dosage forms. Dissolution testing can be useful and valid in a primary quality control procedure to demonstrate differences among products of various manufacturers, as well as in product development studies. With the growing interest and potential for modified-release formulations, the subcommittee on modified-release dosage forms was asked to develop and propose policy regarding dissolution testing of such dosage forms. The policies first appeared in 1982 (55) and later were introduced in official compendia and adopted as official standards (56). The compendia established general standards involving three specific cases and have now provided procedures for their dissolution. In essence they are as described below.

Case 1. All articles are subject to specific dissolution requirements employing 900 mL of water and apparatus 1 at 100 rpm or apparatus 2 at 50 rpm, and the portions of labeled drug dissolved are:

1. At time equal to *0.25D*: 20–50% dissolved ($Q_{0.25}$)
2. At time equal to *0.5D*: 45–75% dissolved ($Q_{0.5}$) and thereafter at
3. Any time up until *1.0D*: not less than 75% dissolved ($Q_{1.0}$) where D is the labeled usual dosing frequency or interval.

Case 2. If the chemistry or the physical properties of the formulation do not allow compliance with case 1, and if no medically significant bioavailability problem is documented, then the monograph sets out details of a specific dissolution test and a specification. Similar in vivo extent of bioavailability is presumed among a group of products. Examples of this case are (58): (a) that the drug release characteristics are over a time period less than the dosing interval D; (b) that the dissolution medium be changed from water to any other medium, e.g., 0.1 N hydrochloric acid or 0.05 M phosphate buffer.

Case 3. If the chemistry or physical properties of the drug formulations among a group of products from different manufacturers differ to such an extent that a single selection of a dissolution test, times, and specifications is not acceptable to the Committee of Revision, and if no medically significant bioequivalence problem is documented, then each manufacturer of an article shall include in the product labeling a graphic or tabular portrayal of either the release profile, using the procedure specified in the monograph, or the documented plasma level profile.

In Vitro–In Vivo Association Considerations

The primary objective of modified-release dosage forms, particularly, controlled-release preparations is to deliver the active ingredient over a longer time interval so as to maintain sustained drug plasma levels. This is accomplished by lowering the elimination rate (or elimination rate constant k_{el}) considerably in comparison to the absorption rate (or absorption rate constant k_a). In fact, for controlled-release products, the drug release rate is reduced such that the rate of absorption is slower than the rate of elimination, thereby prolonging the absorption process. Thus, for most controlled-release dosage forms, the in vivo dissolution and release from undissolving matrices, hydrostatic pumps, and so on, becomes the most important rate-limiting step (59).

The plethora of physiological factors that influence the dissolution process assume great importance because the residence time of these dosage forms in the biological system is significantly long. Thus, the controlled-release products that have virtually similar rates of dissolution over time in the same media are not necessarily equivalent when tested for bioavailability. They may exhibit significantly different bioavailability profiles (54,60). Consequently, discriminating dissolution procedures were developed by the Food and Drug Administration's Division of Biopharmaceutics Research Laboratory. Two quinidine gluconate formulations exhibiting almost identical dissolution profiles were found to be bioinequivalent (54) (refer to Fig. 8.6). It was then concluded that conventional dissolution testing was not a reliable predictor for all controlled-release products. However, it was also proposed that lack of bioequivalence could possibly have been recognized if the dissolution profile was constructed considering the pH gradient as well. The three-dimensional

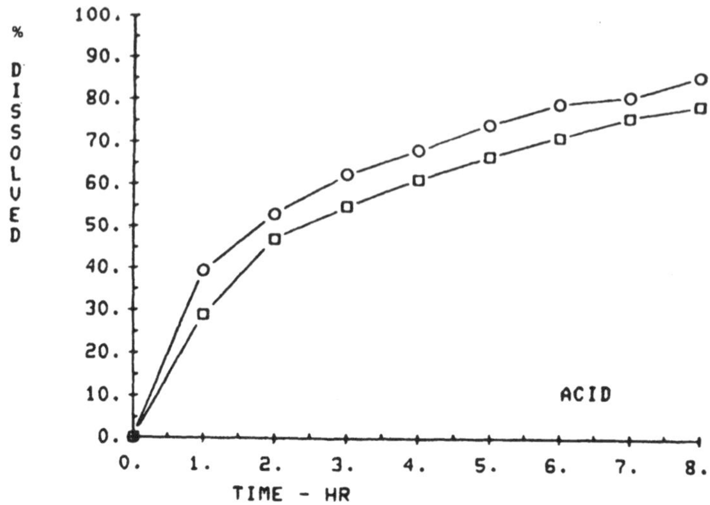

Fig. 8.6 Dissolution of quinidine gluconate from two sustained-release products. ○, Innovator-Berlex Quinaglute; □, dosage form marketed without approval.

topographical plot of amount released as a function of time as well as pH illustrates such a relationship, as shown in Fig. 8.7 (61,62). It can be seen that following an initial rapid dissolution phase there is a gradual increase in percent released as a function of time, as shown in Fig. 8.6. A slight decrease in dissolution rate at about pH 4 can be noted. However, this is in stark contrast to the topographical dissolution behavior of the second quinidine product, as shown in Fig. 8.8. On superimposing Fig. 8.8 on Fig. 8.7, it is evident that although the two products show somewhat similar dissolution characteristics at lower pH and during initial time on a two-dimensional graph, they are significantly different at later time and pH conditions, thus becoming clearly uncomparable at intermediate pH values.

It is also possible that a good predictive in vitro–in vivo correlation of a controlled-release product from the standpoint of dissolution and absorption considerations could be valid only for a specific set of conditions and not for any other (e.g., under fasted and fed conditions). This correlation might not hold true for certain types of food (e.g., fatty meal), since the effects of bile salts, pancreatic secretions, pH gradient, gastric emptying, and so on, change significantly. Figure 8.9 illustrates the changes evidenced in the dissolution topography of a theophylline controlled-release preparation under the influence of a fat meal and under fasted conditions (63,64). Although reproducible 12-h dissolution profiles are obtained at pH values less than 6.6, increased rates of

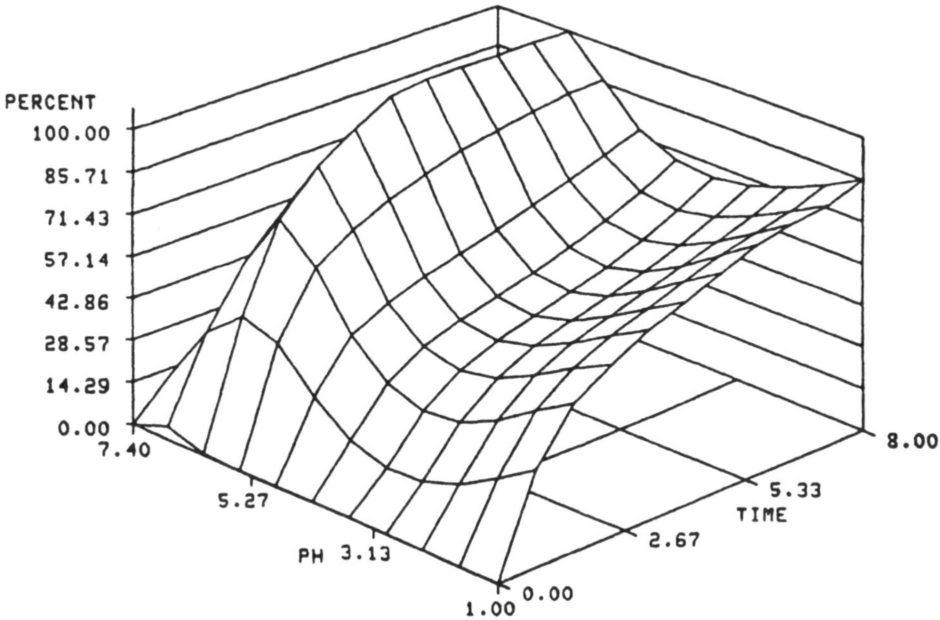

Fig. 8.7 Topographical dissolution characterization of Berlex's Quinaglute brand of quinidine gluconate as a function of time and pH.

dissolution in 8 h were obtained as the pH of the media was raised incrementally from pH 6.6 to 8. On the other hand, dissolution topography of Theodur tablets does not exhibit significant changes under different feeding states (refer to Fig. 8.10). Hence, it is apparent that further investigations are necessary to determine the extrapolation potential of these effects to other products and to assess the validity of the relationship between the dissolution–pH profiles and observed differences in food effects. It can be stated that a steep gradient in the pH–dissolution profile is indicative of potential variability as a result of the pH variability existent in the physiological environment.

It is apparent that in order to adequately and appropriately describe the in vitro–in vivo association of controlled-release products, a multidimensional approach involving pH as the most important factor, particularly for orally administered products, must be considered. Changes in the hydrodynamic conditions (agitation) can lead to changes in absorption properties due to shifts in dissolution rates. On the other hand, an increase in rate of dissolution with an increase in the pH of the dissolution medium can induce changes in the absorption potential. Products that are insensitive to changes in agitation condition and/or pH would not be affected by such changes, as shown in Fig.

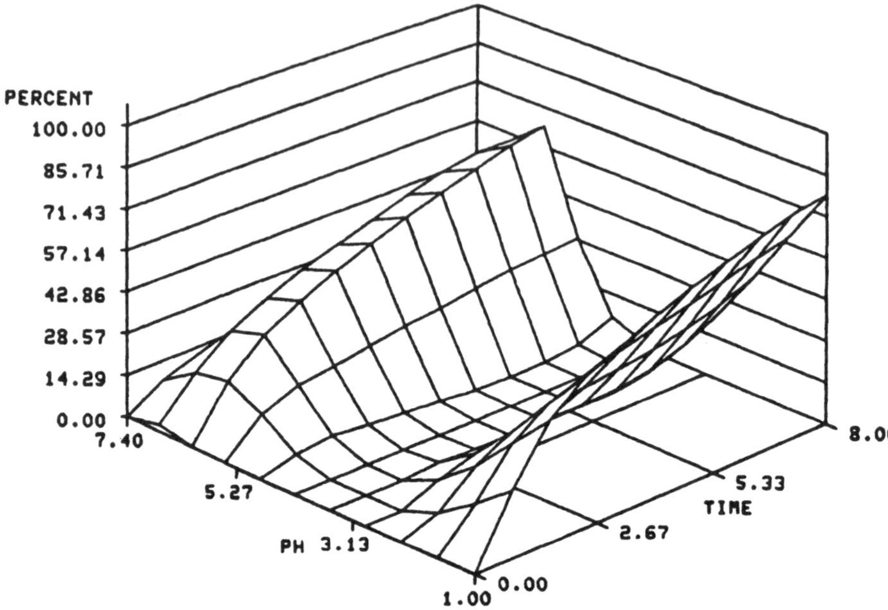

Fig. 8.8 Topographical dissolution characterization of unapproved marketed sustained-release preparation of quinidine gluconate as function of time and pH.

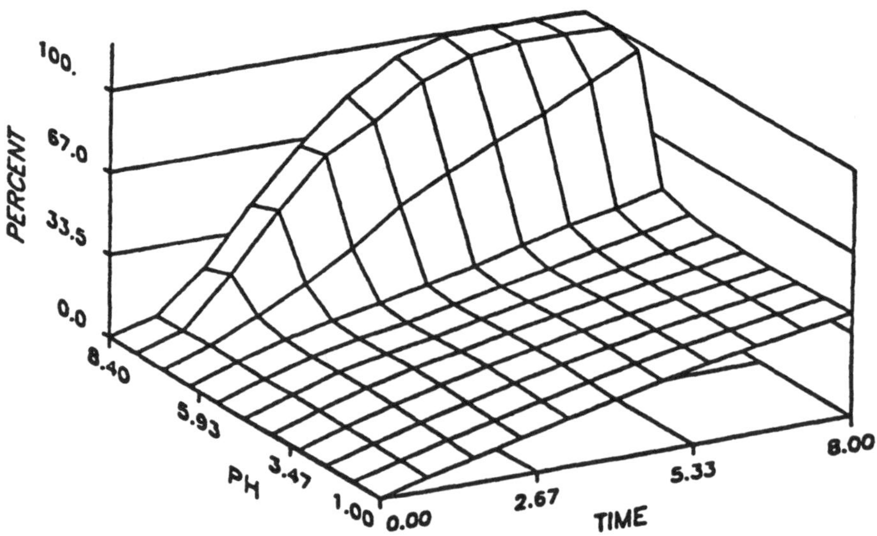

Fig. 8.9 Topographical dissolution performance of theophylline controlled-release product as a function of time and pH.

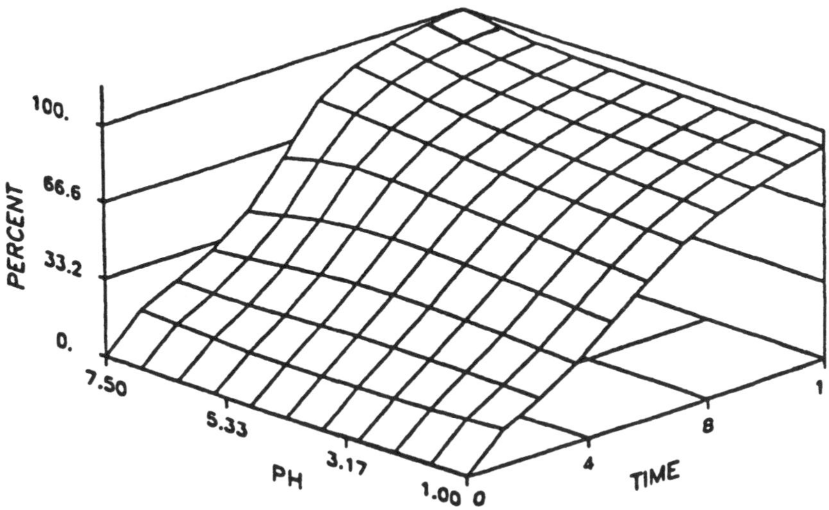

Fig. 8.10 Topographical dissolution performance of theophylline controlled-release product as a function of time and pH (refer to the text for details).

8.11. It is clear that it would be inappropriate to rely on a single dissolution test to predict probable in vivo availability of modified-release and controlled-release products. The perturbation of the system to the flatness or the sloping nature of the topographic surface needs to be assessed in order to arrive at more meaningful in vitro dissolution tests that predict bioavailability more reliably.

In viewing the importance of the foregoing discussion, it is clear that a multifactorial graphical characterization of the relevant dissolution variables is essential as a better predictor of in vivo performance of a controlled-release preparation. Such a characterization can provide assurance of batch-to-batch uniformity as well as bioequivalence characterization of a formulation, provided the bioavailability and controlled-release characteristics are of a single-dose or steady-state bioavailability study. Dissolution testing in lieu of bioavailability data for regulatory processes can be employed only when such in vitro–in vivo relationships are rigorously and completely characterized. Minor changes in a variable are likely to have a negligible effect on other variables, provided that one is within the limits of the plateau as seen in Fig. 8.11. Repeat measurements or duplicative studies are seriously recommended if one is operating on the "slope" portion of the topograph. Such situations can arise while evaluating a product manufactured at two different locations. It is understood that in order to characterize a specific dissolution system or test specifications for a product, several tests must be conducted to recognize and

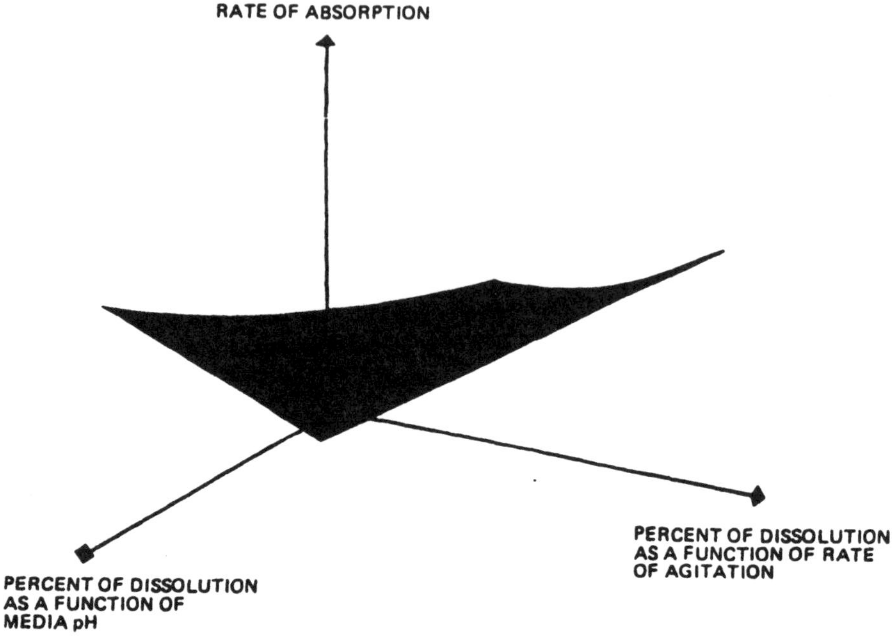

Fig. 8.11 In vitro–in vivo correlation. (From Ref. 59.)

determine the sensitive variables critical to effective characterization of the dosage form in question.

Each controlled-release drug product must be treated separately from the standpoint of developing discriminating dissolution specifications as warranted by the dissolution topograph. A dissolution window at 1 h should be included in the specification to detect possible "burst effects" reflective of dose dumping. A following series of two to three dissolution windows must be included to assure controlled release performance. The terminal sampling window should be a minimum dissolution specification of about 75–80% of the active ingredient, as recommended for phenytoin extended-release preparations by the FDA (65).

The USP proposes that dissolution windows be established at 25, 50, and 75% of the dosage interval, with the awareness that a few good controlled-release products will be unable to meet these specifications. In such cases, it permits adherence to cases 2 and 3, which provide for different methods and/or more individualized specifications. Figure 8.12 depicts that a specification of 20–50% of drug dissolved at 25% of the dosage interval for a BID product would allow up to 50% of the drug dosage to be dissolved and available for absorption within minutes of dosing (59). The FDA requires that a 1-h dissolution window be employed for all controlled-release dosage forms to ensure against this possibility. Table 8.4 provides for continuous testing through three

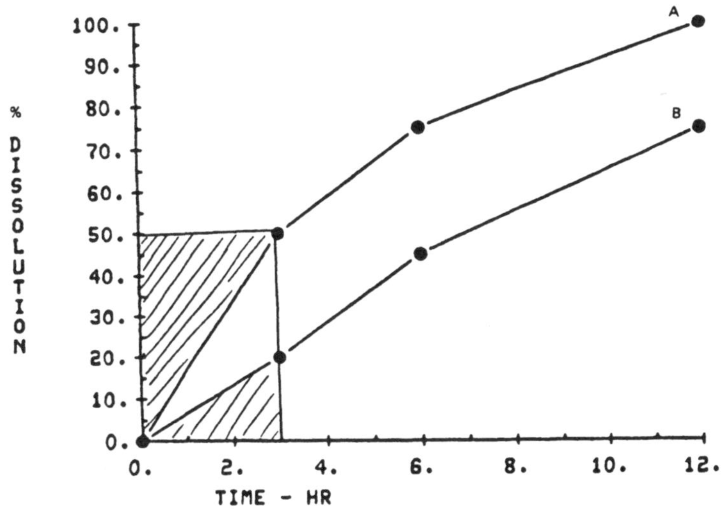

Fig. 8.12 First interval USP limit on controlled-release dissolution. A, USP low; B, USP HI; dissolution range: Q_1 to Q_2 (e.g., 20–50). (From Ref. 59.)

Table 8.4 In Vitro Dissolution Acceptance Levels for Modified-Release Dosage Forms as Recommended by USP

Level	Number tested	Criteria
L_1	6	No individual value lies outside the stated range and no individual value is less than the stated amount at final test time.
L_2	6	The average value of the 12 units ($L_1 + L_2$) lies within the stated range, none is more than 10% of labeled content outside the stated range, and none is less than the stated amount at the final test time.
L_3	12	The average of the 24 units lies within the stated range, not more than 2 of the 24 units are more than 10% of the labeled content outside of the stated range, not more than 2 of the 24 units are less than the stated amount at final test time, and none of the units is more than 20% of labeled content outside the stated range or less than 20% of the stated amount.

levels (L_1 through L_3) to assure conformity as outlined in the modified USP proposal. This can further assure lot-to-lot reproducibility.

Current official dissolution methodology (USP method 1 and USP method 2) does not account for dissolution of an erodible component. Methodology needs to be developed that can efficiently and simultaneously test both erosion and dissolution, especially for products that do not dissolve readily (e.g., matrix-type tablets), but dissolve and release the drug in the gastrointestinal tract.

DISSOLUTION OF CONTROLLED-RELEASE TRANSDERMAL PRODUCTS

Interest in drug delivery through the skin is not new for the pharmaceutical scientist. The enormous amount of activity in the area of transdermal drug delivery can be gauged by the number of articles published in various journals. The passage of a molecule through the various layers of the skin presents unique opportunities for delivering drugs to desired sites. Additionally, it provides a means for noninvasive, continuous administration of various types of drugs. The current favoritism in research toward development of noninvasive drug delivery systems such as transdermal products is based on the lower cost and decreased trauma associated with such systems.

Systemic drug administration by the transdermal route is now an important part of therapeutics. In the United States and various European countries, preparations of nitroglycerin (65,66), etofenamate (67), and 17-beta-estradiol (68,69) are now available for application to the skin for systemic treatment. When the intact skin is used as a port for the entry of drug, a transdermal therapeutic system can deliver medication(s) to the systemic circulation more conveniently and effectively than can currently available dosage form(s).

The controlled-release transdermal systems currently available fall into two main categories: those in which the drug is stored in a membrane-sealed reservoir (reservoir-type systems) and those in which the drug is stored in a matrix (matrix-type systems) (refer to Fig. 8.13).

The last decade has witnessed the successful employment of in vitro dissolution procedures assuring lot-to-lot and batch-to-batch bioequivalence reproducibility of oral solid dosage forms that have been shown to be bioavailable. Additionally, dissolution tests have also been employed to assure the bioequivalence of solid oral drug products for which bioavailability studies are not necessary. Currently, there is a trend toward development of novel drug delivery systems. The emphasis in the area of transdermal controlled medications is increasing rapidly. There is no elaborate information available in the literature on the in vitro dissolution methodology for transdermal patches.

The various manufacturers of transdermal nitroglycerin patches (Ciba, Key, Searle) employ different dissolution methods from the standpoint of quality

(a)

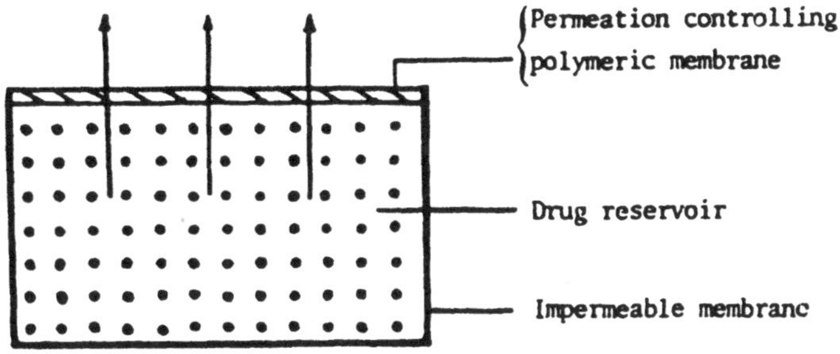

(b)

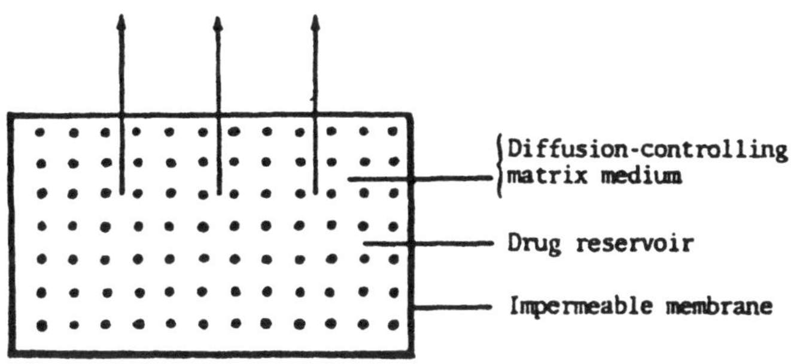

Fig. 8.13 Schematic representation of reservoir-type (a) and matrix-type (b) transdermal drug delivery systems.

control and quality assurance requirements. There is a definite need for development and implementation of a single, probably universal, dissolution method to assure batch-to-batch uniform release which can be utilized for the current available patches as well as for the future patches for regulatory purposes.

In response to this need, the FDA developed an in vitro dissolution method that will assure batch-to-batch in vitro release reproducibility (70). The method, an adaptation of USP apparatus 2 (FDA paddle method), can be employed with relative ease. Various other designs to measure the in vitro dissolution of drug from such transdermal systems have also been devised. Several designs are illustrated in Fig. 8.14a–g and classified according to type in Table 8.5. The horizontal-type designs are more prevalent in various dimensions from the standpoint of the volume of the receptor cell unit. The various designs available and currently in use are illustrated in Fig. 8.15a–e. It is

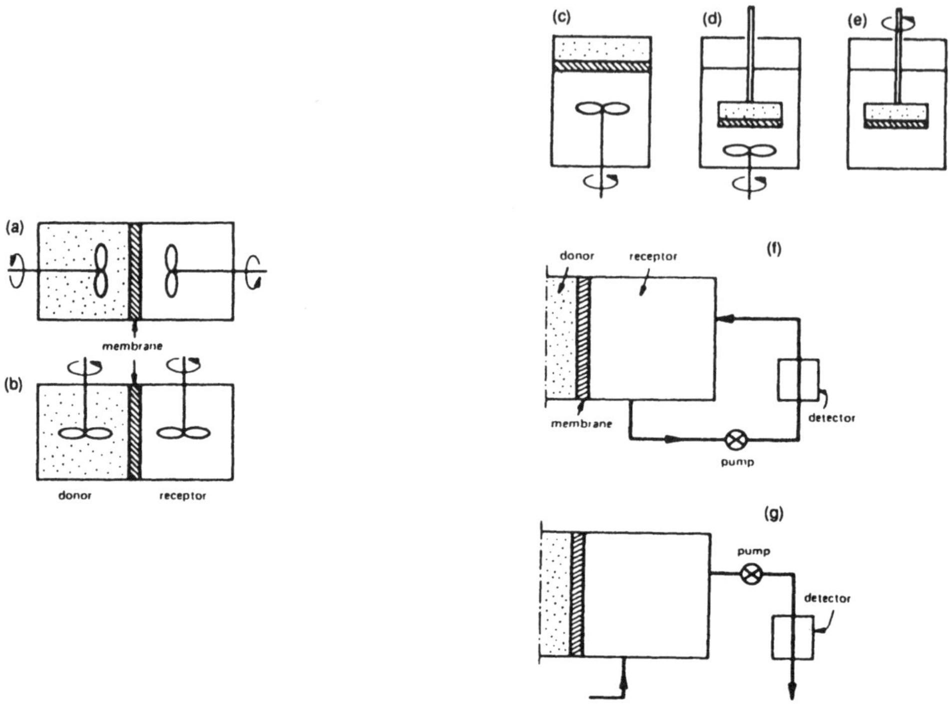

Fig. 8.14 Schematic illustrations of in vitro membrane permeation systems. (a,b) Horizontal type; (c–e) vertical type; (f,g) flow-through type.

Table 8.5 Classification of Various Types of In Vitro Dissolution Systems for Evaluation of Drug Release from Transdermal Drug Delivery Systems

Type	System name	Fig.
Horizontal		8.14a,b[a]
Small volume	Valia–Chien cell	8.15a
Large volume	Ghannam–Chien cell	8.15b
	Franz cell	8.15c
	Keshary–Chien cell	8.15d
	Jhawer–Lord cell	8.15e
Vertical		8.14c–e[a]
Flow-through		8.14f,g
Continuous system		
Fluid circulation		8.14f
Noncirculation		8.14g

[a] These systems are also categorized as intermittent systems: rotating agitation type.

beyond the scope of this book to present elaborate discussions on the rationale and development of these apparatus. However, in the following discussion we focus on the FDA's apparatus in the in vitro dissolution testing of transdermal patches.

The stepwise setup of the transdermal patch dissolution apparatus is illustrated in Fig. 8.16. Transdermal patch holders were prepared from aluminum window screen (-18 mesh) cut and molded to fit a watchglass with 9 cm diameter. The transdermal patch without the protective package and the adhesive tape was placed between the watchglass and the screen with the exposed drug surface of the patch facing the screen. Binder clips (0.75 in.) were used to hold the watchglass–patch–screen sandwich assembly. The entire assembly was placed at the bottom of a dissolution vessel containing 900 mL of deionized distilled water at 32°C [temperature of the skin (71)]. The assembly was also centered in the vessel with the aid of a glass rod. Plastic clips are recommended over binder clips because they are inert to aqueous dissolution media within a pH range of 1–8. Also, it is claimed that the type of clip does not influence the rate of dissolution.

The dissolution apparatus was calibrated using USP prednisone and salicylic acid calibrators and also employing CDA performance standards, before initiating the patch dissolution studies and also at the end of the study. Dissolution was accomplished using a six-spindle USP apparatus 2 employing glass vessels, a paddle speed of 50 rpm, and 900 mL of deaerated water. The height of the paddle was adjusted to 2.5 cm from the surface of the watchglass–patch–screen sandwich assembly. In a few experiments, this height was varied within 2.5 and 3.5 cm. The dissolution was conducted over a 23-h period.

The investigators (70) reached a few important conclusions about the numerous variables that influence the dissolution process of these products. The temperature at which the dissolution was conducted was close to the skin temperature (32°C) rather than 37°C, the temperature employed in case of oral solid dosage forms. Second, the height of the paddle from the surface of the watchglass–patch–screen sandwich assembly, though varied, did not seem to significantly influence the drug release (dissolution) rate from the patch. This observation suggests that the geometrical arrangement of the patch assembly does not have a significant effect on its release rate. Also, sampling from various locations at the same time revealed no difference in drug concentrations, indicating uniform mixing in the dissolution container. It is expected that with an increase in agitation with an increase in the rotational speed of the paddle, there will be an increase in dissolution rate of the drug from the patches. On the other hand, a major mechanistic problem that can be encountered will be the possibility of collision between the patch and the paddle, resulting in damage to the characteristics of the releasing surface. However, the sandwich assembly as described above appears to avert this possibility. This study does make the scientist aware of the possible complexities that

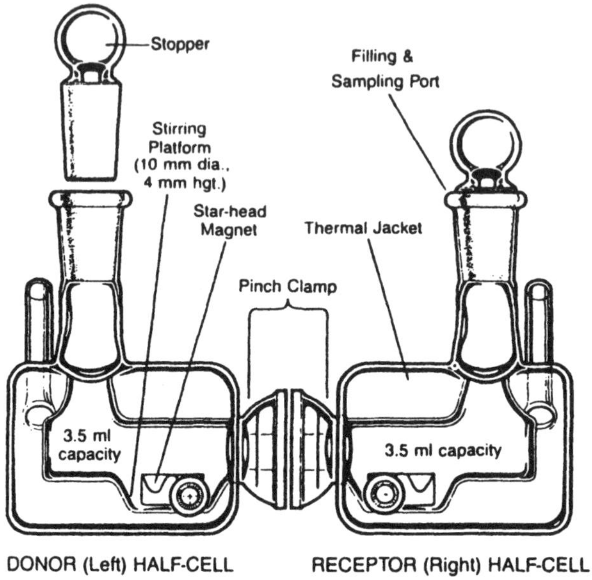
Stopper
Filling & Sampling Port
Stirring Platform (10 mm dia., 4 mm hgt.)
Star-head Magnet
Thermal Jacket
Pinch Clamp
3.5 ml capacity
3.5 ml capacity
DONOR (Left) HALF-CELL
RECEPTOR (Right) HALF-CELL

(a)

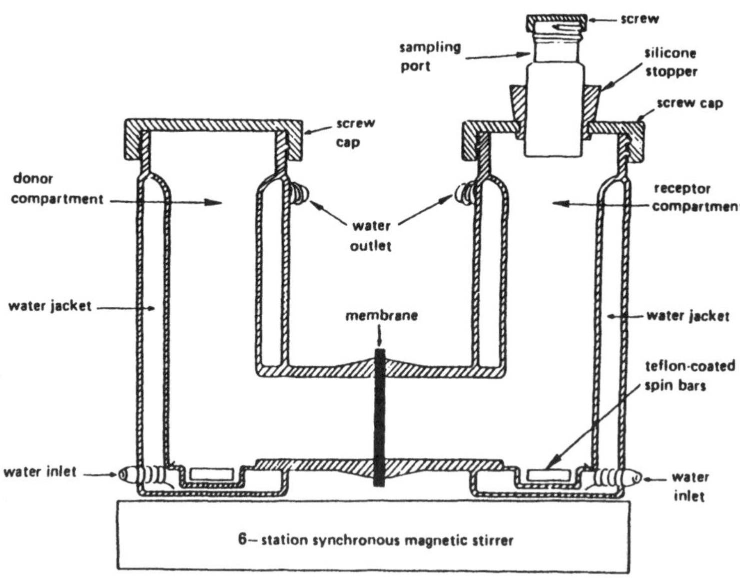
screw
sampling port
silicone stopper
screw cap
screw cap
donor compartment
receptor compartment
water outlet
water jacket
water jacket
membrane
teflon-coated spin bars
water inlet
water inlet
6– station synchronous magnetic stirrer

(b)

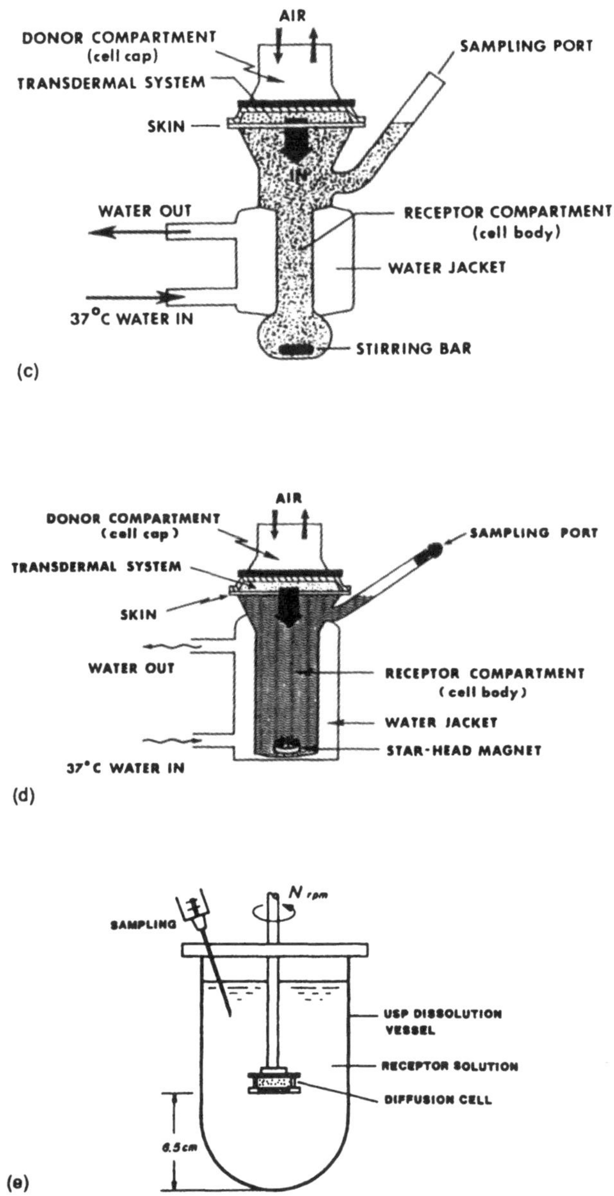

Fig. 8.15 Schematic Illustrations of in vitro membrane permeation systems with fully investigated hydrodynamic conditions. (a) Valia–Chien skin permeation cell; (b) Ghannam–Chien membrane permeation cell; (c) Franz diffusion cell; (d) Keshary–Chien skin permeation cell; (e) Jhawer–Lord rotating-disk system.

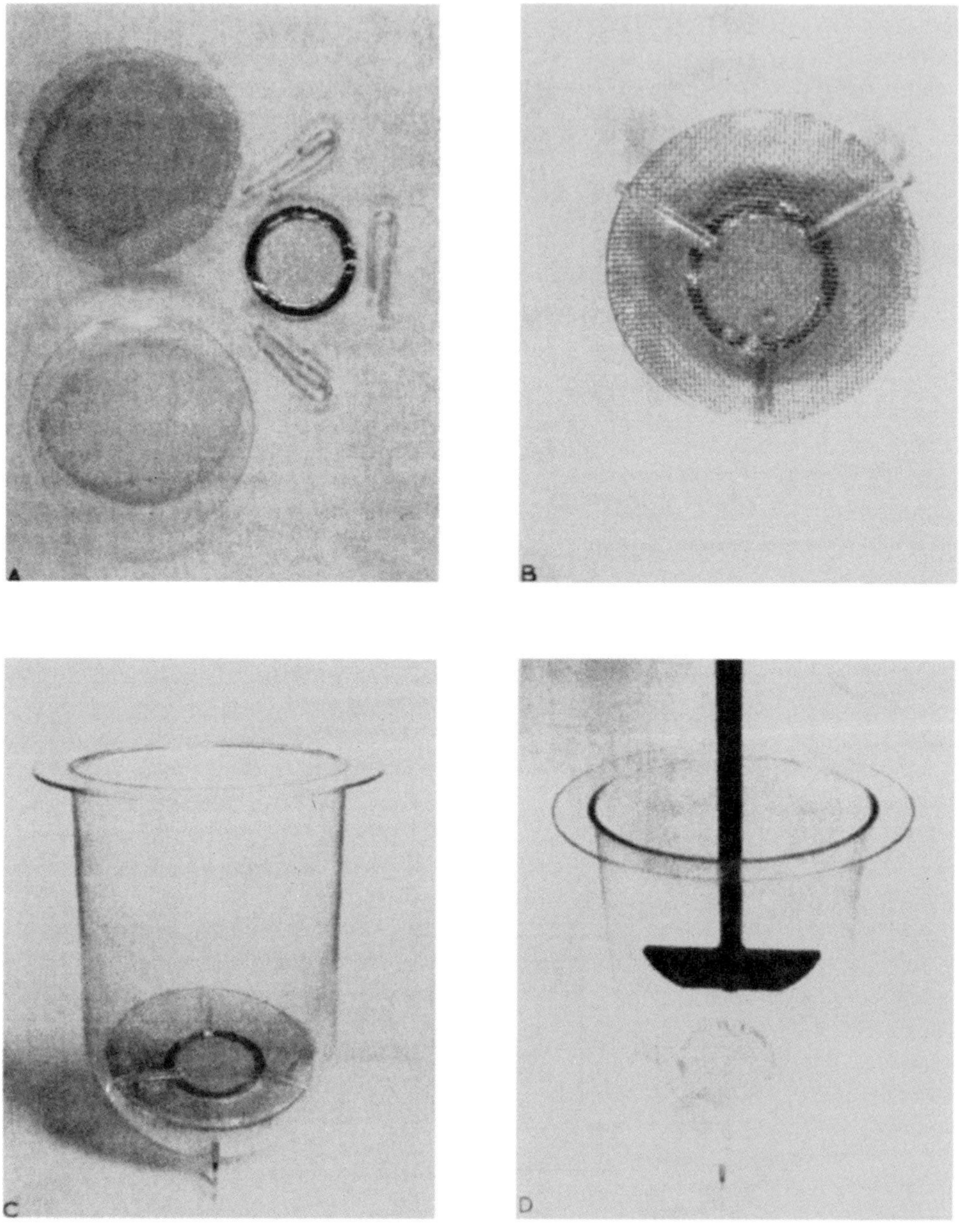

Fig. 8.16 Transdermal patch dissolution setup. (A) Watchglass–patch–wire mesh screen and clips; (B) assembly; (C) assembly in dissolution flask; (D) final setup with paddle apparatus. (From Ref. 71.)

could be associated with efficient dissolution testing as well as the possibilities of a number of variables that could influence the dissolution process of these products.

The results of this study (refer to Fig. 8.17) show that the paddle method developed for dissolution of transdermal patches is simple, reasonably reliable, and reproducible. After rigorous evaluation and careful attention to various factors influencing the efficiency of this system, this method could eventually be adopted as a tool to assure batch-to-batch release uniformity. Since different manufacturing technologies are employed to develop these specialized products with differing release rates, separate specifications should be established for each system.

CONCLUDING REMARKS

The era of conventional drug delivery via traditional rapid-releasing dosage forms is coming to an end. Conventional drug delivery is being replaced by various forms of modified-release dosage technology. More and more nonconventional dosage forms are being introduced and the concepts of extended-release, controlled-release, and prolonged-release medication units are being increasingly accepted. The importance of extended-release dosage forms in contemporary therapy has increased significantly over the last decade, and the tendency toward "once-a-day medicine" has become common. Goyan (72), in his lecture "Drugs of the Future," delivered at the 44th International Congress of the FIP in Budapest, Hungary, stated, "Many changes are expected in drug delivery systems. Many new drug delivery systems will be developed, some with zero-order delivery characteristics, and some with other characteristics depending on therapeutic requirements." New technology for controlled-release dosage forms is currently permitting application of the formulation principle to drugs with varying solubility characteristics, as well as modification of formulation giving changeable drug release characteristics within broad limits. The results of the experiments modifying the rate of dosage form transport through the gastrointestinal tract may be significant for the oral extended- or controlled-release dosage forms.

The distinct advantages of modified-release dosage forms over conventional dosage forms are obvious. Currently, there is a significant emphasis on research and development of new drug delivery systems with controllable as well as predictable drug release characteristics for old drugs as well. More and more techniques are being developed to decrease the dosage frequency and alter the drug release patterns which are closely congruent with the human biological system. There is also a push to develop alternate dosage forms that not only serve the purpose of sustained-, controlled-, or prolonged-drug delivery

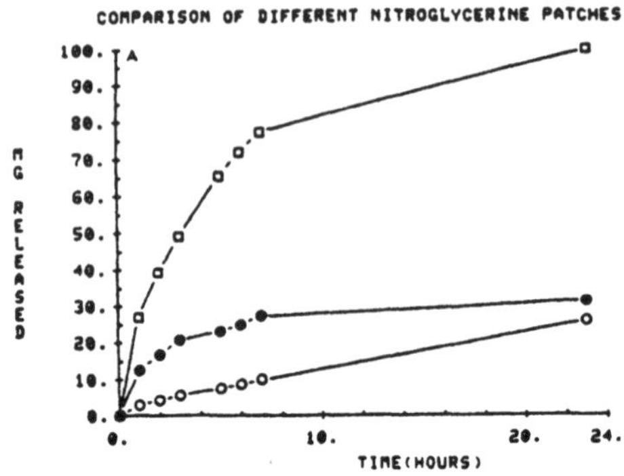

(a)

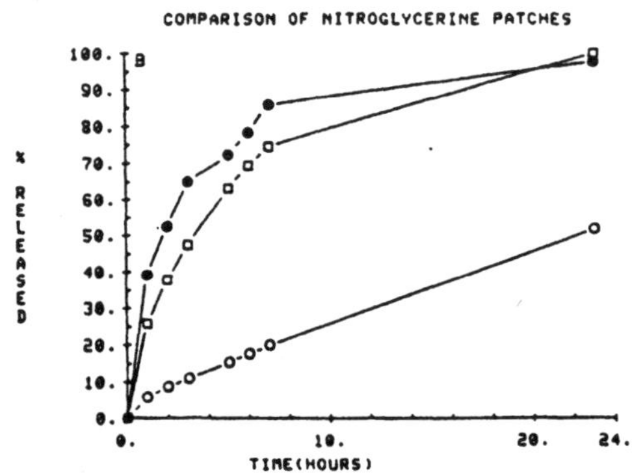

(b)

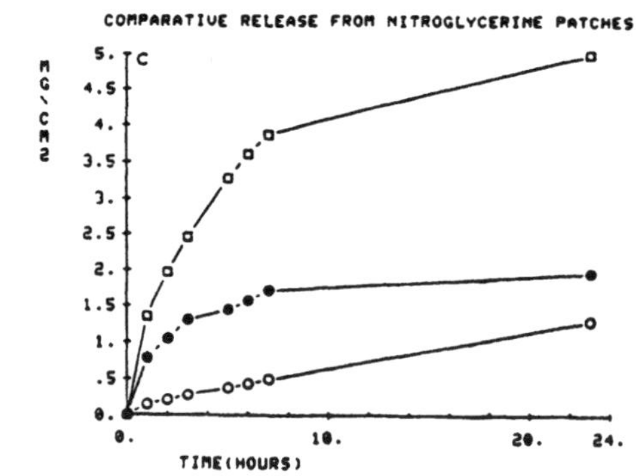

(c)

Fig. 8.17 Comparative dissolution data of three marketed nitroglycerin patches. (a) mg of drug released; (b) % label claim released; (c) mg/cm drug released. ○, CIBA 10 mg (20 cm^2); □, Key 10 mg (20 cm^2); ▲, Searle 10 mg (16 cm^2).

at the site, but also provide a means for noninvasive administration of the drug entity.

In so doing, numerous diversified and successful attempts have resulted in elevation of the technological knowledge base as well as making great strides in drug delivery technology. This advancement, however, has significantly affected the quality assurance as well as quality control departments of the drug industry. A variety of variables, previously unknown, that influence the drug release characteristics have surfaced with even more force than usual. In vitro dissolution testing, one of the most powerful quality control tools, has changed significantly and many new modifications are currently underway which, hopefully, will assist in addressing the various problems associated with modified-release technology.

Recently, the USP Drug Research and Testing Laboratory (DRTL) was involved in an evaluation of an alternative dissolution apparatus—the Bio-Dis Dissolution Apparatus—by testing several extended-release dosage forms (74). The primary objective of this investigation was to determine how this apparatus, reported useful for testing bead-type extended-release products, compared to the standard USP apparatus. The different products tested and the description of the applied test conditions are summarized in Table 8.6. In this apparatus, a dosage unit is held within a clear inner tube, the ends of which are covered with mesh disks. In operation, the inner tube reciprocates vertically within a thermostated outer tube containing the dissolution medium (74). The medium is thus forced through the inner tube, promoting dissolution of the dosage unit. The assembly of six reciprocating inner tubes moves at specified times (programmable to a maximum of six intervals) to adjacent rows of outer tubes (74). USP-DRTL reported that disopryamide phosphate extended-release capsules, nitroglycerin extended-release capsules (product A), and erythromycin delayed-release tablets showed comparable drug release characteristics under the two sets of conditions. However, nitroglycerin extended-release capsules (product B) and pseudoephidrine hydrochloride extended-release capsules exhibited significantly higher drug release at each sampling interval for the Bio-Dis method. Prochlorperazine maleate extended-release capsules, on the other hand, showed significantly higher drug release by the Bio-Dis method only at the 2- and 6-h testing intervals (74).

The rapidly expanding use of sustained-release and patch-type transdermal dosage forms may lead to problems resulting from excipient and polymer interference as well as degradation products with molecular variations. Such problems will require sophisticated analytical procedures, which are tied in with the dissolution assessment of these dosage forms.

Transdermal dissolution, although not new, is definitely an expanding field. Hanson (73) states, "It is easy to picture a list of uncontrolled variables plagu-

Table 8.6 Description of Test Conditions Applied to Different Products Tested for Dissolution Employing Conventional Method and Bio-Diss Apparatus

Name of Product	Test conditions	
	Conventional method	Bio-Dis method
Disopyramide phosphate extended-release capsules	1000 mL of pH 2.5 phosphate buffer; USP apparatus 1 at 100 rpm; sampling at 1, 2, 4, 6, and 8 h; assay by UV absorbance at 264 nm	175 mL of pH 2.5 phosphate buffer; program 5; 420- μm disks; 25 strokes/min; sampling at 1, 2, 4, 6, and 8 h; assay by UV absorbance at 264 nm
Prochlorperazine maleate extended-release capsules	1000 mL of water; USP apparatus 1 at 100 rpm; sampling at 1, 2, 6, 10, and 22 h; assay by UV absorbance at 256 nm	175 mL of water; program 4; 420- μm disks; 25 strokes/min; sampling at 1, 2, 6, 10, 14, and 22 h; assay by UV absorbance at 256 nm
Pseudoephedrine hydrochloride extended-release capsules	1000 mL of water; USP apparatus 1 at 100 rpm; sampling at 1, 2, 6, 10, and 22 h; assay by HPLC	175 mL of water; program 4; 420- μm disks; 25 strokes/min; sampling at 1, 2, 6, 10, 14, and 22 h; assay by HPLC
Nitroglycerin extended-release capsules	900 mL of SGF without enzymes; USP apparatus 2 at 75 rpm; sampling at 1, 2, 4, 6, and 8 h; assay by HPLC	175 mL of SGF; program 5; 420- μm disks; 25 strokes/min; sampling at 1, 2, 4, 6, and 8 h; assay by HPLC
Erythromycin delayed-release tablets	*Acid stage:* 1000 mL of SGF; 1 h; no analysis at the end of *Acid stage; Buffer stage:* 1000 mL of pH 6.8 phosphate buffer; 1 h; colorimetric assay	175 mL of SGF in first row of tubes; 175 mL of pH 6.8 phosphate buffer in second row; program 3; 420- μm disks; 25 strokes/min; colorimetric assay

Source: From Ref. 74.

ing this field of endeavor—just as was once the case with oral dosage forms. The growing use of such dissolution devices as the Franz diffusion cell and the side-by-side cell in percutaneous absorption studies brings back the same problems with uncontrolled variables that the pharmaceutical industry was agonizing over ten years ago."

The coming decade is going to witness even more interesting, if not intriguing, changes in the dissolution testing of these dosage forms. It is just a matter of time before there will be solutions addressing the numerous variables to be successfully implemented.

REFERENCES

1. R. Huttenrauch, *Pharmazie, 30,* 3 (1975).
2. F. A. Maurina, *5th Pan-American Congress of Pharmaceutics and Biochemistry,* Santiago de Chile, Nov. 12–19 (1960).
3. J. Lazarus and J. Cooper, *J. Pharm. Sci., 50,* 715 (1961).
4. A. A. Noyes and W. R. Whitney, *J. Am. Chem. Soc., 19,* 930 (1897).
5. W. Nernst and E. Brunner, *Z. Phys. Chem., 47,* 52 (1904).
6. E. Nelson, *J. Am. Pharm. Assoc. Sci. Ed., 47,* 297 (1958).
7. A. W. Hixson and J. H. Crowell, *Ind. Eng. Chem., 23,* 923 (1931).
8. J. G. Wagner, *Drug Stand., 27,* 178 (1959).
9. J. G. Wagner, *Drug Stand., 28,* 30 (1960).
10. T. Higuchi, *J. Pharm., Sci., 52,* 1145 (1963).
11. R. G. Weigand and J. D. Taylor, *Drug Stand., 27,* 165 (1959).
12. R. C. Rowe, P. H. Elworthy, and D. Ganderton, *J. Pharm. Pharmacol., 234,* 137 (1972).
13. T. J. Roseman and S. H. Yalkowski, *J. Pharm. Sci., 63,* 1639 (1974).
14. F. N. Christensen, F. Y. Hansen, and H. Bechgaard, *J. Pharm. Sci., 71,* 694 (1982).
15. F. Langenbucher, *Pharm. Ind., 38,* 472 (1976).
16. R. Gurny, C. Revillard, and E. Deolkar, *Pharm. Ind., 38,* 913 (1976).
17. J. A. Goldsmith, N. Randall, and S. D. Ross, *J. Pharm. Pharmacol., 30,* 347 (1978).
18. F. N. Christensen, F. Y. Hansen, and H. Bechgaard, *J. Pharm. Pharmacol., 32,* 580 (1980).
19. M. Nakano, K. Juni, and T. Arita, *J. Pharm. Sci., 65,* 710 (1976).
20. A. K. Brodin, D. R. Kavaliunas, and S. G. Frank, *Acta Pharm. Suec., 15,* 1 (1978).
21. B. C. Lippold, in *Formulation and Preparation of Dosage Forms,* J. Polderman, ed., Elsevier, Amsterdam (1977), p. 215.
22. J. Sjögren, *Dan. Tidsskr. Farm., 34,* 189 (1969).
23. E. O. Krueger and E. B. Vliet, *J. Pharm. Sci., 51,* 181 (1962).
24. J. Sjögren and M. Ervik, *Acta Pharm. Suec., 1,* 219 (1964).

25. A. Dominici and M. Marconi, *Boll. Chim. Farm.*, *104*, 648 (1965).
26. C. F. Lerk, *Pharm. Weekbl.*, *111*, 1157 (1976).
27. E. J. Tingstad, *Pharm. Ztg.*, *122*, 1997 (1977).
28. P. Buri, *Schweiz Apoth. Ztg.*, *116*, 55 (1978).
29. L. Krowczynski, *Pharmazie*, *33*, 241 (1978).
30. D. J. Campbell and J. G. Theiragt, *Drug Stand.*, *26*, 73 (1958).
31. J. C. Souder and W. C. Ellenbogen, *Drug Stand.*, *26*, 77 (1958).
32. D. Chiaramonti, C. Giani, F. Innocenti, and A. D. Segre, *Farmaco Ed. Prat.*, *25*, 257 (1970).
33. E. O. Kreuger and E. B. Vliet, *J. Pharm. Sci.*, *51*, 181 (1962).
34. G. Levy and B. A. Hayes, *N. Engl. J. Med.*, *262*, 1053 (1960).
35. G. Levy and L. E. Hollister, *J. Pharm. Sci.*, *54*, 1121 (1965).
36. H. Pernarowaski, W. Woo, and R. O. Searl, *J. Pharm. Sci.*, *57*, 1419 (1968).
37. J. E. Tingstand and S. Riegelman, *J. Pharm. Sci.*, *59*, 692 (1970).
38. F. Langenbucher, *J. Pharm. Sci.*, *58*, 1265 (1969).
39. A. C. Cartwright and C. Shah, *J. Pharm. Pharmacol.*, *29*, 367 (1977).
40. J. H. G. Jonkman, R. Schoeumaker, M. Grinberg, and R. A. De Zeeuw, *Int. J. Pharm.*, *8*, 153 (1981).
41. T. R. Bates, D. A. Lambert, and W. H. Johns, *J. Pharm. Sci.*, *58*, 1468 (1969).
42. J. J. Marty and J. J. Hersey, *J. Pharm. Pharmacol.*, *27*, 437 (1975).
43. M. Berzegar-Jalali and J. H. Richards, *Int. J. Pharm.*, *2*, 195 (1979).
44. J. W. Poole, *Drug Inf. Bull.*, *3*, 8 (1969).
45. Z. Zakrzewski and E. Klepaczewska-Saluda, *Farm. Pol.*, *24*, 229 (1978).
46. N. B. Shah and B. B. Sheth, *J. Pharm. Sci.*, *65*, 1618 (1976).
47. M. Berzegar-Jalali and J. H. Richards, *Int. J. Pharm.*, *4*, 171 (1979).
48. J. J. Windheuser, M. I. Best, and J. H. Perrin, *Bull. Parenter. Drug Assoc.*, *24*, 286 (1970).
49. C. Melis-Decerf and M. van Ooteghem, *J. Pharm. Pharmacol.*, *31*, 12 (1979).
50. M. Chalabala and L. Straha, *Pharmazie*, *25*, 535 (1970).
51. J. H. Fincher, J. G. Adams, and H. M. Beal, *J. Pharm. Sci.*, *54*, 704 (1965).
52. R. Tawashi and J. Piccolo, *Pharm. Acta Helv.*, *45*, 653 (1970).
53. V. K. Prasad, V. P. Shah, P. Knight, H. J. Malinowski, B. E. Cabana, and M. C. Meyer, *Int. J. Pharm.*, *13*, 1 (1983).
54. *Pharm. Forum*, *6*(5), 510 (1980).
55. *Pharm. Forum*, *8*(5) (1982).
56. *United States Pharmacopeia*, XXI rev., United States Pharmacopeial Convention, Rockville, Md. (1985).
57. R. Baweja, *Drug Dev. Ind. Pharm.*, *12*, 2431 (1986).
58. J. P. Skelly and W. H. Barr, in *Controlled Drug Delivery*, J. R. Robinson and V. H. Lee, eds., Marcel Dekker, New York (1987), pp. 293–334.
59. M. C. Meyer, A. B. Straughn, P. Leiberman, and J. T. Jacob, *J. Clin. Pharmacol.*, *22*, 131 (1982).
60. J. P. Skelly, L. A. Yamamoto, V. P. Shah, M. K. Yau, and W. H. Barr, *Drug Dev. Ind. Pharm.*, *12*, 1159 (1986).

61. J. P. Skelly, M. K. Yau, J. S. Elkins, L. A. Yamamoto, V. P. Shah, and W. H. Barr, *Drug Dev. Ind. Pharm.*, *12*, 1177 (1986).
62. L. Hendeles, M. Weinberger, G. Milavetz, M. Hill, and L. Vaughn, *Chest*, *87*, 758 (1985).
63. J. P. Skelly, *APhA/APS Meeting*, Minneapolis, Minn. (1985).
64. V. Shah, V. K. Prasad, C. Freeman, J. P. Skelly, and B. E. Cabana, *J. Pharm. Sci.*, *72*, 309 (1983).
65. P. W. Armstrong, J. A. Armstrong, and G. S. Marks, *Am. J. Cardiol.*, *46*, 670 (1980).
66. P. R. Keshary and Y. W. Chein, *Drug Dev. Ind. Pharm.*, *10*, 883 (1984).
67. I. Heindl, D. Lorenz, S. Seibers, and W. Blumberger, *Arzneim.-Forsch.*, *27*, 1357 (1977).
68. S. Lyrenas, K. Carlstrom, T. Backstrom, and B. von Schoultz, *Br. J. Obstet. Gynaecol.*, *88*, 181 (1981).
69. K. H. Valia, Y. W. Chein, and E. C. Shinal, *Drug Dev. Ind. Pharm.*, *10*, 951 (1984).
70. V. P. Shah, N. W. Tymes, L. A. Yamamoto, and J. P. Skelly, *Int. J. Pharm.*, *32*, 243 (1986).
71. E. A. Pinson, *Pharmacol. Rev.*, *32*, 123 (1952).
72. J. E. Goyan, *Fed. Int. Pharm. Newsl.*, p. 6 (Aug. 1984) (Suppl. to *Pharm. Int.*).
73. W. A. Hanson, *Pharm. Technol.*, *10*(6), 31 (1987).
74. *Pharm. Forum*, USP Conv., Inc. (1989), pp. 4984–4992.

ADDITIONAL READING

Abdallahy, O. Y., N. A. Boraie, and V. F. Naggar, *S T P Pharma.*, *4*, 15–2 (1988).
Acarturk, F., *Pharmazie*, *44*, 547 (1989).
Aiache, J. M., N. Pierre, E. Beyssac et al., *J. Pharm. Sci.*, *78*, 261 (1989).
Anders, R. and H. P. Merkle, *Int. J. Pharm.*, *49*, 231 (1989).
Beerbaum, H., K. Kulpe, K. H. Seidel et al., *Pharmazie*, *43*, 325 (1988).
Bodmeier, R., K. H. Oh, and Y. Pramar, *Drug Dev. Ind. Pharm.*, *15*, 1475 (1989).
Marin Bosca, M. T., J. Sanchez Morcillo, and A. Cerezo Galan, *Rev. Soc. Esp. Farm. Hosp.*, *13*, 199 (1989).
Buckton, G., A. E. Beezer, S. M. Chatham et al., *Int. J. Pharm.*, *56*, 151 (1989).
Capan, Y., S. Senel, and S. Calis, *Pharm. Ind.*, *51*, 443 (1989).
Chang, R. K. and C. Hsiao, *Drug Dev. Ind. Pharm.*, *15*, 187 (1989).
Chu, S. L., H. C. Wang, and X. Y. Chen, *Yaoxue Xuebao*, *23*, 623 (1988).
Das, S. K. and B. K. Gupta, *Drug Dev. Ind. Pharm.*, *14*, 537 (1988).
De Barochez, B. H., F. Lapeyre, and A. Cuine, *Drug Dev. Ind. Pharm.*, *15*, 1001 (1989).
Dey, M., R. Enever, and M. Marino, *Int. J. Pharm.*, *49*, 121 (1989).
Devay, A., I Racz, *Acta. Pharm. Hung.*, *58*, 166 (1988).
Garcia Diaz, B., M. A. Mangues Bafalluy, R. Farre Riba, *Farm. Clin. Spain*, *5*, 590 (1988).

DiLuccio, R. C., M. A. Hussain, and D. Coffin Beach, et al., *Pharm. Res.*, *6*, 844 (1989).
Fassihi, A. R. and D. L. Munday, *J. Pharm. Pharmacol*, *41*, 369 (1989).
Gai, M. N., R. Pezoa, J. Corbeaux et al., *Farmaco*, *44*, 1119 (1989).
Georgarakis, M., A. Panagopoulou, P. Hatzipantou et al., *Drug Dev. Ind. Pharm.*, *16*, 315 (1990).
Ghali, E. S., G. H. Klinger, and J. B. Schwartz, *Drug Dev. Ind. Pharm.*, *15*, 1455 (1989).
Ghali, E. S., G. H. Klinger, and J. B. Schwartz, *Drug Dev. Ind. Pharm.*, *15*, 1311 (1989).
Gurnasinghani, M. L., H. R. Bhatt, and J. K. Lalla, *J. Controlled Release*, *8*, 211 (1989),
Harland, R. S., C. Dubernet, and J. P. Benoit, *J. Controlled Release*, *7*, 207 (1988).
Hirayama, F., H. Hirashima, K. Abe et al., *J. Pharm. Sci.*, *77*, 233 (1988).
Huguenin, P. N., H. W. Zulliger, and R. Niederer, *Arzneim Forsch*, 38, 305 (1988).
Hussain, M.A., R. C. DiLuccio, and E. Shefter, *Pharm. Res.*, *6*, 49 (1989).
Jain, N. K. and A. N. Misra, *Drug Dev. Ind. Pharm.*, *15*, 825 (1989).
Jain, N. K. and S. U. Naik, *Drug Dev. Ind. Pharm.*, *15*, 117 (1989).
Jalal, I., E. Zmaily, and N. Najib, *Int. J. Pharm.*, *52*, 63 (1989).
Jonkman, J. H., W. I. Van Der Boon, and G. Grasmeijer, *Pharm. Weekbl. Sci. Ed.*, *10*, 17 (1988).
Junginger, H. E., J. Verhoeven, and M. Danhof, *Drug Dev. Ind. Pharm.*, *15*, 1059 (1989).
Lin, S. Y. and L. L. Cheng, *Pharm. Ind.*, *51*, 528 (1989).
Lin, S. Y. and J. C. Yang, *Pharm. Acta. Helv.*, *64*, 236 (1989).
Macheras, P., M. Koupparis, and S. Antimisiaris, *Int. J. Pharm.*, *54*, 123 (1989).
Marano, C. G., H. M. Chechile, and P. Lufrano, *Acta. Farm Bonaerense*, *7*, 15 (1988).
Nigalaye, A. G., P. Adusumilli, and S. Bolton, *Drug Dev. Ind. Pharm.*, *16*, 449 (1990).
Pongpaibul, Y., K. Maruyama, and M. Iwatsuru, *J. Pharm. Pharmacol.*, *40*, 530 (1988).
Pena Romero, A., M. Poncet, J. C. Jinot et al., *Pharm. Acta. Helv.*, *63*, 309 (1988).
Pena Romero, A., M. Poncet, J. C. Jinot et al., *Pharm. Acta. Helv.*, *63*, 333 (1988).
Roy, S., S. K. Das, M. Pal et al., *Pharm. Res.*, *6*, 945 (1989).
Ghebre Sellassie, I., U. Iyer, D. Kubert et al., *Pharm. Tech.*, *12*, 96 (1988).
Seta, Y., F. Higuchi, Y. Kawahara et al., *Int. J. Pharm.*, *41*, 245 (1988).
Seta, Y., T. Otsuka, H. Tokiwa et al., *Int. J. Pharm.*, *41*, 263 (1988).
Seta, Y., F. Higuchi, T. Otsuka et al., *Int. J. Pharm.*, *41*, 255 (1988).
Shah, A. C., N. J. Britten, L. S. Olanoff, et al., *J. Controlled Release*, *9*, 169 (1989).
Shah, V. P., N. W. Tymes, and J. P. Skelly, *J. Controlled Release*, *7*, 79 (1988).
Shah, V. P., N. W. Tymes, W. Ment et al., *Pharmacopeial Forum*, *14*, 3458 (1988).
Shah, V. P., N. W. Tymes, and J. P. Skelly, *Pharm. Res.*, *6*, 346 (1989).
Shah, A. C., N. J. Britten, L. S. Olanoff, et al., *J. Controlled Release*, *9*, 169 (1989).
Snaselova, M., and K. Madlova, *Farm. Obz.*, *57*, 227 (1988).
Snaselova, J. Pokorny, and V. Hofschneider, *Farm Obz.*, *58*, 395 (1989).

Skelly, J. P., G. L. Amidon, W. H. Barr, et al., *Pharm. Res.*, *7*, 975 (1990).
Sprockel, O. L. J. C. Price, R. Jennings et al., *Drug Dev. Ind. Pharm.*, *15*, 1393 (1989).
Takeuchi, H., T. Handa, and Y. Kawashima, *Drug Dev. Ind. Pharm.*, *15*, 1999 (1989).
Wang, G. H., *Yaoxue Tongbao*, *24*, 198 (1989).

NINE

Dissolution and Bioavailability

INTRODUCTION

It has now been recognized with certainty that the knowledge of dissolution behavior and of the factors affecting such performance are of paramount importance in the design, evaluation, control, and therapeutic efficacy of solid dosage forms. Furthermore, it has been accepted that the biological activity of a given drug can be related to the rate at which the drug becomes available to the biological system postadministration. As early as 1955, Parrott and coworkers (1) stressed that the release of a drug from the primary particle and its subsequent availability to the body is governed by the dissolution rate of the particle. In 1969, Poole (2) added that the properties of the dosage form that modify the dissolution rate must of necessity influence the blood levels of the drug, and thus may function as the controlling factor in determining the magnitude of the pharmacological response elicited—and sometimes even of determining whether or not such a response is exhibited at all.

The pharmaceutical and medical literature is replete with reports showing variability in clinical response among orally administered drug products that contain chemically equivalent amounts of a drug (3). Those drugs are usually of limited aqueous solubility and the variation has generally been attributed to differences in their rate of dissolution. Additionally, it has often been asked, whether bioequivalence data per se ensure both product equivalence and appropriateness for substitution. In answer to that, one must say that even though the bioavailability data provided may appear to be adequate, the pharmacist must be aware of the limitations of such information. Bioavailability determinations often involve a single study performed on just one batch of a product. Thus unless the data obtained are correlated with in vitro quality control procedures that are employed to monitor all subsequent batches of the product, such data alone cannot ensure batch-to-batch bioequivalence (4).

There is adequate evidence to conclude that the rate at which a drug dissolves (dissolution rate) from its intact or fragmented dosage forms in the human gastrointestinal tract or in a parenteral injection site, often partially or completely controls the rate at which the drug appears in blood (absorption rate). Additionally, adequate evidence alludes to the fact that in many instances in vitro dissolution rate test results can be employed to "explain" observed differences in results obtained in animals and humans. Also, seemingly trivial changes in drug product formulations, manufacturing processes, or inadvertent variations in materials or manufacture can influence bioavailability significantly. It is thus apparent that correlation between in vitro dissolution performance of a drug and its bioavailability must be demonstrated convincingly to guarantee reproducible biological response from batch to batch of a given drug product.

It is recognized that bioavailability testing of drug products in humans can provide the most reliable means for evaluating in vitro dissolution. However, it is impractical to perform the extensive (in both time and personnel involvement) and expensive human testing that might be routinely required. Furthermore, if such studies are conducted, a large number of human subjects would be placed at risk. The position of the FDA is that bioavailability testing in which humans are used as test subjects be minimized by the development and implementation of in vitro dissolution standards that reflect in vivo drug performance (5).

To date, in vitro dissolution tests seem to be the most sensitive and reliable predictors of in vivo availability. Until recently, attempts to estimate physiological availability of a drug from a solid dosage form by in vitro methods have been confined to the measurement of the rates of disintegration and ultimate dissolution. Although official tests have great practical value, the fact that there is still a need for a test more directly related to bioavailability has been pointed out repeatedly. Since dissolution of a dosage form in vivo is often the rate-limiting factor determining the physiologic availability of a drug, measurement of the in vitro dissolution rate or a related parameter is more likely to offer a meaningful indication of physiologic availability (4). If a correlation of "good," "definite," "likely," or "poor" exists between this parameter and some parameter of bioavailability, the relatively simple procedure of monitoring the dissolution profile should permit the prediction of in vivo availability.

The logic and interest behind the correlation of in vitro and in vivo dissolution parameters is twofold (6): first, in the use of in vitro values to evaluate different lots of a particular pharmaceutical product as a quality control check to ensure a desired physiologic performance and second, as a developmental tool for a series of dosage forms to obtain a desired in vivo performance. These objectives can best be fulfilled when a relationship between the in vitro and in vivo parameters can be confirmed, but not when dissolution is merely defined under a random set of in vitro specifications.

The means to assess and develop methods of correlating in vitro and in vivo performance parameters—thus permitting effective means of prediction of biological response—is the subject of this chapter. We discuss briefly not only the importance of such correlations for specific drugs but also the development of various concepts employed in the past in determining in vitro–in vivo correlations. Additionally, specific methods for correlating in vitro–in vivo data will be presented that are more general in nature and have the potential for employment under more universal conditions. It is our intention in this chapter to provide the reader with adequate background necessary for developing specifications for a product under development and/or existing product(s) that demonstrate such a need. Furthermore, this attempt should provide a critical mass of information necessary to address possible currently existing limitations, thus providing an insight into strategies for improved means of correlating in vitro–in vivo data in the future.

Historical Background

In the late 1960s the Academy of Pharmaceutical Sciences recognized the chaos existing in the field of dissolution methodology and so established a Committee on Dissolution Methodology for Solid Dosage Forms in 1970. This involved performing collaborative research work to develop more meaningful, definitive, and sensitive dissolution procedures for solid dosage forms to be performed both by university laboratories and pharmaceutical companies. Gradually, determination of the in vitro dissolution rate evolved to represent a standard procedure for quality control of finished dosage forms (7). As a result of the FDA's commitment to ensuring the bioavailability of active ingredient(s) from a given dosage form, the investigation of dissolution rate of solid dosage forms has also become of prime importance to the industry.

In January 1977, the FDA issued final regulations on bioavailability and bioequivalency, which included a list of drug entities described as having "known or potential bioavailability or bioequivalency problems" (8). In those regulations, the FDA distinctly pointed out that "a bioequivalence requirement for the majority of products should be an in vitro test in which the drug product is compared to a reference material. Preferably, the in vitro test should be an in vitro bioequivalence standard, i.e., a test that has been correlated with human in vivo data. In most instances, the in vitro test should be a dissolution test." Later, Cabana and O'Neil (9), reviewing FDA literature and NDA files, revealed that the two principal causes of documented bioinequivalence are product instability and poor dissolution behavior. Furthermore, approximately 80% of the problems of documented bioequivalence that the FDA had identified resulted primarily from failure of the drug product to dissolve quickly and adequately. The need to establish in vitro–in vivo correlation (5) was clear.

Several reports have been published in the literature describing various attempts to correlate in vitro dissolution data and some in vivo availability parameter (3,4,10,11). Quantitative correlations between in vivo and in vitro data were presented as part of a series of papers for such drugs as penicillin, amphetamine, erythromycin, aspirin, tolbutamide, griseofulvin, and salicylamine (12). Following this series, a plethora of information focusing on attempts to predict effective in vitro–in vivo correlations of various solid dosage forms appeared in the literature. Few attempts have been made to categorize this superabundance of information by classifying it according to the type of investigation, nature of the study, and so on. Table 9.1 briefly illustrates various in vitro–in vivo correlation attempts conducted over the past two decades.

Although there are reports in the literature describing correlations between selected in vitro and in vivo parameters, there are many other reports in which such a correlation is not observed. Additionally, many studies do not attempt to establish such a correlation. On the other hand, when such a correlation does exist between an in vitro parameter and the relevant in vivo parameter, it is of limited value only, for there is no unequivocal relationship between such parameters. Furthermore, while such attempts at correlating in vitro–in vivo data have value in drawing attention to those drugs where variations in clinical response can occur, they are not all to be regarded as deliberate attempts to obtain correlation. Most of these reports, especially those reported during the early years, were the result of clinical observations and were obtained after the fact, so to speak, with no conscious effort to vary the formulation or a drug moiety in a particular manner so as possibly to produce changes in the rate of dissolution and thereby, biological availability. A complete discussion of all such correlations is not within the scope of this chapter. Emphasis will be placed on the reported theoretical hypotheses reported so far while correlating in vitro–in vivo data, thus providing the reader with possible approaches to choose from.

In the late 1960s, Levy classified in vivo–in vitro correlations as follows (85):

Table 9.1 Attempts to Correlate In Vitro–In Vivo Data for Various Medicaments Reported in the Literature, 1962–1987

Drug	Dosage form(s)	References
Acetohexamide	Tablets	13
Aminorex	Sustained release	14
Aminosalicylic acid	Tablets	15
Ampicillin	Capsules	16
Amylobarbitone	Tablets	17
Aspirin	Coated tablets	18
	Tablets	19–21
	Sustained release	22
	Tablets, capsules, and timed-release tablets	23
Bacampicillin	Microcapsules	24
Carbocromene hydrochloride	Soft-gelatin capsules, sugar-coated tablets, sustained-release tablets	25
Chloramphenicol	Capsules	26
	Tablets	27
Chlorpromazine	Tablets	28
Cinoxacin	Capsules	29
Dicumarol	Tablets	30
Diethylcarbamazine	Sustained-release tablets	31
Digitoxin	Tablets	32
Digoxin	Tablets	33–41
	Soft-gelatin capsules	42
Doxantrazole	Tablets, suspension	43
Doxycycline	Capsules	44
Erythromycin stearate	Tablets	45
Furosemide	Tablets	46
Griseofulvin	Tablets	47, 48
	Tablets, capsules	49
Hydrochlorothiazide	Tablets	50
Indomethacin	Microcapsules	51
Lithium carbonate	Tablets, capsules	52
Mefenamic acid	Capsules	53
Methaqualone	Tablets	54
Molsidomine	Controlled-release tablets	55
Nitrofurantoin	Tablets	56
	Tablets, capsules	57

Table 9.1 (continued)

Drug	Dosage form(s)	References
Nitroglycerin	Prolonged-release tablets	58
Oxytetracycline and tetracycline	Tablets, capsules	59
Phendimetrazine	Sustained-release products	60
Phenobarbitol	Tablets	61, 62
Phenylbutazone	Tablets	63–65
Phenylpropanolamine–HCl	Sustained-release beads	66
Phenytoin	Tablets, suspension	67
	Capsules, tablets	68
Prednisone	Tablets	69–72
Quinine–HCl	Enteric-coated tablets	73
Riboflavin	Sugar coated	74
	Sustained-release formulation	75
Sodium *p*-aminosalicylate	Enteric-coated tablets	73
Sodium sulfanilate	Enteric-coated tablets	73
Spironolactone	Tablets	76
Sulfadiazine	Tablets	77,78
Tetracycline	Tablets	79
Tetracycline hydrochloride	Tablets	80
Theophylline	Sustained-release tablets	81
Triple sulfa	Tablets	82
	Suspension	83
Warfarin	Tablets	84

1. Pharmacological correlations: based on clinical observations
2. Semiquantitative correlations: based on blood levels or urinary excretion data
3. Quantitative correlations: the result of absorption kinetics

While most of the published correlations fall within the second class, the most valuable are those based on absorption kinetics. The techniques employed today when one is attempting to establish the existence of a relationship have improved over those of several decades ago. In the following sections we concentrate on the various techniques developed and employed in correlating in vitro dissolution and in vivo availability data.

THEORETICAL AND PRACTICAL CONSIDERATIONS

The ultimate challenge to dissolution rate testing per se (and to any particular method) is its ability to reflect (and if possible predict) the in vivo performance of the dosage unit during the absorptive phase following administration (86). This testing invariably involves measurement of the degree of variation in a parameter. This measurement involves assignment of numerical values to observations in such a manner that these values can be manipulated in accordance with certain basic pertinent rules which depend on the level of measurement being used.

Accordingly, there exist four levels or types of measurement, presented here in order from highest to lowest.

1. *Ratio scale*. In this scale the ratio actually measures proportional changes in the quantity measured. Zero measures complete absence of the measured quantity.
2. *Interval scale*. In this type of measurement, the numerical values are assigned such that there are equal amounts between values of the scale.
3. *Ordinal scale*. This type of measurement, which involves a ranking procedure, permits one to define not only equality and inequality but also magnitude, in terms of greater-than or less-than values. However, the interval is not specified.
4. *Nominal scale*. This type of measurement groups objects into separate classes provided that there is similarity between these objects on the basis of some criteria. In this sense they are equivalent in nature; however, there is no numerical basis to the measurement, which prohibits analysis using arithmetical procedures. It is apparent that objects in different classes are unequal. This type of measurement provides a means of classifying data rather than measuring.

Essentially, two basic types of correlations are employed while comparing in vitro–in vivo data:

1. *Quantitative correlation*. An in vivo parameter usually designated as the Y variable is related to some in vitro parameter (some dissolution parameter) as the X variable employing some form of a linear equation(s), such as $Y = mX$, $Y = mX \pm a$, or $\ln Y = mX \pm \ln Y°$. Although, these relationships are informative, they should be based on theoretical reasoning, particularly while relating the two variables. It is often recommended that one should correlate either an interval scale or a ratio scale. The test for significance of

such a correlation is determined by employing Pearson's product correlation using moment analysis (87) designated by the r value. However, the level of significance is determined from a set of values and comparing with the tabled values. High significant r values may be achieved, but the correlation may be poor for predictive purposes. In such cases the coefficient of determination is calculated by determining r^2, which is indicative of the degree of variance in the dependent-variable values (Y values). This can be accounted for by calculating $100r^2$ and further determining the difference in the X values for a regression of the type $Y = mX \pm a$. It has been pointed out that the higher the magnitude of $100r^2$, the higher the predictive power. On the other hand, the confidence limits of the predicted Y value will be large for a given X value in case of low $100r^2$ values. Due to large differences and variations in the tested in vivo parameter, the value of $100r^2$ is often low, those resulting in poor in vitro–in vivo correlations. Such determinations are often used for improving in vitro dissolution specifications and strategies. It should be noted that the validity of the specifications must be based on sound statistical techniques.

2. *Rank-order correlations.* In this approach the dependent and the independent variables, in vivo and in vitro parameters, respectively, are rank ordered. Three possibilities can arise: for example, Y and X both increase, Y increases as X decreases, and Y decreases and X increases. Two types of rank-order correlations can result, such as "perfect" and "imperfect" rank-order correlation. Once the data are rank ordered, standard statistical tests, such as Spearman's rank order correlation, are employed to determine the in vitro–in vivo correlation and thus the prediction capacity.

Over the past three decades, numerous variables have been derived from in vivo and in vitro data, which have, correspondingly, been correlated with in vitro and in vivo data, respectively, as illustrated in Table 9.2.

The question that is often asked is: Which factors (variables) should be correlated from the myriad of available variables? Several investigators have argued over the relative importance of different in vitro dissolution parameters. However, it appears that the time for 50% of the drug to dissolve in vitro (T_{50}) is probably the best in vitro variable to correlate. There are two reasons that contribute to this observation.

1. By employing this value, one is not limiting or biasing the observation to any formal kinetic interpretation of data.
2. Additionally, the T_{50} value indicates the central tendency of the in vitro dissolution performance.

It has been pointed out that instead of confining oneself to a specific observation point (value), it is more optimal to consider the entire dissolution profile from $T = 0$ to $T = \infty$ or some parameter derived therefrom. This parameter

Table 9.2 Variables Derived from In Vivo and In Vitro Data Employed for Correlating with Variables Derived from In Vitro and In Vivo Data, Respectively

In vivo data	In vitro data
Plasma/serum concentration–time profile	Disintegration time
Peak plasma/serum concentrations	Percent drug dissolution profiles
AUC (plasma/serum) concentration profile ($T_{0 \to t}$)	Dissolution rate profiles
Estimated AUC (plasma/serum) concentration profile ($T_{0 \to \infty}$)	Intrinsic dissolution rates
Pharmacokinetic modeling Absorption-rate constant (K_a) Absorption half-life Elimination half-life	Dissolution-rate constants and dissolution-half-lives
Drug excreted in the urine ($T_{0 \to t}$)	Time for a certain percentage of drug to dissolve (e.g., $T_{30\%}$, $T_{50\%}$, $T_{90\%}$, etc.)
Cumulative amount of drug excreted as a function of time	Parameters resulting from determination of dissolution kinetics
Percent drug absorbed–time profiles	First-order percent remaining to be dissolved—time profiles
Amount of drug absorbed per milliliter of the volume of distribution	Logarithmic probability plots—percent drug dissolved–time profiles
Statistical moment analysis Mean residence time (MRT) Mean absorption time (MAT)	Statistical moment analysis Mean residence time (MRT) Mean dissolution time (MDT)

often provides for a better and meaningful indication of how the dosage form will perform in vivo. The author is a proponent of this school of thought. Accordingly, parameters such as area under the dissolution curve $(\mathrm{AUC}_{\text{in vitro}})_{t=0}^{t=\infty}$ or mean residence time ($\mathrm{MRT}_{\text{in vitro}}$) derived from the in vitro dissolution profile can probably provide a better indication of bioavailability performance.

One of the better values used to estimate from bioavailability data such as urinary excretion data or a plasma concentration profile (especially if the absorption is dissolution-rate controlled in vivo) is the absorption-half-life or the time for 50% of the drug to be absorbed in vivo. This parameter is often dependent on the pharmacokinetic model employed in the estimation. By employing simulated data, however, it has been shown that the ratios are nearly correct even though the absolute values of the absorption half-lives may be in error or an incorrect pharmacokinetic model employed. Thus one can relate in vitro and in vivo data which are dissolution dependent as a comparison or correlation of ratios of estimated absorption half-lives from bioavailability data with in vitro dissolution half-lives ($T_{50\%}$). Hence two formulations with differing $T_{50\%}$ values and estimated absorption-half-life values can give essentially identical in vivo/in vitro ratios. It must be noted that enough units of the formulations are tested to arrive at and establish highly significant differences between the in vitro and in vivo parameters. Many investigations have been reported in the literature with few units of dosage form employed for the study. This resultant data have limited value.

The efficiency of absorption relative to the dosage forms is dependent on the dosage strength. The relative absorption efficiency following equal doses as expressed in Eq. (9.1) provides for a means of comparison. If one of the formulations is a rapidly absorbing dosage form such as a solution, often referred to as the *standard preparation*, then Eq. (9.1) can be modified to depict the bioavailability of the test formulation when compared to the standard formulation as given in Eq. (9.2).

$$\begin{array}{c}\text{relative}\\\text{absorption}\\\text{efficiency}\end{array} = \frac{\text{amount absorbed from formulation 1}}{\text{amount absorbed from formulation 2}} \times 100 \qquad (9.1)$$

$$\begin{array}{c}\text{bioavailability of}\\\text{test formulation}\end{array} = \frac{\text{amount absorbed from test formulation}}{\text{amount absorbed from standard formulation}} \times 100 \qquad (9.2)$$

Both Eqs. (9.1) and (9.2) call for the appropriate estimation of the absorption value(s). The absorption value is often based on many assumptions. Hence it is appropriate to determine various measures by which one can estimate the amount absorbed from both plasma-concentration data and urinary excretion data as well. Table 9.3 illustrates various parameters that may be employed to estimate amount absorbed resulting from pharmacokinetic analysis.

The use of areas derived from plasma-concentration profiles involves the assumption that plasma clearance of drug is the same following different treatments. Additionally, the amount of drug absorbed per milliliter of the volume of distribution varies with the pharmacokinetic model applied for analysis. Use of this parameter involves the assumption that the volume of distribution is the same following different treatments. Additionally, estimation of the elimination-rate constants after different treatments is not biased by measurement in a region where absorption is either incomplete or in progress. However, in such instances, when the elimination-rate constant is estimated, absorption has ceased. Such differences and/or inconsistencies should be taken into considerations and thoroughly understood before any inferences can be drawn.

Table 9.3 Parameters Employed to Estimate Bioavailability (Amount Absorbed) from Pharmacokinetic Data

Plasma concentration data	Urinary excretion data
$AUCl_{t=0}$ following administration of single dose of drug	Total amount of unchanged drug excreted to $t = \infty$ following administration of single dose
Area in dosage interval at steady state when multiple doses are administered at uniform time intervals	Amount of unchanged drug excreted in the dosing interval at steady state following multiple doses of drug given at uniform time intervals
Amount of drug absorbed per milliliter of the volume of distribution resultant to pharmacokinetic model analyses	—
Coefficient of exponential nonlinear least-squares analysis of plasma concentration data	—
Mean absorption time (MAT) resultant to pharmacokinetic analysis employing statistical moment analysis	Mean absorption time (MAT) resultant to pharmacokinetic analysis employing statistical moment analysis

The variables cited in Table 9.3 are meaningful in terms of pharmacokinetic theory. It must be pointed out that estimation of relative bioavailability determined from parameters such as amount excreted at a specific time t, especially when t is less than 10 biological-half lives of the drug, cannot be employed for correlation. Also, area-under-the-plasma-concentration-curve values of truncated blood-level profiles following one or multiple doses are inappropriate and should not be employed in correlating in vitro–in vivo data. The resulting correlations may not be valid, in addition to the fact that they have less meaningful values.

Quantitative correlations of appropriate variables derived from in vitro dissolution data with appropriate variables derived from in vivo performance of the dosage form in human subjects must be established and demonstrated to arrive at pharmaceutically efficient dosage forms. Despite the huge number of such investigations undertaken and reports published in the literature, very few good correlations exist in the literature. These include valid and dependable correlations for drugs such as digoxin and prednisone. Studies should be designed such that they allow appropriate statistical procedures from the standpoint of the number of dosage units used in the study or the number of human subjects used in the study. The study protocol should be developed incorporating these procedures. The countless attempts to modify dissolution-rate testing equipment does not help in determining a reasonably good and universal method that can be employed in designing a protocol for such in vitro–in vivo correlation experimentation. Such factors and many others have contributed to the development of varied and diversified theoretical as well as practical approaches to testing and correlating in vitro and in vivo data. In the following sections we focus on the different measures reported in the literature that are employed while correlating in vitro–in vivo data.

METHODS FOR CORRELATING IN VITRO AND IN VIVO DATA

Many articles describing different methods for evaluating and correlating in vitro dissolution parameters with some in vivo parameters have been published. Most of these methods can be classified as either a predictive or an after-the-fact type of observation. Methods that set out with the aim of predictive conversion of in vitro data and speculating on in vivo performance followed by the determination of goodness of fit from the standpoint of correlation have a more meaningful value. Other methods also have significance; nonetheless, their ability for universal application is very limited.

Disintegration and Bioavailability of Drugs

Tablet disintegration tests have served a useful purpose and have resulted in improvements in the bioavailability of drugs in oral dosage forms. In vitro disintegration tests have been employed in the past as one of the primary in vitro evaluation parameters for predicting and/or determining the extent of bioavailability of a drug. However, these tests have certain inherent faults that limit their usefulness as measures of physiological availability of drugs.

Chapman and co-workers (88) reported that the bioavailability of riboflavin and *p*-aminosalicylate tablets in humans could be predicted from their in vitro disintegration time employing a modified USP XIV disintegration test. Tablets with a disintegration time of more than 60 min were not fully bioavailable. However, Endicott and Kirchmeyer (89), using different disintegration test procedures, reported that tablets which took more than 60 min to disintegrate were completely bioavailable. Later, Nair and Bhatia (90) observed that merely altering the mesh of the screen in the USP disintegration apparatus could markedly affect the disintegration times of tablets. These studies indicate the specificity of the relationship between in vitro disintegration time and bioavailability.

Later, Campagna et al. (91) unequivocally indicated that an in vitro disintegration test may not distinguish between fast- and slow-dissolving particles as was inherently present in earlier studies with tolbutamide products (92,93).

Additionally, it can also be pointed out that disintegration tests may not be able to distinguish between tablets with dissolution rates that differ because of the presence of different crystalline structures of polymorphic compounds.

The aforementioned aspects imply that in vitro disintegration tests apparently have certain inherent faults that lead to their eventual replacement or modification by more critical tests of physiological availability. Despite their weaknesses, however, disintegration time tests can still provide valuable information on the in vivo availability of some drugs for which little is known regarding their quantitative relationships between rate of solution and in vivo availability. Such information is essential for the development of meaningful in vitro dissolution time limits.

Variables Derived from Plasma Data

Once a drug formulation is shown to possess potential for further development to a commercial product through evaluation of in vitro dissolution testing, it is routine to evaluate the physiological performance of selected formulations that are promising. This results in the acquisition of plasma profile, urinary excretion profile, or some biological response profile as a function of time. The parameters generated from plasma profile of the drug as a function of time are numerous and can vary depending on the physicochemical properties of the drug molecule. The parameters are subsequently correlated with some parameter generated from the in vitro dissolution profile.

Levy (94) demonstrated a correlation between in vivo absorption data and in vitro dissolution rate for two different aspirin tablet formulations, plain tablets and buffered tablets. An excellent linear correlation was obtained when the amount absorbed at time t, was correlated with the amount dissolved in one-third the respective time period, as shown in Fig. 9.1. The positive intercept on the abscissa is indicative of the lag time before the drug dissolves and appears in systemic circulation. The slope of the line is unity, which indicates that the in vitro dissolution rate is consistently three times as fast as bioavailability of the drug. This factor is referred to as the *intensity factor*. Subsequently, the percent dose of aspirin absorbed at time t, following drug administration was correlated as a function of percent dissolved in vitro at time (t − lag time)/intensity factor. The lag time and intensity factor were the observed delay in the in vivo absorption of the drug and the dissolution-rate constant/absorption-rate constant ratio, respectively. Such a correlation can yield regression lines with unit slopes and zero intercept. In the case of processes that are not first order, the intensity factor can be expressed as the ratio of time for 50% absorption to time for 50% dissolution.

Improper formulation of many important drugs administered orally can lead to poor or incomplete absorption. Serious consequences can result for patients

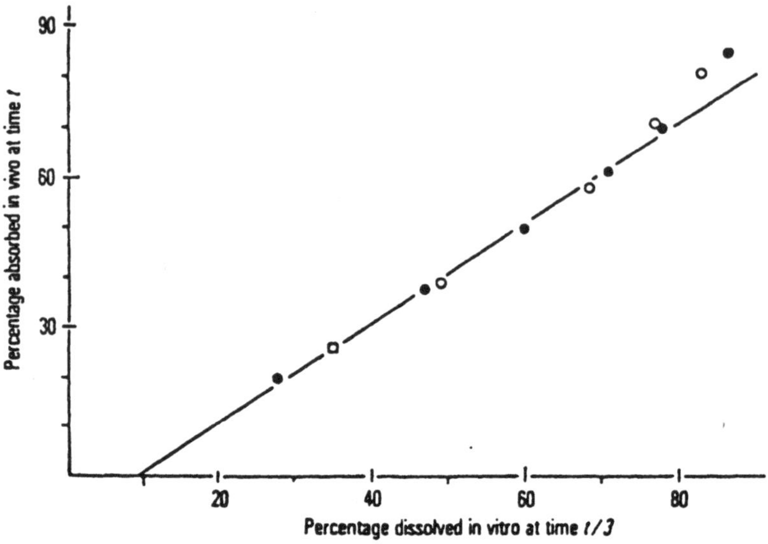

Fig. 9.1 Percent aspirin absorbed at various times post oral administration as a function of percent aspirin dissolved in vitro at one-third the respective times. ●, Plain tablets; ○, buffered tablets. (From Ref. 94.)

due to subsequent misjudgment of appropriate dosage regimens. On the other hand, the acceptance of a model dissolution system is partly by its adaptability to variations in test conditions or variations introduced to optimize in vitro–in vivo correlations. For example, improper agitation conditions can result in the failure of some dissolution tests to predict in vivo performance. The study by Levy et al. (19) involving three types of aspirin formulations—tablets, buffered tablets, and sustained-release tablets—of microencapsulated particles failed to achieve good correlation for agitation other than 50 rpm. This observation indicates that at 50 rpm the existing agitation conditions can reflect more realistically the biological conditions in the gastrointestinal tract. Later, Weintraub and Gibaldi (95,96) demonstrated an excellent correlation between the amount of aspirin dissolved in vitro and the amount absorbed in the same interval from these three formulations, as shown in Fig. 9.2.

Middleton et al. (97) established a correlation between the dissolution rate of seven oral dosage forms of PAS and its sodium salt and biological availability, with the exception of one of the products, as shown in Fig. 9.3. The data show that tablets containing PAS having a half-life in excess of 80 min (employing the stationary basket method) will possess an in vivo availability of less than 85%. This approach has been considered a reasonable criterion for bioavailability.

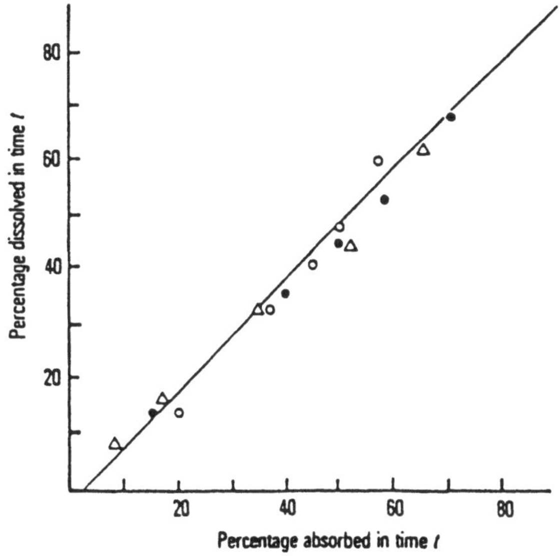

Fig. 9.2 Relationship between the percentage of aspirin dissolved in vitro and percentage of aspirin absorbed in vivo within the the same time *t*. ●, Buffered tablets; ○, plain tablets; △, timed-release tablets. (From Ref. 96.)

Katchen and Symchowicz (49) studied the dissolution and absorption profiles of several different griseofulvin preparations. They reported a good linear correlation between the mean plasma level following a single 500-mg dose and the logarithm of the in vitro dissolution rate. The dissolution studies were conducted employing an oscillating tube method and were expressed as the weight in milligrams dissolved in 30 min.

Sullivan et al. (70) evaluated the bioavailability of three commercial prednisone tablets—two generic brands and an innovator's product—in standard preparation form. The rate of systemic availability differed between the products but not in the amount of prednisone that reached general circulation. Additionally, the results indicated that differences in the systemic availability rates in humans correlated with in vitro dissolution rates and with reported clinical failure in prednisone use. Later, the same group demonstrated that the average time to reach the half-maximal plasma concentration of prednisolone (the bioactive form of prednisone) and the average plasma concentrations of prednisolone at 0.5 and 1 h obtained from three crossover bioavailability tests, involving 10 commercial prednisone tablets, correlated very well with parameters generated from in vitro dissolution testing employing spin-filter apparatus (72). Dissolution parameters used were times required to dissolve 16% or 50%

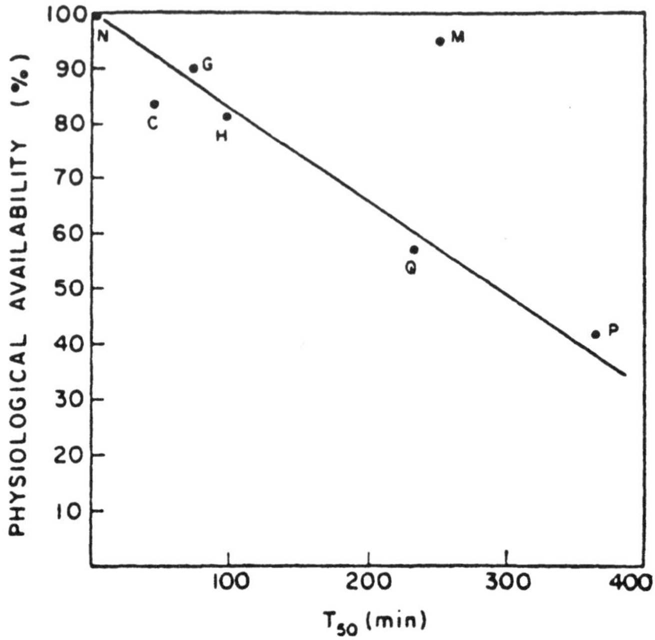

Fig. 9.3 Correlation between physiological availability and in vitro dissolution half-life for seven PAS formulations. N, P, Q, plain PAS; C, G, H, NaPAS; M, CaPAS. (From Ref. 97.)

of label or the percent of label dissolved in water in 20 min. Figure 9.4 illustrates the in vitro–in vivo correlation based on the time taken to reach half-maximal plasma concentration of prednisolone and the time required to dissolve 16% of labeled amount of prednisone. Figure 9.4 illustrates that six of the formulations (S, U, L, B, Me, and N) have the same in vivo parameter in magnitude, indicating obeyance to the theory that there will be some range of in vitro dissolution rates for which the in vivo parameters will not differ significantly. Thus, any further decrease in dissolution rates below some critical value will result in a progressive change in the bioavailability parameters. Overall, it can be concluded that predisone tablets differ primarily in the rate of prednisolone in plasma rather than in the amount of prednisolone that reaches circulation, the latter parameter being a measure of the extent of availability (71).

Nelson evaluated a series of erythromycin esters for their dissolution rate, dissolution media effects, and bioavailability. The area under the plasma concentration–time curve, a reflection of degree of bioavailability, was plotted semilogarithmically as a function of in vitro dissolution rates, as shown in Fig.

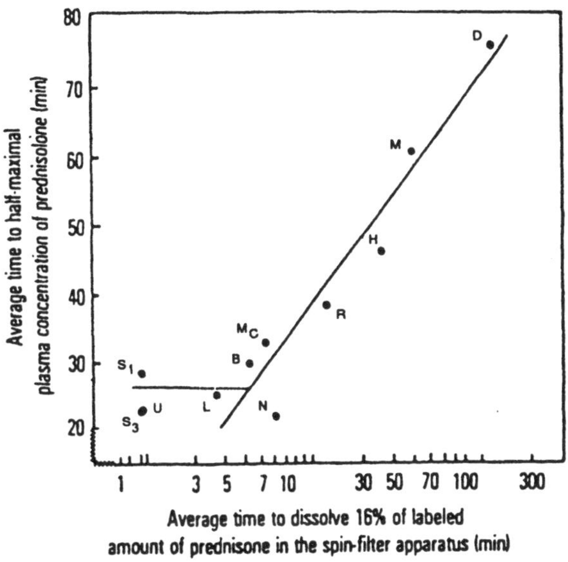

Fig. 9.4 Average time to half-maximal plasma concentration of prednisolone as a function of average time to dissolve 16% of labeled amount of prednisone in spin-filter apparatus. (From Ref. 72.)

9.5. The relationship indicates that the more slowly dissolving esters had the greatest bioavailability, contrary to what one can expect. In the case of erythromycin, however, this observation is not out of place since erythromycin rapidly degrades in acidic medium. Thus the degree to which the compound breaks down essentially determines the extent of bioavailability.

Shinkuma et al. (53) evaluated five commercial mefanamic acid capsules for in vitro dissolution. Of the five, three products (one fast dissolving and two slow dissolving) were subsequently evaluated for bioavailability in healthy human volunteers against a suspension formulation as a standard. Bioavailability parameters, C_{max}, T_{max}, and AUC, were calculated from the plasma concentration–time curves. Significant differences were observed among the products. No correlation was observed between in vitro dissolution rate of the drug from capsules and the in vivo data, possibly due to the dispersing effect of the capsules, which markedly influenced the dissolution rate. A good correlation was found between the bioavailability and the rate of dissolution of the drug from the capsule contents. Overall, the dissolution test results for the drug from the capsule contents reflected the bioavailability data and a correlation was found between T_{50} and AUC values.

The area under the plasma concentration–time curve generated from the bioavailability data has been employed to determine the correlation between

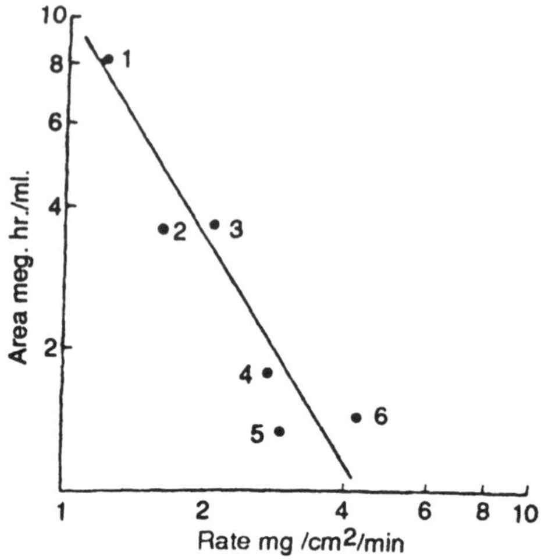

Fig. 9.5 Relationship between area under erythromycin blood-concentration-time curves and in vitro dissolution rate of various salts of the drug. [From E. Nelson, *Chem. Pharm. Bull.*, *10*, 1099 (1962).]

biological availability and the area under the in vitro dissolution-time curve. The correlation between these two parameters can be illustrated schematically as shown in Fig. 9.6. The characteristic of the dosage form, such as rapidly dissolving or slowly dissolving, can significantly influence these areas. Accordingly, their position on the correlation profile can be anticipated. Additionally, the areas will vary depending on the route of administration as well. Consequently, one would have a family of curves for each value of AUC after administration. One of the more prominent advantages of this approach is that if the area under the dissolution-time curve were known, AUC for blood levels at various times thereafter could be predicted (98).

Cressman et al. (14) developed an oral dosage form of aminorex which would produce prolonged and stable plasma levels of total drug. Since no definite set of dissolution conditions existed then for the evaluation of bioavailability, an arbitrary set of dissolution conditions was chosen. It was assumed that a correlation existed between in vitro dissolution and in vivo availability, a priori. If this were true, changes in dosage form characteristics could be evaluated in vitro before going to human or animal testing. Bioavailability was determined in human subjects by determination of the total plasma radioactivity following administration of [^{14}C] aminorex. In vivo absorption rates of intact drug were calculated from the plasma data for total radioactivity, employing a one-compartment open model. An estimate of the degree of correla-

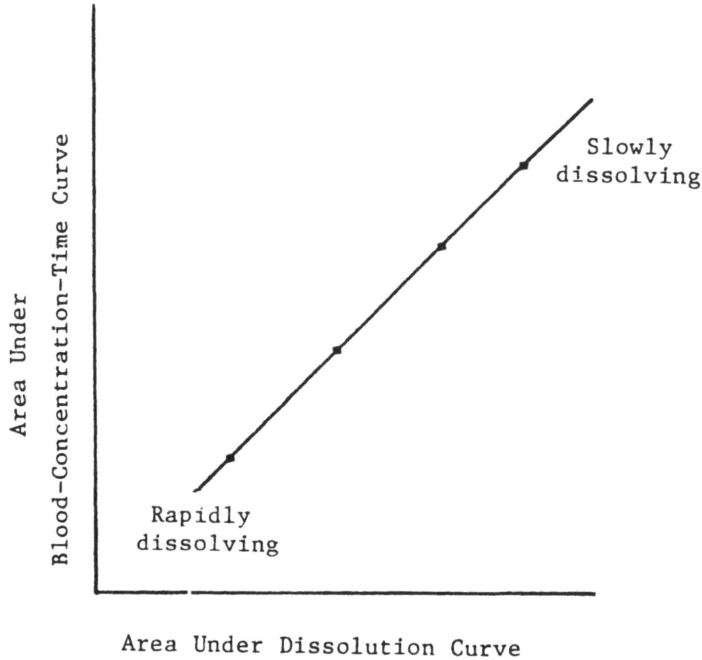

Fig. 9.6 Correlation between area under blood-concentration-time curve and area under in vitro dissolution-time curve.

tion obtained between dissolution and bioavailability data is illustrated in Fig. 9.7, where the lines for 25 and 50% absorption are plotted as a function of 25 and 50% dissolution. A good linear correlation was obtained with correlation coefficients of 1.0 and 0.99 for the 25 and 50% values, respectively.

It is important to recognize that differences in the in vitro rates of dissolution of various formulations of a drug may not necessarily be paralleled by differences in the bioavailability or physiological response. In the case of a drug with a good absorption profile and possessing a long biological half-life, such an effect may be observed (99). No significant differences were observed in the bioavailability of various sulfamethazine tablets having dissolution half-lives of approximately 1.5 and 15 to 20 min and 15 to 20 and 40 to 50 min, respectively. However, a significant difference in bioavailability, was observed between tablets having dissolution half-lives of 1.5 and 40 to 50 minutes. Similar results have been reported by other investigators for other drugs as well (100,101). The question that arises is: How large a difference in in vitro dissolution must be obtained before a significant change in bioavailability effect can

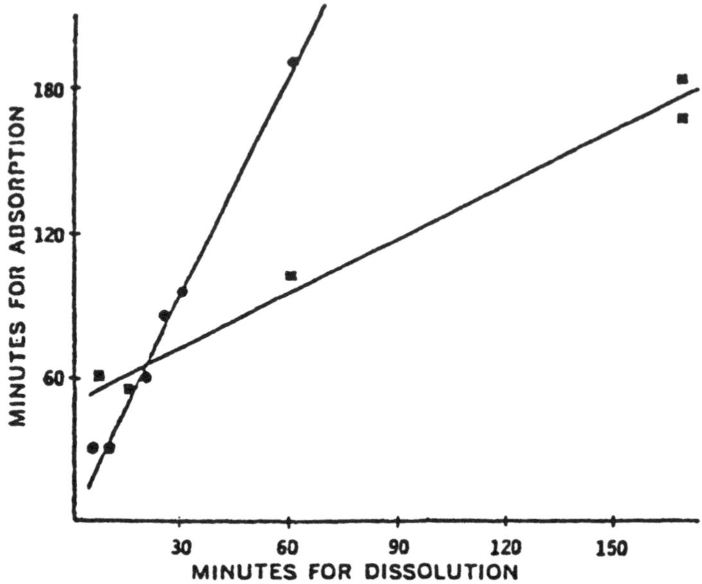

Fig. 9.7 Linear correlations between the times of 25% dissolution versus 25% absorption (●) ($r = 1.0$), and for the times of 50% dissolution versus 50% absorption (■) ($r = 0.99$) for various dosage forms of aminorex. (From Ref. 14.)

be expected? Ideally, it has been pointed out that one should employ an in vitro test that has the same sensitivity as that found in vivo.

Variables Derived from Urinary Excretion Data

Urinary excretion data are also an indication of the physiological performance of a drug formulation. The urinary excretion profile of the drug and/or the metabolite can provide an insight into the biological handling of the drug molecule. Urinary excretion data can be employed successfully to simulate blood/plasma data. Additionally, pharmacokinetic profiling via determination of urinary excretion of a drug is often preferred, wherever possible, over plasma data since this pathway provides a noninvasive method of evaluation of the bioavailability of the drug as well as the drug product. One of the major disadvantages of this method is that if the drug's pathway of excretion is not predominantly via urine, one is forced to determine the pharmacokinetics and thereby bioavailability via other modes, such as plasma data, pharmacological response, and so on.

The absorption and excretion of nitrofurantoin are affected by differences in the particle size of the drug (99). The USP has included a dissolution rate specification as well as a disintegration test since both adverse effects and bioavailability are influenced by the rates of dissolution and absorption of nitrofurantoin. The modified dissolution standard (between 25.0 and 60.0% of nitrofurantoin in the tablets dissolves in 1 h) was designed to overcome, if not prevent, rapid drug release, thereby reducing nausea augmented by rapid absorption as well as to obviate situations in which formulations exhibiting much lower bioavailabilities than control could be accepted in the absence of a lower limit (100). USP XX, finally, specified the lower limit only for the dissolution standard of nitrofurantoin tablets. Meyer et al. (101) conducted dissolution rate and bioavailability determinations of 19 commercial nitrofurantoin tablet products. Correlation between USP $T_{60\%}$ and numerous in vivo parameters was attempted. However, no useful correlation was found from the standpoint of predictability. A higher correlation was observed when the amount of nitrofurantoin excreted in 1 h was plotted as a function of the amount of nitrofurantoin dissolved in the first hour, as shown in Fig. 9.8. However, the curve was not useful for predicting bioavailability. Inter- and intralot variations, presumably caused by poor quality control during manufacturing process or by changes in formulations, were reflected from the dissolution test. Several other studies have been reported evaluating the dissolution and bioavailability of nitrofurantoin (56,101,102).

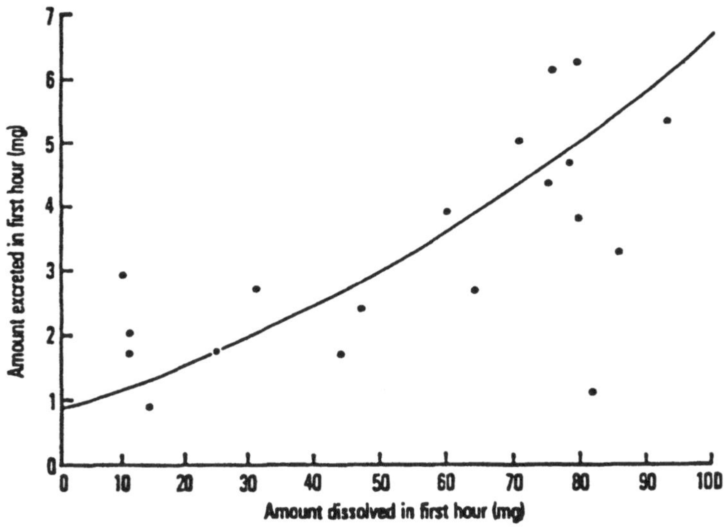

Fig. 9.8 Correlation of in vitro dissolution and urinary excretion of commercially available nitrofurantoin products (multiple regression analysis: $100r^2 = 68$). (From G. L. Mattock et al., *Can. J. Pharm. Sci.*, *7*, 84 (1972).]

Levy (21) determined the absorption rates of several types of commercial aspirin tablets employing a urinary excretion method. The results indicate that the bioavailability is proportional to the in vitro dissolution rate determined by the beaker method. A linear relationship was observed between the amount of salicylate excreted within 1 h of administration of two 300-mg aspirin tablets and the in vitro dissolution of one tablet after 10 min, as illustrated in Fig. 9.9. In the same study, Levy found that no relationship whatsoever could be determined between disintegration times of different aspirin products and their bioavailability. In a later report, Levy and Sahli established a rank-order correlation between amount of apparent salicylate excreted in the urine postadministration of equivalent oral doses of 1 g of aspirin and in vitro dissolution rates determined by the rotating pellet method, as illustrated in Table 9.4. Later, Bates et al. (103) demonstrated a correlation between the mean cumulative percent of the dose of salicylamide excreted in the urine of four human volunteers in 1 h and the percent salicylamide in solution after 15 and 20 min in vitro. Three different dosage forms of salicylamide were employed: a commercial tablet, a commercial suspension, and an experimental tablet formulation. The results are illustrated in Fig. 9.10.

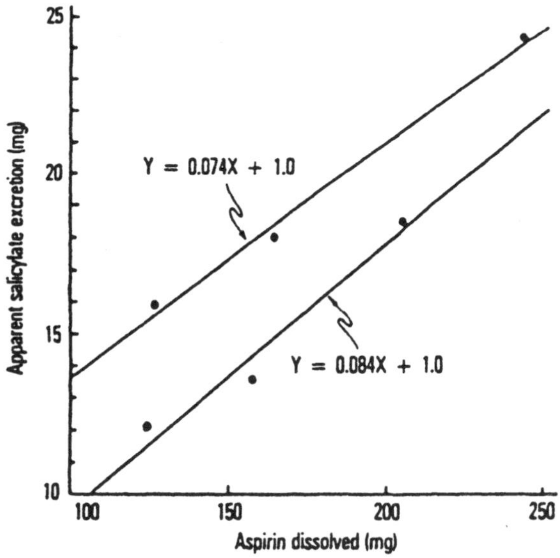

Fig. 9.9 Mean amount of apparent salicylate excretion (1 h post oral administration of 300-mg aspirin tablets) as a function of in vitro dissolution rate (mean amount of aspirin dissolved from one tablet in 10 min). (From Ref. 21.)

Table 9.4 Rank-Order Correlation

Form administered	Average amounts of apparent salicylate (mg) excreted in the urine of nine subjects: 1h	2 h	In vitro rate of dissolution ($mg/cm^2/h$)
Acetylsalicylic acid	14.7	50.9	65.1
Aluminum acetylsalicylate	5.23	19.7	8.88
Ratio: $\frac{\text{ASA}}{\text{Al ASA}}$	3.07	2.77	7.44

Shah and Needham (50) prepared four different hydrochlorothiazide formulations and determined cumulative urinary hydrochlorothiazide excretion in a crossover study. In vitro dissolution was conducted employing the flask, USP basket, and magnetic basket methods at agitation speeds of 50, 100, and 150 rpm. One of the formulations consistently showed significantly different results in both in vitro dissolution parameters and in vivo parameters. Regression analysis and an F test was used to determine in vitro–in vivo correlations. Significant correlations were observed as shown in Table 9.5. With a correlation coefficient and a 95% confidence interval, the USP basket method with an agitation intensity at 150 rpm proved to be the best predictor of urinary hydrochlorothiazide excretion among the dissolution methods evaluated. Several studies indicate a significant influence of formulation factors on the dissolution performance of hydrochlorothiazide tablets (104,105). However, other data indicate that such tablets apparently are not particularly susceptible to bioavailability deficiencies (106–109).

MacDonald et al. (109) evaluated the bioavailability (serum concentrations and urinary excretion) of four tetracycline hydrochloride capsule formulations prepared by four different manufacturers. The in vitro dissolution rate testing was performed using a special V-shaped transparent cylindrical chamber oscillating freely about its center. Using their data, Wager calculated the relative area and relative urinary excretion values from the areas and urinary excretion, respectively. An estimate of the relative in vitro dissolution rates from various capsules was obtained from the reciprocals of the $T_{50\%}$ values. Table 9.6 illustrates the relationship between both serum concentrations and urinary excretion of tetracycline hydrochloride and in vitro dissolution data. The relative in vitro $1/T_{50\%}$ values are rank-order correlated with both the relative areas and relative urinary excretion values. An almost linear relationship exists

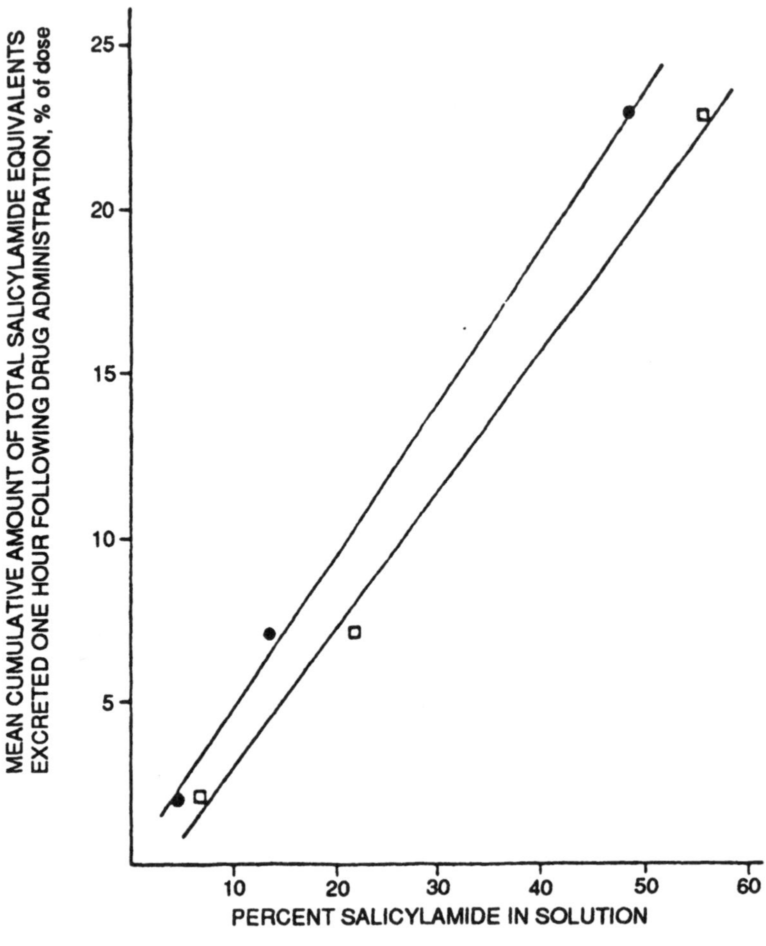

Fig. 9.10 Linear relationship between the mean cumulative percent of the dose of salicylamide excreted in the urine of four human subjects in 1 h and the percent salicylamide in solution after 15 min (●) and 20 min (□) in vitro. Three formulations of salicylamide were employed for this study: an experimental tablet, a commercial tablet, and a commercial suspension. (From Ref. 109.)

Table 9.5 Significant Correlations Based on Regression Analysis and *F* Test

Method	Agitation speed (rpm)	In vivo time (h)	In vitro time (min)	Slope	Intercept	Correlation coefficient[a]
Flask	50	14	80	2.29	−1.90	0.748
Flask	100	14	30	2.07	−1.54	0.698
Flask	150	14	20	1.33	−0.21	0.644
Magnetic basket	50	2	60	1.88	−1.09	0.630
Magnetic basket	100	2	60	2.02	−0.48	0.672
Magnetic basket	150	2	60	2.13	−0.17	0.604
USP basket	50	2	60	2.36	−0.33	0.609
USP basket	100	2	60	2.18	−0.69	0.656
USP basket	150	8	10	1.18	−0.25	0.649

[a] Significant at 0.99 level.

Table 9.6 Relationship between Serum Concentrations and Urinary Excretion

	In Vitro		Average serum concentration (μg/ml) at indicated time (h)						Area under serum curve		Urinary excretion	Relative
Prep.	$T_{50\%}$[a] (min)	Relative $1/T_{50\%}$	0	½	1	2	3	6	$\left(\frac{\mu g}{ml} \times h\right)$	Relative area	0–8 h (mg)	urinary excretion
A[b]	5.1	1.00	0	0.43	1.09	1.80	1.61	1.10	7.70	1.00	54.1	1.00
B[c]	41	0.12	0	0.27	0.78	1.28	1.19	0.83	5.63	0.73	38.5	0.71
C[c]	107	0.048	0	0.19	0.57	1.14	1.09	0.86	5.13	0.67	35.9	0.66
D[c]	244	0.021	0	0.08	0.29	0.76	0.69	0.53	3.19	0.41	22.2	0.41

[a] Time for 50% of tetracycline hydrochloride to dissolve in pH 1.0 aqueous medium.
[b] Preparation A was acchromycin (Lederle Laboratories).
[c] Preparations B, C, and D were other commercial forms of tetracycline hydrochloride capsules.

between relative urinary excretion or relative areas and the logarithms of the reciprocal of relative $T_{50\%}$ values.

Other Methods

Methods other than those that directly involve the measurement of the plasma-concentration profile or urinary-excretion profile are used to correlate with in vitro dissolution performance. Some of these methods include measurement of a pharmacological response, measurement of physiological residence time, and simulation methods involving convolution and deconvolution approaches. All of these methods have the same basis: they attempt to establish a definite correlation between the bioavailability parameter and an in vitro dissolution parameter, thereby determining the predictability of in vivo behavior from in vitro–in vivo correlation. Not all methods can be described. However, some of the more prominent ones will be described.

Lethal Time of Death and Dissolution

As early as 1962, Morozowich et al. (110) demonstrated a correlation between in vitro dissolution rates and the appearance of drug in vivo. A series of salts of benzphetamine and etryptamine were used. They were able to demonstrate a good correlation between the median lethal time of death (LT_{50}) and the in vitro dissolution rate of pH 7.2 determined by the hanging pellet method as illustrated in Fig. 9.11. From the figure it is apparent that those salts with low rates of dissolution had the highest $LT_{50\%}$ values following oral intubation of a

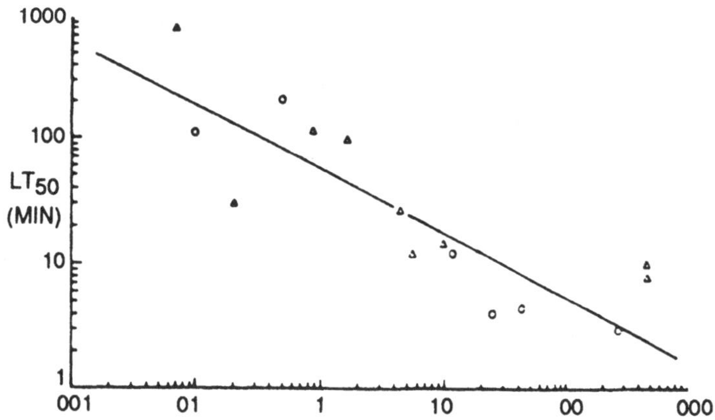

Fig. 9.11 Relationship between LT_{50} in mice and equivalent dissolution rate at pH 7.2 for etryptamine (○) and benzphetamine (△) salts. (From Ref. 117.)

lethal dose in starved mice. Conversely, lower LT_{50} values were exhibited by salts with faster rates of dissolution.

The original data from this study were modified by excluding the data points for benzphetamine hydrochloride and etryptamine acetate. The regression line was determined with the remaining data. The theory developed by DiSanto and Wagner (111) can explain the reasons for excluding these data points. These two salts had the highest dissolution rates; thus the availability of active bases to the receptors may not have been dissolution-rate limited.

Convolution–Deconvolution and In Vitro–In Vivo Correlations

Smolen and Erb (112) described a method that allowed for the predictive conversion of in vitro dissolution data into in vivo data. This method involves a mathematical approach to computing the in vivo drug-response profiles, such as pharmacological response, plasma concentration, and urinary excretion as a function of time, corresponding to the observed in vitro dissolution of drug dosage form as a function of time. The profiles of rate or extent of dissolution as a function of time are mathematically transformed into computationally predicted biological or response-output profiles.

The method involves a transfer function relationship between the drug's dissolution–time profiles and the average drug's biological-response-time profiles resulting from a bioavailability study of the dosage form in a panel of human subjects. The weighing or transfer function then permits in vivo pharmacological response, blood level, or urinary recovery-rate-time profiles for other dosage forms to be predicted computationally from their observed dissolution profiles. Updating of the mathematical relationship can be performed as more in vitro and in vivo data become available, thus improving the fidelity of the predictions. This black-box linear systems-analysis approach involves determining a weighing function, $G(t)_{BD}$ [transfer function, $G(\omega)_{BD}$ in the frequency, ω, domain] between in vitro dissolution data and in vivo drug response data for one or more reference dosage forms (113). The $G(t)_{BD}$ is obtained by the mathematical operation of deconvolution of the known in vivo data profile, $Q_B(t)$, with the in vitro dissolution profile, $Q_D(t)$, for the reference dosage forms. The inverse mathematical operation of convolution of the observed in vitro dissolution profile with the weighing function of the in vitro predicted blood curve for a dosage form under test is obtained once the weighing function is established. This approach employing convolution–deconvolution techniques in pharmacokinetics has been reported in literature (114,115). Smolen and Erb (112) exemplified this method for warfarin tablets, for which the observed in vivo plasma profiles were compared to corresponding predicted profiles computed from in vitro dissolution data. Figure 9.12 illustrates the comparison of in vitro dissolution rates to corresponding in vivo observed plasma concentrations. The multiple correlations are obviously non-

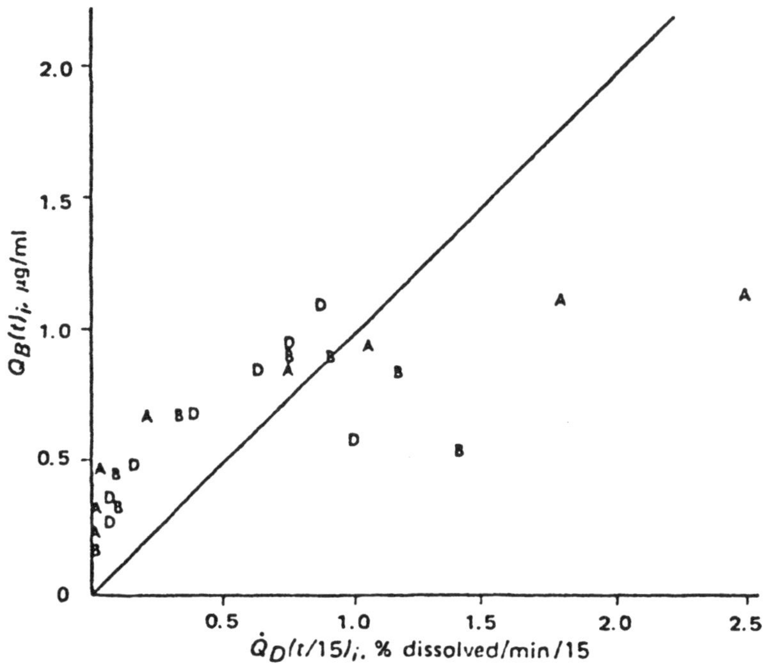

Fig. 9.12 Linear relationship comparing in vitro dissolution rates for tablets A (two 5 mg), D (two 5 mg), and B (one 25 mg) to corresponding plasma concentrations. [From V. F. Smolen and R. J. Erb, *J. Pharm. Sci.*, *66*, 297 (1977).]

linear. This is observed even when the rates of dissolution are properly time scaled. Consequently, in the case of warfarin, this approach proves to be a poor predictor of in vivo response from in vitro dissolution performance. However, in contrast, the use of in vitro predicted plasma concentrations obtained by the computational conversion of observed in vitro dissolution data does provide a theoretically rational, meaningful, and more reliable means of judging the bioavailability performance of drug products from the results of in vitro dissolution testing. One of the major disadvantages of this approach, as indicated by the authors themselves (112), is that these computations are not readily performed since a relatively uncommon computer with Fourier analysis capability is required.

Statistical Moments in In Vitro–In Vivo Correlations

One of the earliest applications of statistical moments to biological systems was provided in a report concerned with the kinetics of body cholesterol in humans (116). Since then, statistical moments have become increasingly popular and have been widely employed in different areas of bioavailability determinations, in vivo–in vitro correlations in particular (4,117,118).

The theory of statistical moments is based on the preliminary assumption that movement of the individual drug molecules through the body compartment is governed by probability. Furthermore, the time course of drug concentrations in plasma can usually be regarded as a statistical distribution curve (117). Thus the residence time of the drug in the body can be conceived as a frequency distribution with the mean and variance about the mean (119).

As defined by Dost (120), mean residence time (MRT) is the statistical mean of the times the individual molecules in the system at $t = 0$ are retained within that system before elimination (biological system) or liberation (dosage form dissolution in vivo). According to von Hattingberg and co-workers (121), cumulative dissolution and in vivo disposition curves may be viewed as frequency distribution curves of the individual times the drug molecules for a specific dose reside within the respective system—that is, within the in vitro dissolution medium and the test subject. Using Pearson's concept of statistical moments to characterize frequency distributions, one can evaluate in vitro–in vivo experimental data (121). Hence if a good correlation exists between the MRT for in vitro dissolution and MRT for a suitable in vivo disposition parameter, the relatively simple procedure of monitoring the dissolution profile should allow the prediction of in vivo availability.

The mean of all individual occupancy (or residency) times (MRT) is given by the equation

$$\text{MRT} = \frac{\int t\,dM(t)}{\int dM(t)} \tag{9.3}$$

where t is the elapsed time and m is the mass of drug (number of molecules) within the system. Partial integration and rearrangement of Eq. (9.3) yields

$$\text{MRT} = \frac{\int_0^\tau [M(\tau)\,dt - M(t)]dt}{\int_0^\tau dM(t)} \tag{9.4}$$

Since $M(\tau)$ and $M(t)$ are continuous within the interval, Eq. (9.4) can be further simplified as follows:

$$\text{MRT} = \frac{\int_0^\tau M(\tau)\,dt - \int_0^\tau M(t)\,dt}{\int_0^\tau M(t)}$$

or

$$\text{MRT} = \frac{M(\tau) - \int_0^\tau M(t)\,dt}{\int_0^\tau dM(t)} \tag{9.5}$$

$M(\tau)$ from Eq. (9.5) is the value of the integrand at the end of the integration interval; $dM(t)$ is the total mass of the drug under consideration (dose).

The physical meaning of the foregoing relationships may be more evident from an examination of Fig. 9.13, in which system response (whether in vitro dissolution or in vivo response) is portrayed as a function of time elapsed in the in vitro or in vivo system (MRT_{sys}). The numerator in Eq. (9.5) reflects the amount of drug that has not yet dissolved, or, consequently, the pharmacokinetic response yet to be observed. As a result, the numerator is nothing more than the area between the curve and the plateau (ABC), corresponding to 100% response (see Fig. 9.13). Thus

$$\text{MRT} = \frac{\text{ABC}}{\text{total mass of drug}} \tag{9.6}$$

If $M(t)$ is defined as the mass of the drug within an in vivo system (i.e., the amount of the drug remaining in the system or the amount of drug yet to be eliminated), then ABC is identical to the area under the curve (AUC) since $M(\tau)_{t=\infty} = 0$. Thus

$$\text{MRT} = \frac{\text{ABC}}{\text{AUC}} \tag{9.7}$$

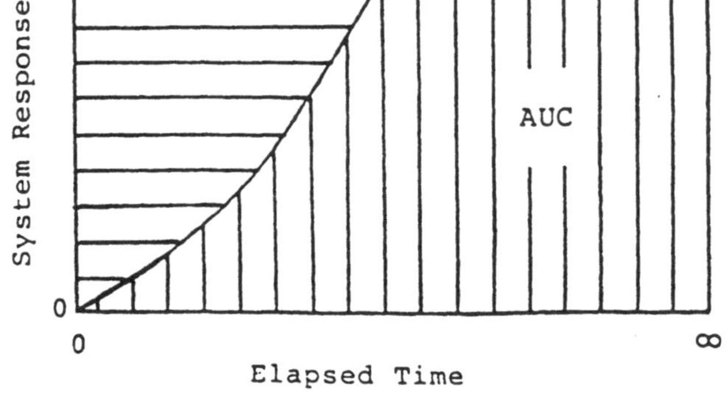

Fig. 9.13 Schematic representation of system response as a function of elapsed time.

If $M(\tau)$ is defined as the mass of drug that has yet to undergo dissolution, Fig. 9.14 is typical as well of in vitro dissolution curves. Thus the mean residence time for dissolution ($MRT_{in\ vitro}$) must be similar to the mean residence time in vivo ($MRT_{in\ vivo}$).

Exemplification of the MRT principle involves cumulative urinary excretion data for which the representation of "system response" as a function of time is relatively straightforward. For plasma drug concentration–time data, however, this may not be the case realistically.

When interpreting plasma drug concentration–time data, it must be noted that in accord with the mean residence time concept, system response corresponds to the AUC as a function of time. The distinction between the AUC of system response as a function of time and the AUC of an in vivo drug concentration–time plot may be difficult to envisage unless one examines a graph such as that in Fig. 9.14. Upon examination of the AUC as a function of the time segment of Fig. 9.14, it is evident that

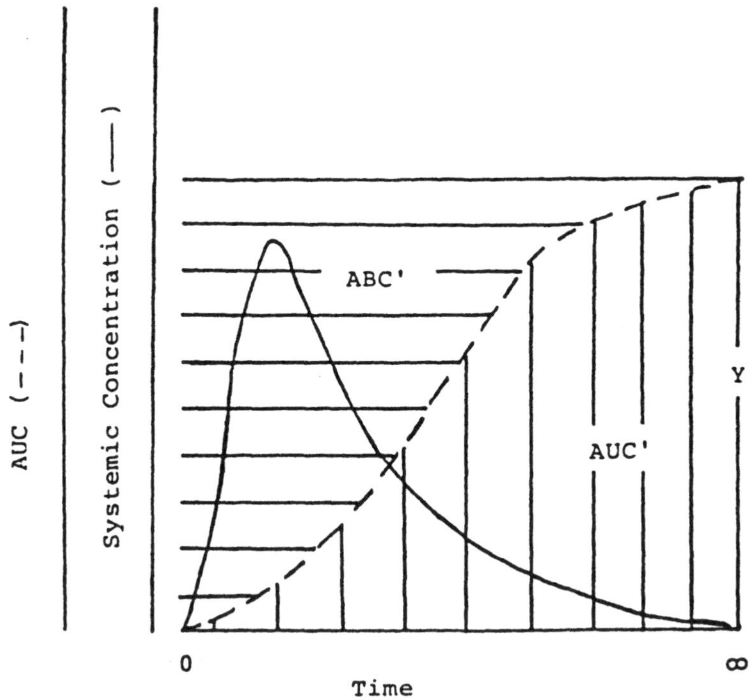

Fig. 9.14 Schematic illustration of transformation of blood–concentration–time data for determination of mean residence time (MRT).

$$MRT_{\text{in vivo}} = \frac{ABC'}{AUC'}$$

or simply,

$$MRT_{\text{in vivo}} = \frac{ABC'}{Y} \tag{9.8}$$

Demonstration of a good correlation (high coefficient of correlation accompanied by a p value < 0.05) is indicative of high predictability. The utility and inherent simplicity of this model-independent approach to in vitro–in vivo data correlation can be illustrated by transforming data, reported to possess poor correlation between in vitro and in vivo parameters.

McNamara et al. (122) evaluated the in vitro dissolution and in vivo availability relationship for six furosemide tablet formulations to evaluate bioequivalency. The dissolution studies were conducted in acetate buffer at pH 4.6 and pH 5.6 employing USP apparatus 2 at 50 rpm. Bioavailability was determined by characterizing plasma concentration—time profiles as well as cumulative urinary-excretion-time profiles. The investigators reported poor correlation when in vitro dissolution parameters such as T_{30} at pH 4.6 or T_{30} at pH 5.6 and urinary excretion data were compared with plasma-level data (r ranging between -0.67 and 0.62 accompanied by a p value > 0.1).

Three of the six formulations yielded data that were acceptable from the standpoint of essentially complete dissolution data as well as the attainment of a plateau for urinary excretion data and essentially complete characterization of plasma profile. Examining these data using the mean-time concept, one can transform the data for the determination of mean residence time both in vitro and in vivo (urinary excretion and plasma data). Correlating $MRT_{\text{in vitro}}$ and $MRT_{\text{in vivo}}$ for urinary excretion data yielded an improved correlation ($r = 0.99$, $p < 0.05$), as shown in Table 9.7. Also, significantly improved correlation was obtained when $MRT_{\text{in vitro}}$ and $MRT_{\text{in vivo}}$ for plasma data (employing the method for the computation of mean time as described earlier) were compared ($r = 0.98$, $p < 0.05$), as shown in Table 9.7.

In another study, Meyer and co-workers (101) observed significant differences in bioavailability as determined from crossover urinary excretion studies of 14 nitrofurantoin products. They were unable to make any useful correlation between the extent of excretion and the disintegration or dissolution characteristics of the products tested. They reported a correlation of $r = 0.45$ when mean percent nitrofurantoin dissolved after 90 min was compared with cumulative percent nitrofurantoin excreted after 12 h. When data are omitted for those products for which dissolution data were incomplete (i.e., for which the dissolution-time profile was incompletely characterized), one is left with acceptable data for five nitrofurantoin products. Even these data provide only a limited improvement in correlation with $r = 0.80$, as

Table 9.7 Correlation of $MRT_{in\ vitro}$ and $MRT_{in\ vivo}$ Computed from Data

Factor	Furosemide tablet formulation A	C	D	Correlation coefficient[a]
$MRT_{in\ vivo}$ (urinary excretion data)	0.74	1.18	1.12	0.99
$MRT_{in\ vitro}$ (dissolution data)	1.26	1.34	1.33	0.98
$MRT_{in\ vivo}$ (plasma data)	10.72	11.46	11.20	

Source: Ref. 122.
[a] $p < 0.05$.

shown in Fig. 9.15. Using the mean residence time concept and examining these data, one can transform the data sets to calculate $MRT_{in\ vitro}$ and $MRT_{in\ vivo}$. When the calculated in vitro and in vivo mean residence times are plotted for the five products selected (see Fig. 9.16), the correlation improves from 0.80 to 0.94 with a p value < 0.01.

The simplicity and utility of this approach (mean time) and its employment in correlating in vitro–in vivo data is obvious. The ease of data transformation, as demonstrated, can assist in facilitating data correlation, thus improving the prospects for reproducibility in in vivo performance of a formulation from batch to batch.

Mixing-Tank Model

Recently, Dressman and Fleisher (123) have developed a mixing-tank model for predicting dissolution rate control of oral absorption. This model is used to simulate gastrointestinal absorption of nonionized drugs. This model, as opposed to a two-tank model (124), provides a simple but useful picture of intestinal absorption. The following assumptions are inherent to this model (123):

1. Gastrointestinal flow patterns can be approximated by a one-tank mixing-tank model.
2. Drug is delivered as a bolus at time, $t = 0$.
3. Solid drug is transported at the same rate as dissolved drug.
4. Solid drug is composed of spherical particles of uniform size.
5. Drug is in a nonionized state at gastrointestinal pH, and absorption and transit are first-order processes.

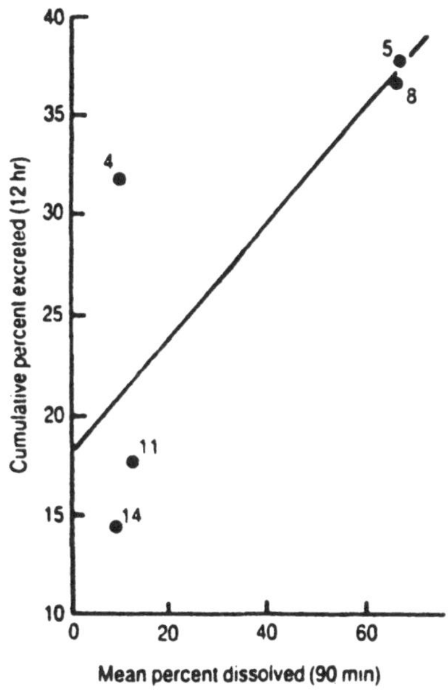

Fig. 9.15 Correlation between cumulative percentage of nitrofurantoin excreted after 12 h and the mean percentage of nitrofurantoin dissolved after 90 min for five of the nitrofurantoin products evaluated by Meyer et al. (106) ($r = 0.80$, $p > 0.05$). The numbers adjacent to the points indicate product code numbers.

The schematics of the mixing-tank model are illustrated in Fig. 9.17. The model is developed from mass balance considerations in which the nonsink dissolution term is a function of the remaining surface area and the concentration gradient across the boundary layer. This model predicts circumstances under which dissolution rate dominates membrane transport and drug transit rate, thus limiting the extent of absorption.

The authors demonstrate that the model correctly predicts bioavailability as a function of particle size for griseofulvin and digoxin. Other dissolution parameters include initial particle radius, dose, diffusivity, density, and boundary layer thickness, which were also incorporated in the study. This model can be applied successfully to drugs that are sparingly soluble and remain nonionized at gastrointestinal pH. This model, although in its infancy, has the potential for application for a spectrum of drugs having a wider range of aqueous solubilities. Readers interested in the details of this model are referred to the original work (123).

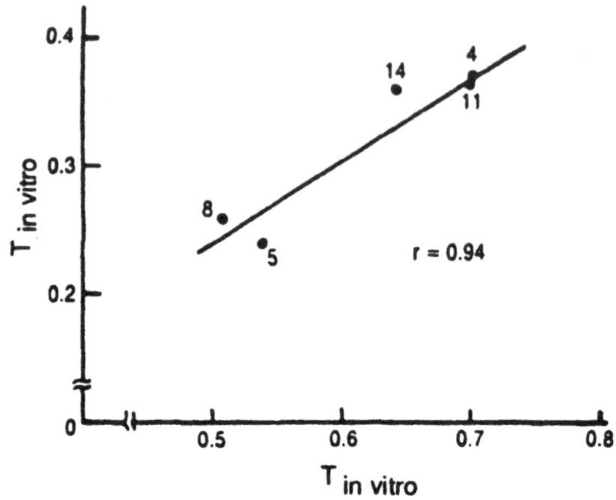

Fig. 9.16 Correlation between $MRT_{in\ vivo}$ and $MRT_{in\ vitro}$ for the five selected nitrofurantoin products evaluated by Meyer et al. (106) ($r = 0.94$, $p < 0.01$). The numbers adjacent to the points indicate product code numbers.

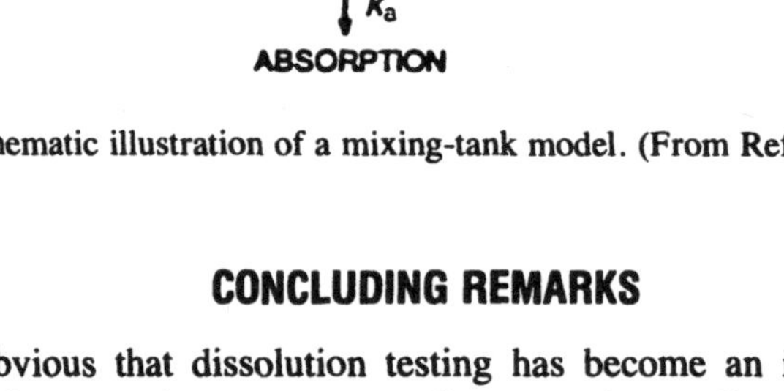

Fig. 9.17 Schematic illustration of a mixing-tank model. (From Ref. 123.)

CONCLUDING REMARKS

It is quite obvious that dissolution testing has become an important tool in solid dosage form development and quality control as well. Even if an in vitro dissolution test cannot replace biavailability assessment, it gives the formulator valuable biopharmaceutical information in a dosage form design program (125). Despite the fundamental relationship between the in vivo availability and in vitro dissolution rate, present evidence suggests that no single dissolution rate test can be applied to all drugs. The possibility that a single test could be applied to drugs possessing similar physicochemical properties remains to be established. If that is not possible, it may be necessary to obtain direct evidence of availability of each drug in each formulation by quantitative objective measurements carried out in vivo (126). Properly designed in vitro tests, dissolution rate tests in particular, would then be required primarily to ensure that products were manufactured under proper pharmaceutical control.

It should also be recognized that one will not always be able to establish a correlation between bioavailability data and those generated by a model in vitro system. Several factors can contribute to this inability. The limitations of the in vitro model systems are among the more predominant ones in in vitro testing of the dosage product in question. In addition, there are in vivo (biological) factors that can either mask or distort possible correlations. Some of these factors include variation in gastric emptying and intestinal transport rate, the potentially differing effects shown by sick patients confined to bed and healthy ambulatory subjects, and the variations arising from the use of a multidose approach as compared to a single-dose approach, still commonly employed to obtain bioavailability data. Phenomena such as in vivo differences observed with a subject who is a rapid absorber may not be present with a slow absorber; in vitro dissolutin rate data might only correlate in the case of rapid absorbers. Such factors need to be rigorously evaluated before a firm inference as to the predictability of an in vitro dissolution test of in vivo behavior of a drug product can be guaranteed.

In 1985, the Pharmaceutical Manufacturers Association's joint committee on bioavailability published an article outlining the role of dissolution testing in drug quality, bioavailability, and bioequivalence testing (127). After elucidating the benefits of dissolution rate testing in the design, development, and quality control of dosage form, the committee came to the conclusion that dissolution testing can be used only as a guide to a formulator in the early stages of drug product design. For some drugs, correlations can be made between in vitro dissolution and in vivo absorption, the report added. However, these correlations can be developed only after biological data have been obtained. Although dissolution rate testing is one of the critical assessments that must be performed to ensure that a formulation proven safe and effective in the clinic is being manufactured with consistent quality, it is not sufficiently predictive biological testing (127). Once a drug product has been designed and has been shown by bioavailability and biological testing to be both safe and efficacious, the quality of the product from lot to lot can be ensured by control of the dissolution rate specifications.

Studies reporting correlations between in vitro dissolution and in vivo availability in humans have, in most instances, been possible retrospectively. Additionally, these correlations have been possible only after a generation of bioavailability data and usually involving agreement with only one of the critical bioavailability parameters (one-point measurement), such as maximum plasma concentration, the time to reach maximum plasma concentration, or the area under the plasma concentration–time profile. Furthermore, these correlations are applicable only to the specific products tested. In other words, a new product may not relate to a correlation established previously.

The issue of in vitro–in vivo correlation becomes more complex for cases in which rapid dissolution is not desirable due to the possibility of toxicity and/or other unwanted symptoms, such as gastric upset. Examples of such products includes tolbutamide and nitrofurantoin. In such instances, an inverse correlation between dissolution and bioavailability would be expected. Also, dissolution-rate studies are unable to predict poor bioavailability for causes stemming from the effect of food, for example, in the case of tetracycline products containing calcium salts. In such cases, a good dissolution rate is observed but poor bioavailability.

Limitations of the in vitro dissolution model to predict explicitly the overall drug-absorption process, coupled with hesitancy on the part of the developer of a new drug product to explore fully the properties of noncommercialized formulations probably speaks for the overall scarcity of published data on in vitro–in vivo correlations. The development and validation of an in vitro dissolution model that can account for biological complexities associated with the absorption process, such as gastric emptying, gastrointestinal pH gradient, or influence of food, could be an extensive undertaking applicable only to a single drug product of interest.

Nonetheless, it is clear that the relation between in vitro dissolution results generated in the laboratory and bioavailability trials conducted in a clinical setting is complex in nature. Although dissolution-rate testing is claimed to be the most sensitive predictor of clinical performance, it is dangerous to assume so. Thus far, dissolution testing has failed to predict reliably the differences among products that are poorly bioavailable or superbioavailable, and those that are absorbed at an equivalent degree but whose clinical response is dependent not only on the absorption rate but on the extent of absorption as well. Dissolution testing can only be employed as a control device to ensure process and batch-to-batch consistency for a particular formulation of a particular manufacturer and as a screening tool in formulation development.

REFERENCES

1. E. L. Parrott, D. L. Wurster, and T. Higuchi, *J. Am. Pharm. Assoc. Sci. Ed.*, *44*, 269 (1955).
2. W. Poole, *Drug Inf. Bull.*, *3*, 8 (1969).
3. A. Dakkuri and A. C. Shah, *Pharm. Technol.*, *6*, 67 (1982).
4. U. V. Banakar and L. H. Block, *Pharm. Technol.*, *7*, 107 (1983).

5. *Federal Register*, vol. 42, part III (1977).
6. W. A. Ritschel, H. P. Koch, and G. J. Alcorn, unpublished report, University of Cincinnati Medical Center, Pharmacokinetics Laboratory, Cincinnati, Ohio (1985).
7. W. H. Barr, *Pharmacology, 8*, 88 (1972).
8. *Federal Register*, vol. 42 (Jan. 7, 1977), pp. 1621–1653.
9. B. E. Cabana and R. O'Neil, *Pharm. Forum, 6*, 71 (1980).
10. D. J. Campbell and J. G. Theivagt, *Drug Stand., 26*, 73 (1958).
11. J. G. Wagner, *Drug Intell., 3*, 198 (1969).
12. J. G. Wagner, *Drug Intell. Clin. Pharm., 4*, 232 (1970).
13. J. F. Nash, J. A. Galloway, A. D. Garner, D. W. Johnson, J. W. Kleber, and B. E. Rodda, *Can. J. Pharm. Sci., 12*, 59 (1977).
14. W. A. Cressman, C. A. Janicki, P. C. Johnson, J. T. Dolvisio, and G. A. Braun, *J. Pharm. Sci., 58*, 1516 (1969).
15. R. E. Schirmer, J. W. Kleber, and H. R. Black, *J. Pharm. Sci., 62*, 1270 (1973).
16. S. A. Khalil, L. M. Mortada, and F. A. Ismail, *Drug Dev. Ind. Pharm., 10*, 929 (1984).
17. W. S. Gledhill and A. P. Westwood, *Aust. J. Pharm., 45*, 512 (1965).
18. J. H. Wood and J. Syarto, *J. Pharm. Sci., 53*, 877 (1964).
19. G. Levy, J. R. Leonard, and J. A. Procknal, *J. Pharm. Sci., 54*, 1719 (1965).
20. H. Derendorf, G. Drehsen, and P. Rohdewald, *Int. J. Pharm., 15*, 167 (1983).
21. G. Levy, *J. Pharm. Sci., 50*, 388 (1961).
22. J. H. Wood, unpublished; through J. H. Wood, *Pharm. Acta Helv., 42*, 129 (1967).
23. T. E. Needham, K. Shah, J. Kotzan, and H. Zia, *J. Pharm. Sci., 67*, 1070 (1978).
24. J. Sjovall, R. Sjoquist, B. Huitfeldt and H. Nyquist, *J. Pharm. Sci., 73*, 141 (1984).
25. D. Voegele, D. Brockmeier, and H. M. von Hattingberg, *Proc. International Symposium on Methods in Clinical Pharmacology*, Frankfurt, West Germany (May 1979).
26. H. Andersgaard, P. Finholt, R. Gjermundsen, and T. Hoyland, *Acta Pharm. Suec., 8*, 403 (1971).
27. H. Ogata, T. Shibazaki, T. Inoue, and A. Ejina, *J. Pharm. Sci., 68*, 712 (1979).
28. P. A. Jablon, G. S. Banker, and V. F. Smolen, *J. Pharm. Sci., 59*, 1143 (1970).
29. J. F. Quay, R. F. Childers, D. W. Johnson, J. F. Nash, and J. F. Stucky II, *J. Pharm. Sci., 68*, 227 (1979).
30. M. J. Akers, J. L. Lach, and L. J. Fischer, *J. Pharm. Sci., 62*, 1192 (1973).
31. S. K. Baveja, K. V. R. Rao, and K. P. Devi, *Int. J. Pharm., 27*, 157 (1985).
32. L. Nyberg, B. Bergdahl and G. Wettrell, *Can. J. Pharm. Sci., 14*, 79 (1979).
33. A. Bertler, A. Redfors, S. Medin, and L. Nyberg, *Lancet, 2*, 708 (1972).
34. J. Lindenbaum, V. P. Butler, Jr., J. E. Murphy, and R. M. Cresswell, *Lancet, 1*, 1215 (1973).
35. B. F. Johnson, H. Greer, J. McCrerie, C. Bye, and A. Fowle, *Lancet, 1*, 1473 (1973).

36. E. Steiness, *Clin. Pharmacol. Ther.*, *14*, 949 (1973).
37. E. J. Fraser, R. H. Leach, J. W. Poston, A. M. Bold, L. S. Culank, and A. B. Lipede, *J. Pharm. Pharmacol.*, *25*, 968 (1973).
38. P. R. Klink, R. I. Poust, J. L. Colaizzi, and R. H. McDonald, Jr., *J. Pharm. Sci.*, *63*, 1231 (1974).
39. P. F. Binnion, *Clin. Pharmacol. Thera.*, *16*, 807 (1974).
40. P. Ylitalo, G. Wilen, and S. Lundell, *J. Pharm. Sci.*, *64, 1264 (1975).*
41. J. H. G. Jonkman, Ch. F. Gusdorf, W. J. V. van der Boon, G. Grassmeijer, and J. N. Jedema, *Arzneim.-Forsch./Drug Res.*, *37*, 62 (1987).
42. J. G. Wagner, R. G. Stoll, D. H. Weidler, J. W. Ayres, M. R. Hallmark, et al., *J. Pharmacokinet. Biopharm.*, *7*, 147 (1979).
43. H. Jones and A. Bye, *J. Pharm. Pharmacol.*, *31*, 730 (1979).
44. E. J. Antal, J. M. Jaffe, R. I. Poust, and J. L. Colaizzi, *J. Pharm. Sci.*, *64*, 2015 (1975).
45. S. Stavchansky, J. T. Doluisio, A. Martin, C. Martin, B. Cabana, S. Dighe, and A. Loper, *J. Pharm. Sci.*, *69*, 1307 (1980).
46. P. J. McNamara, T. S. Foster, G. A. Digenis, R. B. Patel, W. A. Craig, P. G. Welling, R. S. Rapaka, V. K. Prasad, and V. P. Shah, *Pharm. Res.*, *4*, 150 (1987).
47. S. Symchowicz and B. Katchen, *J. Pharm. Sci.*, *57*, 1383 (1968).
48. B. Katchen, *Acta Pharmacol. Toxicol.*, *29* (Suppl. 3), 88 (1971).
49. B. Katchen and S. Symchowicz, *J. Pharm. Sci.*, *56*, 1108 (1967).
50. K. A. Shah and T. E. Needham, *J. Pharm. Sci.*, *68*, 1486 (1979).
51. J. S. Rowe and J. E. Carless, *J. Pharm. Pharmacol.*, *33*, 561 (1981).
52. T. E. Needham, P. Javid, and W. Brown, *J. Pharm. Sci.*, *68*, 952 (1979).
53. D. Shinkuma, T. Hamaguchi, Y. Yamanaka, and N. Mizuno, *Int. J. Pharm.*, *21*, 187 (1984).
54. R. G. Stoll, G. C. Chao, H. J. Hoyt, and A. Yacobi, *J. Pharm. Sci.*, *67*, 1328 (1978).
55. A. G. Cassella and H. Aktiengesellschaft, *Pharm. Ind.*, *47*, 524 (1985).
56. R. Gronig, *Drug Dev. Ind. Pharm.*, *6*, 475 (1980).
57. R. W. Mendes, S. Z. Masih, and R. R. Kanumuri, *J. Pharm. Sci.*, *67*, 1616 (1978).
58. J. Ipsen, *Curr. Ther. Res.*, *13*, 193 (1971).
59. T. Bergan, B. Oydvin, and I. Lunde, *Acta Pharmacol. Toxicol.*, *33*, 138 (1973).
60. A. H. Beckett, D. H. Staniforth, and A. Raisi, *Drug Dev. Ind. Pharm.*, *6*, 121 (1980).
61. M. F. Sylvestri and C. Ueda, *Int. J. Clin. Pharmacol. Biopharm.*, *17*, 492 (1979).
62. D. Steinbach, K. Thoma, H. Moller, and G. Stenzhorn, *Int. J. Pharm.*, *4*, 327 (1980).
63. E. G. Lovering and C. A. Manville, *Can. J. Pharm. Sci.*, *12*, 48 (1977).
64. R. O. Searl and M. Penarowski, *Can. Med. Assoc. J.*, *96*, 1513 (1967).
65. R. J. Withey, H. Feng, D. Cook. G. R. van Petten, and H. F. Lettau, *J. Clin. Pharmacol.*, *11*, 187 (1971).

66. I. Yamakawa, M. Shimomura, T. Hattori, S. Watanabe, J. Tsutsumi, A. Shinoda, and Y. Miyake, *J. Pharmacobiodyn.*, *9*, 947 (1986).
67. P. J. Neuronon, P. J. Pentikainen, and S. M. Elfving, *Int. J. Clin. Pharmacol.*, *15*, 84 (1977).
68. S. Sved, D. Hossie, I. J. McGilveray, N. Beaudoin, and R. Brien, *Can. J. Pharm. Sci.*, *14*, 67 (1979).
69. A. R. DiSanto and K. A. DeSante, *J. Pharm. Sci.*, *64*, 109 (1975).
70. T. J. Sullivan, E. Sakmar, K. S. Albert, D. C. Blair, and J. G. Wagner, *J. Pharm. Sci.*, *64*, 1723 (1975).
71. T. J. Sullivan, M. R. Hallmark, E. Sakmar, D. J. Weidler, R. H. Earhart, and J. G. Wagner, *J. Pharmacokinet. Biopharm.*, *4*, 157 (1976).
72. T. J. Sullivan, E. Sakmar, and J. G. Wagner, *J. Pharmacokoinet. Biopharm.*, *4*, 173 (1976).
73. S. Rasmussen, *J. Pharm. Sci.*, *57*, 1360 (1968).
74. H. M. Ingani, J. Timmermans, and A. J. Moes, *Int. J. Pharm.*, *35*, 157 (1987).
75. E. J. Middleton, J. M. Davies, and A. B. Morrison, *J. Pharm. Sci.*, *53*, 1378 (1964).
76. J. M. Clarke, L. M. Ramsey, J. R. Shelton, M. J. Tidd, S. Murray, and R. F. Palmer, *J. Pharm. Sci.*, *66*, 1429 (1977).
77. M. C. B. van Oudtshoorn and F. J. Potgieter, *Pharm. Wkbld.*, *105*, 409 (1970).
78. W. A. Ritschel, G. Ritschel, C. R. Buncher, and J. Rotmensch, *Drug Intell. Clin. Pharm.*, *10*, 402 (1976).
79. K. A. DeSante, A. R. DiSanto, D. J. Chodor, and R. G. Stoll, *J. Am. Med. Assoc.*, *232*, 1349 (1975).
80. E. J. Lovering, I. J. McGilveray, I. McMillan, W. Tostowaryk, T. Matula, and G. Marier, *Can J. Pharm. Sci.*, *10*, 36 (1975).
81. D. Brockmeier, H. J. Dengler, and D. Voegele, *Eur. J. Clin. Pharmacol.*, *28*, 291 (1985).
82. R. J. Withey, G. R. van Petten, and H. F. Lettau, *J. Clin. Pharmacol.*, *12*, 190 (1972).
83. L. K. Mathur, J. M. Jaffe, R. I. Poust, H. Barry III, T. J. Goehl, V. P. Shah, and J. L. Colaizzi, *J. Pharm. Sci.*, *68*, 699 (1979).
84. J. G. Wagner, P. G. Welling, K. P. Lee, and J. E. Walker, *J. Pharm. Sci.*, *60* 666 (1971).
85. G. Levy, Indus. *Pharmaceuticals Section Symposium*, APha *Meeting*, Dallas (1966), p. 233.
86. F. Langenbucher and H. Retting, *Drug Dev. Ind. Pharm.*, *3*, 241 (1977).
87. H. M. von Hattingberg, D. Brockmeier and D. Voegele, How to Test for in vitro-in vivo correlation, *Biopharm. Pharmacokinet.* Workshop, Univ. of Cincinnati Medical Center, Cincinnati, OH (1982).
88. D. G. Chapman, R. Crisafio, and J. A. Campbell, *J. Pharm. Sci.*, *45*, 374 (1956).
89. C. J. Endicott and F. J. Kirchmeyer, *Drug Stand.*, *24*, 193 (1956).
90. A. D. Nair and V. N. Bhatia, *J. Pharm. Sci.*, *46*, 131 (1957).
91. F. Campagna, et al., *J. Pharm. Sci.*, *52*, 603 (1963).

92. F. C. Lu, W. B. Rice, and C. W. Mainville, *J. Pharm. Sci.*, *54* (1965).
93. A. K. Carter, *Can. Med. Assoc. J.*, *88*, 98 (1963).
94. G. Levy, *Arch. Int. Pharmacodyn.*, *152*, 59 (1964).
95. H. Weintraub and M. Gibaldi, *J. Pharm. Sci.*, *59*, 1792 (1970).
96. M. Gibaldi and H. Weintraub, *J. Pharm. Sci.*, *59*, 725 (1970).
97. E. J. Middleton, H. S. Chang, and D. Cole, *Can. J. Pharm. Sci.*, *3*, 97 (1968).
98. W. D. Walking, *Bioavailability Testing*, seminar presented to Duquesne University School of Pharmacy (1974).
99. H. E. Paul, J. H. Kenyon, M. F. Paul, and A. R. Borgmann, *J. Pharm. Sci.*, *56*, 882 (1967).
100. I. J. McGilveray, G. L. Mattock, and R. D. Hossie, *J. Pharm. Pharmacol.*, *235*, 2465 (1971).
101. M. G. Meyer, G. W. A. S. Slywka, R. E. Dann, and P. L. Whyatt, *J. Pharm. Sci.*, *63*, 1693 (1974).
102. R. Groning, *Dtsch. Apoth. Ztg.*, *119*, 2044 (1979).
103. T. R. Bates, D. A. Lambert, and W. H. Johns, *J. Pharm. Sci.*, *58*, 1468 (1969).
104. D. Cook, H. S. Chang, and C. A. Mainville, *Can. J. Pharm. Sci.*, *1*, 69 (1966).
105. P. Seth, *Pharm. Acta Helv.*, *47*, 457 (1972).
106. R. D. Hossie, G. L. Mattok, and I. J. McGilveray, *Rev. Can Biol.*, *32* (Suppl.), 85 (1973).
107. I. G. McGilveray, R. D. Hossie, and G. L. Mattok, *Can. J. Pharm. Sci.*, *8*, 13 (1973).
108. M. C. Meyer, A. P. Melikian, P. L. Whyatt, and G. W. A. Slywka, *Curr. Ther. Res.*, *17*, 570 (1975).
109. H. MacDonald, F. Pisano, J. Burger, A. Dornbush, and E. Pelcak, *Drug Inf. Bull.*, *3*, 76 (1969).
110. W. Morozowich, T. Chulski, W. E. Hamlin, P. M. Jones, J. I. Northam, A. Purmalis, and J. G. Wagner, *J. Pharm. Sci.*, *51*, 993 (1962).
111. A. R. DiSanto and J. G. Wagner, *J. Pharm. Sci.*, *58*, 1077 (1969).
112. V. F. Smolen and R. J. Erb, *J. Pharm. Sci.*, *66*, 3 (1977).
113. V. F. Smolen, L. Ball, and M. Scheffler, *Pharm. Technol.*, *2*, 89 (1979).
114. V. F. Smolen, *J. Pharmacokinet. Biopharm.*, *4*, 337 (1976).
115. V. F. Smolen, *J. Pharmacokinet. Biopharm.*, *4*, 355 (1976).
116. W. Perl and P. Samuel, *Circ. Res.*, *25*, 191 (1969).
117. K. Yamaoka, T. Nakagawa, and T. Uno, *J. Pharmacokinet. Biopharm.*, *6*, 547 (1978).
118. D. J. Cutler, *J. Pharm. Pharmacol.*, *30*, 476 (1978).
119. S. Riegelman and P. Collier, *J. Pharmacokinet. Biopharm.*, *8*, 509 (1980).
120. F. H. Dost, *Klin. Wochenschr.*, *36*, 655 (1958).
121. H. M. von Hattingberg, D. Brockmeier, and D. Voegele, in *Methods in clinical Pharmacology*, N. Riedbrock, B. Woodcock, and G. Neuhaus, eds., Friedr Viewig, Wiesbaden (1980), pp. 85–93.
122. P. J. McNamara, T. S. Foster, G. A. Digenis, R. B. Patel, W. A. Craig, P. G. Welling, R. S. Rapaka, V. K. Prasad, and V. P. Shah, *Pharm. Res.*, *4*, 150 (1987).

123. J. B. Dressman and D. Fleisher, *J. Pharm. Sci., 75*, 109 (1986).
124. J. B. Dressman, G. L. Amidon, and D. Fleisher, *J. Pharm. Sci., 73*, 1274 (1984).
125. M. Nicklasson, B. Wennergren, J. Lindberg, C. Persson, R. Ahlhgren, B. Palm, A. Pettersson, and L. Wenngren, *Int. J. Pharm., 37*, 195 (1987).
126. A. B. Morrison and J. A. Campbell, *J. Pharm. Sci., 54*, 1 (1965).
127. PMA's Joint Committee on Bioavailability, *Pharm. Technol., 9*, 62 (June 1985).

ADDITIONAL READING

Audran, M., Y. Lasserre, J. Rambaud et al., *Pharm. Acta. Helv., 63, 343 (1988).*

Banakar, U. V., L. H. Block and A. M. Galinsky, Proc. 9th Pharm. Technol. Conf., *Vol 1,* 135 (1990).

Beerbaum, H., K. Kulpe, K. H. Seidel et al., *Pharmazie, 43*, 325 (1988).

Block, L. H. and U. V. Banakar, *Drug Dev. Ind. Pharm., 14*, 2143 (1988).

Bosca, M. T., M. J. Sanchez Morcillo, and A. Cerezo Galan, *Rev. Soc. Esp. Farm. Hosp., 13*, 199 (1989).

Capan, Y., S. Senel, and S. Calis, Pharm. Ind., *51*, 443 (1989).

Chattaraj, S. C. and S. K. Das, *Drug Dev. Ind. Pharm., 16*, 283 (1990).

Chaumeil, J. C., J. M. Khoury, M. Zuber et al., *Drug Dev. Ind. Pharm., 14*, 2225 (1988).

Das, S. K. and B. K. Gupta, *Drug Dev. Ind. Pharm., 14*, 537 (1988).

Dash, B. H., R. G. Blank, B. P. Schachtel et al., *Drug Dev. Ind. Pharm., 14*, 1629 (1988).

Dey, M., R. Enever, and M. Marino, *Int. J. Pharm., 49*, 121 (1989).

Din, E. E. El, M. H. El Shaboury, and H. A. El Aleem, *Pharm. Ind., 51*, 694 (1989).

Doherty, C., and P. York, *J. Pharm. Pharmacol, 41*, 73 (1989).

Feely, L. C. and S. S. Davis, *Pharm. Res., 6*, 274 (1989).

Gai, M. N., R. Pezoa, J. Corbeaux et al., *Farmaco, 44*, 1119 (1989).

Georgarakis, M., A. Panagopoulou, P. Hatzipantou et al., *Drug Dev. Ind. Pharm., 16*, 315 (1990).

Giron, D., *S T P Pharma., 4*, 330 (1988).

Herman, J., J. P. Remon, R. Lefebvree et al., *J. Pharm. Pharmacol, 40*, 157 (1988).

Hollenbeck, R. G., *Int. J. Pharm., 47*, 89 (1988).

Hsu, H. Y. and J. W. Ayers, *J. Pharm. Sci., 78*, 844 (1989).

Huguenin, P. N., H. W. Zulliger, and R. Niederer, *Arzneim Forsch, 38*, 305 (1988).

Jain, N. K. and A. N. Misra, *Drug Dev. Ind. Pharm., 15*, 825 (1989).

Jain, N. K. and S. U. Naik, *Drug Dev. Ind. Pharm., 15*, 117 (1989).

Jato, J. L. Vila, R. Martinez, and G. Bilbao, *Cienc. Ind. Farm., 7*, 177 (1988).

Jonkman, J. H., W. I. Van Der Boon, and G. Grasmeijer, *Pharm. Weekbl. Sci. Ed., 10*, 17 (1988).

Kaojarern, S., S. Nathakarnkikool, and U. Suvanakoot, *DICP Ann. Pharmacother, 23*, 29 (1989).

Keller, M., *Dtsch. Apoth. Ztg., 128*, 1565 (1988).

Kikuchi, M., and K. Uekama, *Yakugaku Zasshi, 108,* 156 (1988).
Kimura, Y., N. Goto, N. Yoshimura et al., *Yakuzaigaku, 48,* 313 (1988).
Lagas, M. and A. M. Duchateau, *Pharm. Weekbl. Sci. Ed., 10,* 254 (1988).
Liu, G. L., Y. S. Zhang, Q. Y. Cai, et al., *Yaoxue Tongbao, 24,* 343 (1989).
Madhusudan, V., and S. L. Nasa, *East Pharm., 31,* 129 (1988).
Meyer, M. C., G. C. Wood, and A. B. Straughn, *Biopharm. Drug Dispos., 10,* 321 (1989).
Mishra, B. and J. K. Pandit, *Indian J. Pharm. Sci., 50,* 44 (1988).
Patel, N. K., N. R. Poola, A. Babar et al., *Drug Dev. Ind. Pharm, 15,* 1175 (1989).
Runhaar, E. A., J. P. Neijt, J. J. Holthuis et al., *Pharm. Weekbl. Sci. Ed., 11,* 218 (1989).
Serajuddin, A. T., P. C. Sheen, D. Mufson et al., *J. Pharm. Sci., 77,* 414 (1988).
Shaheen, O., H. Mouti, M. Karmi et al., *Curr. Ther. Res., 45,* 517 (1989).
Snaselova, M. and K. Madlova, *Farm. Obz., 57,* 227 (1988).
Sournac, S., J. C. Maublant, J. M. Aiache et al., *J. Controlled Release, 7,* 139 (1988).
Skelly, J. P., G. L. Amidon, W. H. Barr, et al., *Pharm. Res. 7,* 975 (1990).
Sprockel, O. L., J. C. Price, R. Jennings et al., *Drug Dev. Ind. Pharm., 15,* 1393 (1989).
Wang, G. F., Q. Liang, and Y. X. Luo, *Chin. J. Hosp. Pharm., 8,* 4 (1988).
Wilson, C. G. and N. Washington, *Drug Dev. Ind. Pharm., 14,* 211 (1988).
Yu, C. D., S. A. Sweetana, N. I. Chu et al., *Drug Dev. Ind. Pharm., 15,* 609 (1989).
Zuidema, J., F. A. Pieters, and G. S. Duchateau, *Int. J. Pharm., 47,* 1 (1988).

TEN

Dissolution Testing and the Assessment of Bioavailability/Bioequivalence

Santosh J. Vetticaden
International Drug Registration, Inc.
Rockville, Maryland

INTRODUCTION

Dissolution testing has been recognized as a relatively fast and inexpensive in vitro technique that can be utilized in the assessment of the release characteristics of dosage forms under investigation. Over the past 10 to 15 years it has been established that dissolution testing is probably the most important in vitro test that can be used to assess and control variables associated with formulation excipients, design, and manufacturing, which may alter the release characteristics of the active moiety from the formulation. Currently dissolution testing is therefore implemented in the assessment and evaluation of the release rates and bioavailability of a variety of conventional tablet and capsule dosage forms. Further, the advent of controlled-release dosage forms has also resulted in the utilization of dissolution testing in evaluation of the release characteristics of novel controlled-release oral and transdermal dosage forms during dosage form development for screening formulations with the desired release-rate profiles and during the postdevelopment and marketing stages for assurance of batch-to-batch uniformity.

Recognition of the importance of dissolution testing has resulted in dissolution testing requirements being incorporated into official compendia and into regulatory criteria for drug and/or dosage form approval. This is evident in the substantial number of USP monographs that include dissolution testing (1). Further, "in instances where the dissolution test results have been correlated with in vivo performance of the product, in vitro dissolution test criteria are used as part of bioequivalence requirements by the Food and Drug Administration" (2). In these particular cases, satisfying the dissolution requirements often ensures that batch-to-batch variability of in vivo bioavailability is minimized.

A test product is deemed bioequivalent to a reference product when the rate and extent of absorption of the active moiety from the two products do not show a significant difference when administered in a similar fashion and under similar experimental conditions (3). For an in vivo assessment of bioequivalence, traditionally, comparisons of AUC, C_{max} and T_{max} are conducted between the dosage forms. Comparisons of AUC serve as indicators of the relative bioavailability, and comparisons of C_{max} and T_{max} as indicators of the relative rate of release of the active species from the investigational dosage form. Therefore, attempts to assess bioequivalence of dosage forms using dissolution techniques would necessarily involve correlations of dissolution parameters to in vivo bioequivalence parameters (i.e., AUC, C_{max}, and T_{max}). Hence the role of dissolution testing in bioequivalence determinations rests largely on the reliability and predictive value of the foregoing correlations.

The primary aim of this chapter is to elucidate the importance of dissolution testing in the assessment of bioavailability/bioequivalence determinations of dosage forms. The fine line of demarcation between the role of dissolution tests in predicting bioavailability of dosage forms alone (i.e., in vitro–in vivo correlations) and in predicting bioequivalence determinations can sometimes be ignored. This is particularly true for the numerous methods employed to correlate in vitro dissolution data and in vivo parameters for a given product. Consequently, there will be some overlap of information, particularly in the methodology segment, that is inevitable. However, only information that is germane to the objectives of this chapter is presented. The information presented in this chapter is to be viewed in context with the assessment of the bioequivalence and bioavailability of dosage forms.

METHODS FOR INVESTIGATING IN VIVO–IN VITRO RELATIONSHIPS

Establishing bioequivalence criteria based on dissolution testing is achieved primarily by two routes. Under the first approach, for the dosage forms studied, it is possible to identify relationships (usually linear) between the in vitro dissolution parameters and in vivo bioequivalence parameters (approach A,

Fig. 10.1). Having established such a relationship, this relationship can then be used to predict the bioavailability or performance of an investigational dosage form, based on its dissolution characteristics. The alternative approach investigates various formulations (containing the same active moiety) that have been demonstrated to be bioequivalent based on in vivo studies. Dissolution methodology is then modified or developed that results in meaningful in vitro–in vivo correlations or are predictive of in vivo results (approach B, Fig. 10.1). However, both methods mentioned above should involve a large number of investigational or commercially available formulations to verify the appropriateness of criteria that may be established based on observed in vitro–in vivo relationships.

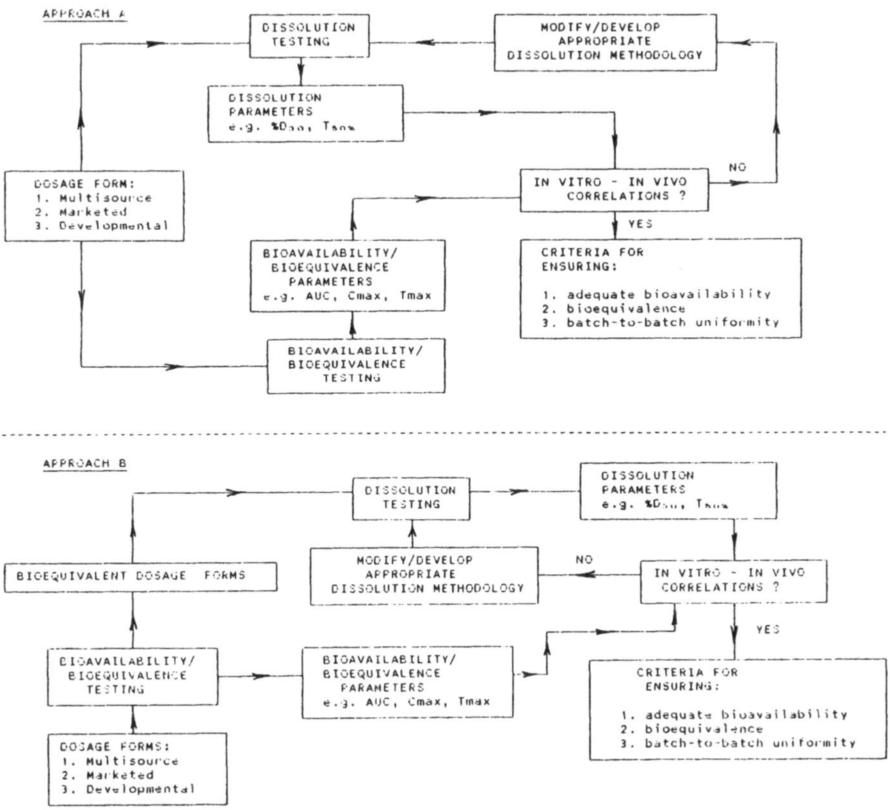

Fig. 10.1 Schematic representing approaches for investigating and establishing the applicability of dissolution testing in bioavailability/bioequivalence determinations.

Various methods have been employed in investigating correlations between in vivo bioavailability/bioequivalence parameters and in vitro dissolution parameters and are discussed in greater detail in one of the preceding chapters. These correlations may be classified into three groups: (a) direct correlation of dissolution parameters, (b) deconvolution techniques, and (c) other techniques.

Direct Correlations

In vitro dissolution parameters utilized in direct correlations to in vivo bioavailability/bioequivalence parameters include percentage of dose dissolved in a fixed time ($\%D_t$), time for a fixed percentage of the dose to dissolve ($\%T_p$), and rate constant for dissolution (k_d) or its transformations. The frequent use of these parameters is evident from Table 10.1 and they are also discussed later in the book. The use of rank-order correlations in bioavailability determinations tends to be extremely limited because such correlations do not normally result in quantifiable numerical estimates of bioavailability. Therefore, in most cases, in vitro dissolution parameters are directly correlated, through linear relationships, to observed in vivo bioequivalence parameters (i.e., AUC, C_{max} and T_{max}).

Deconvolution Techniques

Deconvolution techniques and their application in evaluation of the absorption and release from controlled-release formulations are more recent in nature. Within the constraints of compartmental modeling, the Wagner–Nelson (4) and Loo–Riegelman (5) methods continue to be utilized for estimating the input function characteristic of a dosage form. However, deconvolution techniques are now an important tool in evaluation of the absorption/release characteristics of controlled-release formulations from plasma concentration as a function of time data.

Utilizing deconvolution techniques, the input function is usually generated as

$$I(t) = R(t) * W(t) \tag{10.1}$$

where $I(t)$ is the input function, $R(t)$ the response function, $W(t)$ the weighting function, and $*$ the operation of deconvolution.

If the input function desired is the in vivo absorption/release rate, the response function is generally the observed plasma concentration versus time profile following administration of the dosage form, and the weighting function is the response to an intravenous bolus. Relationships between the predicted $I(t)$ and the in vitro dissolution rate can then be investigated. Conversely, $R(t)$ can be predicted for a known $W(t)$ and $I(t)$. The technique was utilized successfully to predict the in vivo release rates of oxprenolol from osmotic release oral system (OROS) formulations (6). The predicted release rate for oxprenolol was found to correspond well with the in vitro release profiles obtained from dissolution testing. Further, the residual drug content in the shell recovered from the feces was similar to that predicted. However, caution should be exercised when correlating in vitro dissolution data to in vivo results for controlled-release dosage forms because controlled-release dosage forms (e.g., OROS systems) release drug throughout the gastrointestinal tract with varying physiological conditions. In contrast, dissolution testing is normally conducted under fairly constant predetermined conditions. Additionally, deconvolution analysis makes assumptions of linearity and time invariance regarding the absorption processes.

Other Techniques

Other procedures include modifications of the direct method and the deconvolution method. A simple procedure for predicting in vivo availability parameters from in vitro data was employed by El-Yazigi and Sawchuck (7) in evaluation of commercially available theophylline dosage forms. Dissolution data were first obtained and then using in vivo and in vitro correlations between two reference dosage forms, a linear relationship was utilized in predicting in vivo parameters for a theophylline tablet, capsule, and sustained-release capsule. The predicted values of the bioavailability relative to a solution (F) area under the curve from 0 to 6 h postdosing ($AUC_{0\text{-}6}$) and AUC from 0 to infinity (AUC_{inf}) were slightly lower than the values actually observed but were not significantly different. Another procedure involved deconvolution followed by correlation of the fraction of drug released/absorbed in vivo to the fraction of drug released in vitro (referred to by the author as the "Levy plot") and was used with sufficient predictability (8). Good correlation was observed between the in vivo and in vitro release rates.

ASSESSMENT OF BIOAVAILABILITY/BIOEQUIVALENCE

In vivo availability of a test product is normally assessed relative to an equivalent dose administered either intravenously or as an oral solution. However, bioequivalence (from a regulatory standpoint) generally involves comparisons with a previously approved product, usually the innovator product or some other suitable reference standard. Among the various criteria for determining bioequivalence, the Code of Federal Regulations (21 CFR 320) indicates that an in vitro test correlated with bioavailability data and/or currently established dissolution tests may also be used for the purposes of assessing bioequivalence of the test product to the reference (3). However, the preferred use of dissolution testing in assessing bioavailability and bioequivalence remains in those cases where definite relationships to the in vivo performance of the dosage form have been demonstrated.

An observed in vitro–in vivo relationship, if linear, may be expressed as

$$A = mB + c \tag{10.2}$$

where A is the in vitro dissolution parameter (e.g., $\%D_t, \%T_p$), B the in vivo bioavailability/bioequivalence parameter (e.g., AUC, C_{max}, T_{max}), and m and c are constants.

For bioequivalence comparisons it is generally required that the bioavailability of the test dosage form be within p percent of that of the reference formulation. Using Eq. (10.2), the dosage forms would then have to satisfy the dissolution requirement

$$-p \leqslant \frac{A_t - A_r \times 100}{A_r - c} \geqslant p \tag{10.3}$$

where the subscripts t and r denote the test and reference formulations, respectively, and differences are computed relative to the reference formulation. The criteria above may also be utilized in establishing limits for batch-to-batch variability of the manufactured product.

In some cases it may be required that the test formulation satisfy a minimum bioavailability requirement (usually when approach B, Fig. 10.1, is utilized), in which case the following dissolution requirement should be met:

$$A_t \geqslant A_r \tag{10.4}$$

where A_r has been previously established for the reference formulation and/or other products with demonstrated in vivo bioequivalence to the reference. The discussion above assumes that the dissolution tests for both reference and test formulations are conducted under similar experimental conditions. As mentioned earlier, correlations of dissolution parameters to in vivo parameters should attempt to predict both the rate and extent of absorption:

Extent of Absorption

AUC and the amount of unchanged drug (or total drug, i.e., drug + metabolites) excreted in the urine are generally accepted as good indicators for assessment of bioavailability of the dosage form. Correlations of these bioavailability parameters to in vitro dissolution-rate testing usually involves relationships of time to dissolution for a specified amount ($\%D_t$) or amount dissolved until a definite time interval ($\%T_p$).

Correlations Employing AUC

Some of the earlier reported correlations of in vitro dissolution parameters to AUC were for digoxin (9). The amount of digoxin dissolved in 1 h and the reciprocal of the half-life for dissolution ($1/T_{50\%}$) as in vitro parameters were correlated with the extent of digoxin bioavailability. The ability of dissolution testing to discriminate between acceptable and nonacceptable in vivo performance of batches of granules was also demonstrated during the development of acid-resistant granules of omeprazole (10). Omeprazole has a low water solubility and is degraded in an acid environment. Avoidance of dissolution-rate-limited absorption and preabsorption degradation were important. Granules were tested for acid resistance by determining dissolution characteristics in an acid medium. AUC_{inf} for the faster-dissolving granules were 95% and 92%, respectively. The granules with the lowest in vitro dissolution rate were absorbed to a lower extent and had a mean relative AUC of only 73%.

Such correlations need not be restricted to the finished dosage form (i.e., tablets or capsules) but may be used for the purpose of evaluation during the initial stages of dosage form development as demonstrated in the evaluation of omeprazole granules in the example above and in the evaluation of a suspension in the following example. In a four-way crossover study in 12 healthy volunteers administered 400 mg of bacampicillin suspensions with differing polymer content (11), a significant linear correlation was demonstrated between the in vitro dissolution half-life and the observed AUC values. The 95% confidence limits for the regression indicated adequate predictability of the in vivo data from the in vitro dissolution data (Fig. 10.2). The good correlation was attributed to diffusion through the polymer film being the rate-limiting step for both in vitro and in vivo diffusion.

Criteria Based on Correlations to AUC

Evaluation of in vivo–in vitro correlations such as those described above can then be utilized to establish criteria for ensuring bioavailability and/or bioequivalence of dosage forms, and possibly for inclusion as compendial criteria. This predictive ability of dissolution testing has been demonstrated in a number of cases, some of which are outlined below.

A significant linear relationship was demonstrated between the log dissolution rate constant and the individual AUC for four controlled-release (insoluble matrix type) formulations of alaproclate (12). A difference in the rate constant of $0.70\,h^{-1}$ was found to result in a reduction in AUC by 20% (permissible limit set by the FDA), demonstrating the practical applicability of this correlation in discriminating between formulations based on their bioavailability.

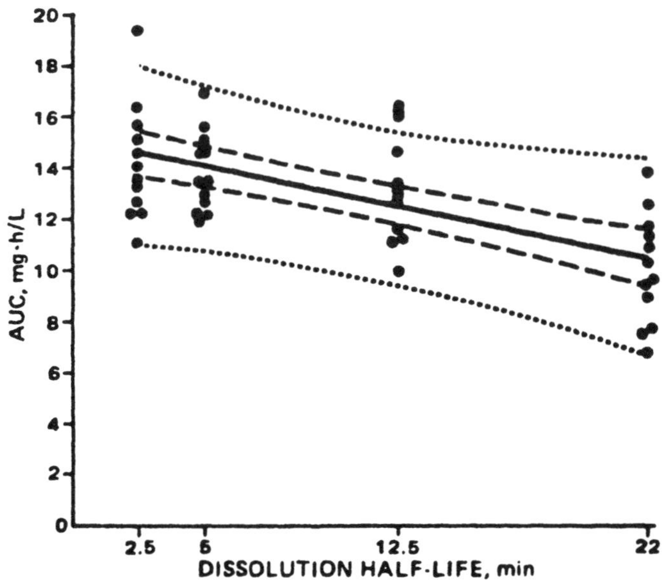

Fig. 10.2 Correlation of an in vitro dissolution parameter (dissolution half-life, $T_{50\%}$) to an in vivo bioavailability parameter (area under the curve from 0 to infinity, AUC_{inf}). The observed relationship follows administration of a single 400-mg dose of microencapsulated bacampicillin hydrochloride suspension in a crossover study in 12 subjects. The 95% confidence intervals for the regression line are represented as dashes, and predictions for a random subject for a suspension with a given dissolution half-life are represented as dots. (From Ref. 11.)

Confidence intervals around the regression line may also be drawn to get a better assessment of the predictive value of the observed relationships, as demonstrated in the evaluation of furosemide tablets (13). A linear relationship was observed between the percentage of the dose dissolved in 30 min and the bioavailability relative to an equivalent solution. The regression was observed to be linear only over the bioavailability range studied (i.e., 76 to 97%) relative to the solution. The *y* intercept corresponded to a bioavailability of 73%. Based on the confidence limits from the regression, the authors observed that if the tablets release at least 60% of their furosemide content in 30 min, there is 97.5% confidence that the relative bioavailability of the tablets would exceed 85%. The authors therefore suggested that the compendial specifications for furosemide tablets be modified to include a requirement of 60% dissolution in 30 min when tested in 900 mL of buffer at pH 5.0 at 37°C employing the USP rotating basket apparatus at 150 rpm.

Correlations to Amount Excreted in the Urine

Where a noninvasive assessment of bioavailability is required, the amount of unchanged drug (if the drug is excreted largely unchanged) or the total drug (drug + metabolite) excreted in the urine may be used as an in vivo indicator of the bioavailability of investigational dosage forms.

Evaluation of conventional and controlled-release terbutaline tablets exhibited good correlations for the linear relationship between the amount of terbutaline excreted in the urine in 72 h and the amount dissolved in 4 h after a single dose, as depicted in Fig. 10.3 (14). However, better correlations were obtained for the amount dissolved in 6 h to the steady-state excretion of terbutaline in the urine. A linear relationship with a negative slope was observed for the ratio of the amount excreted in the urine an hour before the dose at steady state to the 24-h excretion postdosing. The results are indicative of the influence of dissolution characteristics of the dosage form on its ultimate bioavailability. With sustained-release formulations a greater bioavailability was observed at steady state relative to a single dose. The authors attributed it

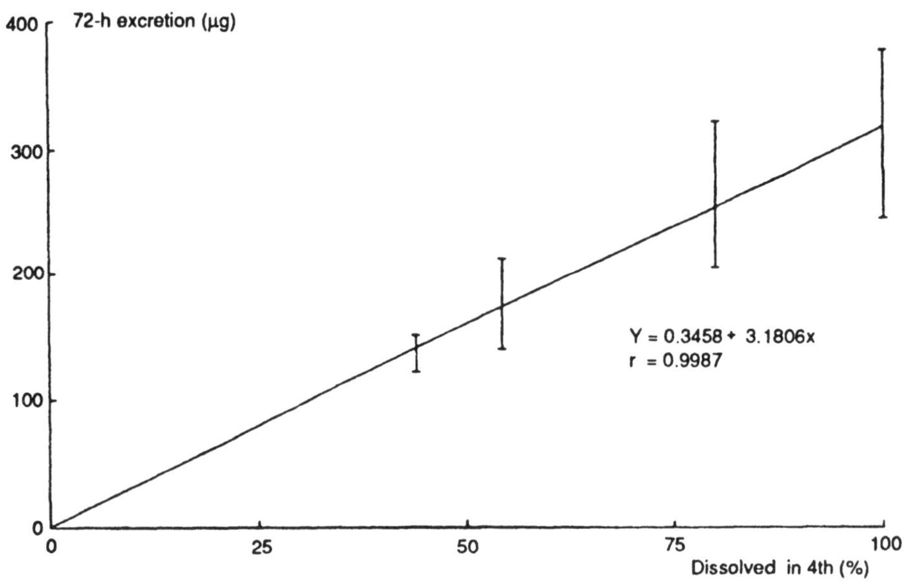

Fig. 10.3 Correlation of an in vitro dissolution parameter (% dissolved in 4 h, $\%D_{4\text{-hr}}$) to an in vivo bioavailability parameter [72-h urinary excretion of terbutaline, $A_e(0\text{–}72\ \text{h})$]. The observed relationship follows administration of single doses of terbutaline SR tablets to 11 subjects. The amounts excreted are normalized to a dose of 7.5 mg of terbutaline sulfate. (From Ref. 14.)

to effects on intestinal motility by terbutaline, since the sustained-release tablets with the slowest dissolution rate were the most affected. However, the results may also be explained by "residual" absorption, or absorption beyond 24 h that is not accounted for in a 24-h urine collection following a single dose.

A good linear relationship was demonstrated between the urinary recovery of bacampillicin 0 to 8 h postdosing and the dissolution half-life, indicating that bioavailability estimates could be obtained from in vitro dissolution data. Similar in vitro–in vivo correlation between the amount excreted in the urine and the percent dissolved was demonstrated for triameterene (15).

The examples above serve to emphasize the utility of correlations of in vitro dissolution parameters to in vivo urinary recovery of drug (unchanged or total as appropriate) as a predictive tool in bioavailability assessment.

Rate of Absorption/Release

Since bioequivalence requirements also require similar in vivo rates of appearance of the active species in the blood, the utility of in vitro parameters in predicting the rate of release needs to be demonstrated by correlations to in vivo parameters that are indicative of the rate of release, the parameters commonly used being C_{max} and T_{max}. The in vivo absorption/release rate computed employing the Wagner–Nelson or Loo–Riegelman methods or those obtained using deconvolution techniques are also appropriate for investigating these in vitro–in vivo correlations.

Correlations to C_{max}

Relatively few studies have attempted to correlate in vitro dissolution parameters to the in vivo rate of release. However, correlations have been observed for nitrofurantoin where the amount dissolved in the first hour was correlated to the amount of nitrofurantoin excreted in the first hour (16). C_{max} has also been shown to be significantly correlated with $1/T_{50\%}$, but not with $T_{50\%}$ in the case of flufenamic acid (17). Significant correlations were also observed in a bioavailability study of seven commercial trisulfapyrimidine suspensions in 14 adult male volunteers (18). Dissolution tests carried out using the USP paddle method revealed correlations between C_{max} for sulfamethazine and percent of the dose dissolved in 30 min ($\%D_{30}$), as illustrated in Fig. 10.4.

In the evaluation of six commercially available theophylline preparations discussed earlier (7), a correlation of greater than 0.9 was observed between dose-normalized peak plasma concentrations and $\%D_{60}$. The predictive ability of the in vitro–in vivo technique utilized also resulted in estimates comparable to the observed values. In one of the studies mentioned earlier (11), good linear correlation was observed between the peak plasma concentration of

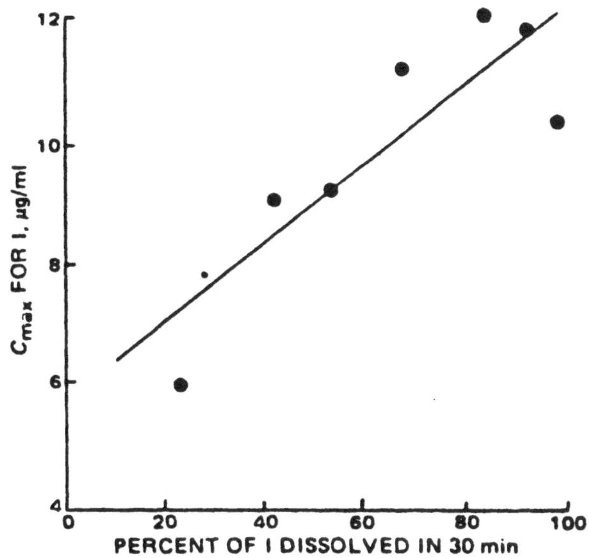

Fig. 10.4 Correlation of an in vitro dissolution parameter (% dissolved in 30 min, $\%D_{30}$) to an in vivo bioavailability parameter [peak plasma concentration, C_{max}, of sulfadiazine (I)]. The observed relationship follows administration of single doses of seven commercial trisulfapyrimidine suspensions in a crossover study in 14 subjects. (From Ref. 18.)

bacampicillin and the dissolution half-life, although a similar correlation could not be demonstrated for the rate constant for absorption (k_a) and the dissolution half-life.

Criteria Based on Correlations to C_{max}

Each of the correlations described could be utilized to promulgate criteria for bioequivalence based on Eqs. (10.3) and (10.4) described earlier. In a recent application of this concept, criteria for predicting (or establishing) limits on the rate of release were derived from evaluation of four controlled-release alaproclate tablets, where a significant correlation between the individual C_{max} and the in vitro dissolution rate constant was observed (12). Based on the regression line, a difference in the dissolution rate of $1.52\,h^{-1}$ was found to reduce the C_{max} by 20% (maximum permissible under FDA requirements), thus demonstrating the predictive applicability of this correlation.

Few of the other instances where correlations between C_{max} and dissolution parameters have been demonstrated are listed in Table 10.1. However, the utility of dissolution testing in predicting C_{max} remains limited, since C_{max} is dependent on release of the active species from the dosage form, dissolution of

Table 10.1 Dissolution Testing Parameters Commonly Used for In Vivo–In Vitro Correlations

In vivo parameter[a]	In vitro parameter[a]	Formulation type	Drug/ active moiety	Reference
AUC $_{(0-\infty)}$	$\%D_{15}$, D_{30}	Tablets	Promethazine	31
	k_d	Granules	Omeprazole	10
	$T_{50\%}$	Microcapsules	Bacampicillin hydrochloride	11
AUC $_{(0-\infty)}$	$\%D_{30}$	Tablets	Hydrocortisone	27
AUC $_{(0-24h)}$	$\%D_{30}$ min	Capsules	Indomethacin	24
AUC $_{(0-6h)}$,	$\%D_{30}$, $\%D_{60}$	Uncoated tablets, capsules (SR), tablets (SR)	Theophylline	7
AUC $_{(0-6h)}$	$\%D_{60}$, $1/T_{50\%}$	Tablets	Digoxin	9
AUC	$\log k_d$	Film-coated tablets and controlled-release tablets (insoluble matrix type)	Alproclate	12
	$\%D_{4\,h}$	Tablet (controlled release)	Quinidine Gluconate	29
$F\%$ (rel. to soln.)	$\%D_{30}$	Tablets	Frusemide	13
F	$T_{50\%}$	Tablets	Nalidixic acid	23
F	$1/T_{50\%}$	Tablets	Digoxin	9
$F\%$ (6 h)	k_s	Uncoated tablets, capsules (SR), tablets (SR)	Theophylline	7
F% (1 h)	$\%D_{60\ \mathrm{mins}}$	Uncoated tablets, capsules (SR), tablets (SR)	Theophylline	7
A_e(0–8 h)	$T_{50\%}$	Microcapsules	Bacampicillin hydrochloride	11
A_e (0–24 h) (steady state)	$\%D_{6\,h}$	Slow-release tablets	Terbutaline	14
A_e (0–48 h)	$\%D_{4\,h}$	Tablets (rapid and slow release)	Metformin	32
A_e (0–48 h)	$\%D_{60}$	Tablets and capsules	Triamterene–hydrochlorthiazide	15

Table 10.1 (continued)

In vivo parameter[a]	In vitro parameter[a]	Formulation type	Drug/ active moiety	Reference
A_e (0–72 h) (single dose)	$\%D_{4\ h}$	Slow release	Terbutaline	14
A_e (0–72 h)	$\%D_{60}$	Tablets	Chlorothiazide	2
C_{max}	$\%D_{30}$	Suspensions	Trisulfapyrimidine	18
C_{max}	D_{60}		Nitrofurantoin	16
C_{max}	$T_{50\%}$	Microcapsules	Bacampicillin hydrochloride	11
C_{max}	$1/T_{50}$		Flufenamic acid	17
C_{max}	$\%D_{60\ min}$	Uncoated tablets, capsules (SR), tablets (SR)	Theophylline	7
C_{max}	k_d		Alproclate	12
In vivo release rate	In vitro release rate	OROS tablets	Oxprenolol	6
Time to invasion	Time for dissolution	Tablets	Molsidomine	8
$MDT_{in\ vivo}$	$MDT_{in\ vitro}$	Film-coated tablets	Alproclate	12
MT (invasion)	MDT (in vitro)	Tablets (extended release)	Theophylline	8

[a] $\%D_n$, percentage of dose dissolved in n minutes; $\%T_p$, time to dissolve p percent of the dose; $F\%$, bioavailability percent (relative to solution or IV); AUC, area under the plasma concentration time curve; C_{max}, peak plasma concentration; A_e, amount of unchanged or total drug excreted in the urine; k_s, rate constant for dissolution; MDT, mean dissolution time.

the active species, and eventual transfer of these species across the gastrointestinal membrane into systemic circulation. Some of the other variables that contribute to a lack of in vitro–in vivo correlations are discussed later in the book. However, in instances where rigorous investigations indicate that correlations do exist, it should be possible to obtain meaningful predictions of C_{max} from dissolution data.

Correlations to T_{max} and Mean Dissolution Time

Since T_{max} is also a parameter indicative of the rate of absorption, it is subject to most of the limitations described earlier for C_{max} in obtaining in vitro–in vivo correlations. Statistical moment theory may also be used to determine the mean dissolution times ($MDT_{in\ vitro}$) and mean residence times ($MRT_{in\ vivo}$) for conventional oral dosage forms. $MDT_{in\ vivo}$ may also be obtained by the relationship

$$MDT_{in\ vivo} = MRT_{tablet} - MRT_{solution} \tag{10.5}$$

However, assumptions of reproducibility of the experimental conditions and time invariance of the pharmacokinetics are inherent in the foregoing methodology. The applicability of the technique above was demonstrated with alaproclate tablets, where a significant linear relationship between the MDT in vitro and in vivo was obtained for four controlled-release formulations (12). Correlations were also obtained for AUC and C_{max} versus the $MDT_{in\ vitro}$. A reduction in AUC of more than 20% was not observed until $MDT_{in\ vitro}$ exceeded a value of 3 h for these tablets. A significant linear relationship was also observed between the MRT and $MDT_{in\ vitro}$.

LIMITATIONS

The discussion above focused largely on the positive aspects of dissolution testing in bioavailability and bioequivalence determinations. However, correlations of in vivo parameters to in vitro dissolution tests may be affected by variables involved in dissolution testing and by physiological and pharmacokinetic variables, which possibly accounts for the lack of such correlations in the case of certain drugs and their dosage forms. Some of these variables are listed in Table 10.2. The extent of influence of these variables places considerable limitations on the role of dissolution in bioequivalence determinations. The method used in dissolution testing may contribute greatly to the observed results due to different rates and levels of agitation, varying concentration gradients due to the size and shape of the vessel, and a host of other reasons (19). The commonly used methods are the basket and paddle method, generally referred to as USP I and USP II methods, respectively, but investigators have often used methods from other compendia. The influence of methodology variables on observed in vitro–in vivo correlations was demonstrated in the case of indomethacin (24), where the $\%D_{30}$ value using the paddle method at 100 rpm (JP X) was significantly correlated with the observed $AUC_{(0-24)}$ (24). However, low correlations between $\%D_{30}$ and the in vivo parameters were observed using oscillating basket or solubility simulator methods, which provide stronger disintegrating forces.

Furthermore, it has been demonstrated using dissolution standards that calibration of these instruments are of vital importance in obtaining reproducible data (20). The dissolution medium and the volume of the dissolution medium used may profoundly affect dissolution (21). Results obtained from dissolution tests utilizing 20 mL of medium were more predictive of in vivo rates of

Table 10.2 Selected Examples of Physicochemical, Physiological, and Methodology Variables That Place Limitations on the Applications of Dissolution Testing in Bioavailability/Bioequivalence Determinations

Variable	Drug	Reference
Instrument/method	Prednisone	20
Medium	Norethindrone–mestranol	32
	Quinidine gluconate	29
	Furosemide	21
Volume of medium	Trichlorthiazide	22
pH of medium	Trichlormethiazide	22
Gastric emptying time	Tetracycline	2
Presystemic metabolism	Prednisone	30
	Hydrocortisone	27
	Metformin	33
Binding to intestinal wall	Metformin	33
Particle size	Indomethacin	24
	Medroxyprogesterone acetate	34
Food-induced changes	Theophylline	26
Matrix and design of dosage form	Theophylline	26

absorption of trichlormethiazide in the presence of magnesium oxide than the JP X procedure utilizing 500 mL of medium (22). However, in another investigation of three commercially available tablets and two experimental tablets of nalidixic acid, the rank order of the bioavailabilities of the tablets was the same as the rank order of their dissolution rates using eight different dissolution methods (23). Particle size is another important physical property to be considered in interpreting results of dissolution testing. In a study investigating the relationship between the dissolution rates and bioavailability (24) of five 25-mg indomethacin capsules (two commercial and three experimental), the dissolution of the capsule containing 74- to 105-μm particles was faster than that of the capsule containing 125- to 177-μm particles (24).

There also exist a host of physiological variables that on occasion possibly detract from the ability of dissolution testing in predicting bioavailability and bioequivalence of certain dosage forms. Some of the salient variables include gastric emptying time, hepatic first-pass metabolism, and splanchnic blood flow rates. Some of these are discussed below.

The effects of gastric emptying may not always be assessed by in vitro dissolution tests. Generally, with dissolution-limited dosage forms, dissolution testing provides an accurate assessment of the bioavailability of the dosage form being evaluated. However, dissolution-enhancing agents such as dioctyl sulfosuccinate have been demonstrated to reduce the bioavailability of tetracycline preparations, although increased dissolution was observed (25). This was ascribed to the slowing of gastric emptying due to the surfactant.

Presystemic metabolism of the drug and binding of the drug to the intestinal wall have been cited as possible explanations for the low bioavailability of metformin tablets and the lack of correlation of AUC to the dissolution rate. Evaluation of food-induced changes in absorption from conventional and especially from controlled-release formulations may not always be detected from dissolution studies, due to consideration of gastric emptying time and that drug release in vivo occurs under varying conditions of pH and varying rates of transfer across the intestinal membrane. Furthermore, drug release may often depend on the matrix or design of the dosage form. Theo-dur Sprinkle, a beaded multiple unit, and Uniphyl, a cellulose matrix single-unit controlled-release formulation, of theophylline were evaluated (26). Although both have pH-independent in vitro dissolution rates, both showed substantial and opposite food-induced absorption changes. Because a high-fat meal delays gastric emptying and increases secretion of bile, pancreatic fluid, digestive enzymes, and gastric hormones, one or a combination of these factors were deemed responsible for the absorption changes. It is apparent from the data that pH dependency in dissolution rate alone does not predict food-induced absorption changes. Innovative in vitro systems that simulate high-fat meal-related in vivo conditions are needed to better predict the food-induced absorption changes from test formulations.

In the case of certain drugs, systemic bioavailability may not depend on the dissolution characteristics of the drug and its formulation (e.g., corticosteroids). Earlier studies have suggested that hydrocortisone is 50 to 60% available to the systemic circulation following 10- to 20-mg tablet or suspension doses. Results of an investigation evaluating five hydrocortisone products (27)—suspension (A) and the four tablets (B–E)—showed similar plasma profiles obtained among tablet dosages, despite a 12-fold range in their dissolution rates, suggesting that the incomplete absorption of hydrocortisone was probably due to intrinsic absorption effect, first-pass hepatic clearance, or both. Similar overall bioavailability of the tablet and suspension formulations was observed, indicating that dissolution was not the rate-limiting step in the absorption of orally administered hydrocortisone.

The foregoing physicochemical and physiological factors that affect the results of dissolution testing also possibly explain the lack of correlation of the in vitro dissolution parameters to observed bioavailability/bioequivalence parameters. In such instances dissolution methodology have to be modified or appropriate methodology has to be developed that take into consideration the foregoing factors and yet give rise to meaningful in vitro–in vivo correlations.

REGULATORY BIOEQUIVALENCE REQUIREMENTS AND DISSOLUTION TESTING

The usefulness of dissolution studies as compendial methods for determining product content, uniformity, and rate and extent of drug release has been discussed earlier for a number of drugs and dosage forms. Although in vivo performance of dosage forms remains the ultimate test of any dosage form, results of in vitro dissolution testing of oral dosage forms are required in submissions of a new drug application (NDA) or abbreviated new drug applications (ANDA) in order to satisfy requirements for drug approval by the Food and Drug Administration (FDA). In the case of certain drugs (e.g., aspirin, phenacetin, and caffeine tablet and capsules, conjugated estrogens with meprobamate, etc.), the bioavailability need only be demonstrated "if the product fails to achieve adequate dissolution when compared to the test standard." Further, certain drug products may also be approved based on dissolution data if the drug product passes the in vitro test approved by the FDA or if it meets an in vitro test correlated with in vivo data. Dissolution data have also been used as the basis of drug approval when no published method for in vivo availability determination exists.

An example is dihydroergotoxamine, where an in vitro dissolution criterion was used in the approval of sublingual tablets (28). Conversely, dissolution tests have also been developed at the FDA to discriminate between products. In the case of evaluation of controlled-release formulations of quinidine gluconate (29), the dissolution in 4 h using acetate buffer at pH 5.4 correlated well with the observed bioavailability parameters (AUC and C_{max}). The unapproved product had only 41% AUC and 35% C_{max} of the reference product, whereas the reformulated product was comparable to the reference product (Fig. 10.5). In the case of controlled-release formulations, dissolution-rate profiles are also evaluated for indications of dose dumping by the formulation, pH dependency in its release, and total percentage of the dose released from the dosage form.

Important applications of dissolution testing in the realm of drug approval process are in those cases where multiple strengths of the formulation containing the same therapeutic moiety is the subject of a new drug application. In certain of these cases, the intermediary strengths may be approved based on in vitro dissolution tests if approval of the lowest and highest marketed strengths

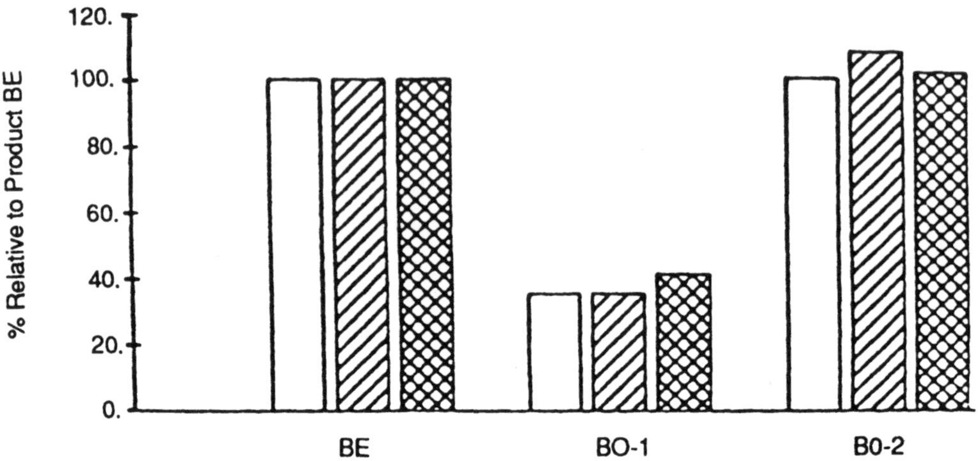

Fig. 10.5 Predictive ability of dissolution testing in bioavailability/bioequivalence determinations. Depicted is an in vitro–in vivo relationship for quinidine gluconate following administration of a single 324-mg tablet in crossover studies in healthy volunteers. The unapproved product BO-1 was observed to be bioinequivalent to the reference product BE. However, the reformulated product BO-2 was observed to be bioequivalent to BE. □, Dissolution in pH 5.4 acetate buffer in 4h; ▨, C_{max}; ⊠, AUC. (From Ref. 29.)

are based on evaluations of in vivo data submitted as part of a new drug application.

The dissolution requirements of the FDA have played constructive roles in rectifying observed product variability in the marketplace or clinical setting. Prednisone is an example where reports indicated treatment failures with several generic prednisone products. The paddle method developed by the National Center for Drug Analysis was found to provide greater reproducibility and resulted in good correlation between the in vivo and in vitro data obtained and was adopted as the official USP method. Since then, a recent evaluation of five of the commercially marketed prednisone products revealed that the products that passed the official in vitro dissolution requirements were also bioequivalent to each other (30).

Perhaps the most important application of dissolution testing is in ensuring adequate control of process and manufacturing variables and for purposes of quality control, with the express intent of minimizing batch-to-batch variability. In this regard the FDA maintains that the manufacturer conduct those in vitro tests specified in the bioequivalence requirements (usually, dissolution testing) on a sample of each batch of the product to assure batch-to-batch uniformity (21 CFR 320.56).

CONCLUSIONS

The ability to reliably predict in vivo performance of a dosage form is the ultimate objective of all in vitro dissolution testing. The foregoing discussion has amply demonstrated correlations between in vitro dissolution parameters and in vivo availability parameters and evolving criteria for bioavailability/bioequivalence based on such correlations. Although some of the techniques reported earlier have demonstrated the ability to detect differences of 20% in AUC and C_{max}, the power associated with detecting these differences has not been investigated and is an aspect that merits further investigations.

However, the various in vitro–in vivo correlations used are indicative of the arbitrary selection of dissolution parameters. Also, various physicochemical, design, process, and physiological variables place limitations on the ability of dissolution criteria in predicting bioavailability and bioequivalence. However, to date, dissolution testing remains the single most important in vitro test that when applied and evaluated correctly ensures quality, batch-to-batch uniformity, and consistency in developed and marketed oral dosage forms. In those cases where adequate in vitro–in vivo correlations exist, it is predictive of bioavailability and bioequivalence. Considerations of ease, cost, and minimization of the use of human subjects for bioequivalence investigations are attractive reasons for advocating an increasing role of dissolution testing for bioavailability/bioequivalence determinations.

REFERENCES

1. *United States Pharmacopeia*, XXth rev., Mack Publishing, Easton, Pa. (1980).
2. V. P. Shah, P. Knight, V. K. Prasad, and B. E. Cabana, *J. Pharm. Sci.*, *71*(7), 822 (1982).
3. *Code of Federal Regulations*, 21 CFR 320, Office of the Federal Register, National Archives and Records Administration, Washington, D.C. (1987), pp. 148–166.
4. J. G. Wagner and E. Nelson, *J. Pharm. Sci.*, *53*, 1392 (1964).
5. J. C. K. Loo and S. Riegelman, *J. Pharm. Sci.*, *57*, 918 (1968).
6. F. Lagenbucher and J. Myscika, *Br. J. Clin. Pharm.*, *19*, 151S (1985).
7. A. El-Yazigi and R. J. Sawchuk, *J. Pharm. Sci.*, *74*(2), 161 (1985).
8. D. Voegle, *Methods Find. Exp. Clin. Pharmacol.*, *6*(10), 597 (1984).
9. E. J. Fraser, R. H. Leach, J. W. Poston, A. M. Bold, L. S. Culank, and A. B. Lipede, *J. Pharm. Pharmacol.* *25*, 968 (1973).
10. A. Pilbrandt and C. Cedenberg, *Scand. J. Gastroenterol.*, *20*(Suppl. 108), 113 (1985).
11. J. Sjovall, R. Sjoqvist, B. Huitfeldt, and H. Nyqvist, *J. Pharm. Sci.*, *73*(2), 141 (1984).
12. C. Graffner, M. Nicklasson, and J. E. Lindgren, *J. Pharmacokinet. Biopharm.*, *12*(4), 367 (1984).

13. M. Kingsford, N. J. Eggers, G. Soteros, T. J. B. Maling, and R. J. Shirkey, *J. Pharm. Pharmacol.*, *36*, 536 (1984).
14. L. Nyberg and B. M. Kennedy, *Eur. J. Respir. Dis.*, *65* (Suppl. 134), 119 (1984).
15. V. P. Shah, M. A. Walker, V. K. Prasad, J. Lin, G. Knapp, and B. E. Cabana, 11 (1984).
16. G. L. Mattok, R. D. Hossie, and I. J. McGilveray, *Can. J. Pharm. Sci.*, *7*, 84 (1972).
17. N. Kaniwa, H. Ogata, N. Aoyagi, T. Shibazaki, A. Ejima, Y. Watanabe, K. Motohashi, K. Sasahara, E. Nakajimi, T. Morioka, and T. Nitanai, *Int. J. Clin. Pharmacol. Ther. Toxicol.*, *21*, 56 (1983).
18. L. K. Mathur, J. M. Jaffe, R. I. Poust, H. Barry III, T. J. Goehl, V. P. Shah, and J. L. Colaizzi, *J. Pharm. Sci.*, *68*(6), 699 (1979).
19. D. C. Cox, C. C. Douglas, W. B. Furman, R. D. Kirchhoefer, J. W. Myrick, and C. E. Wells, *Pharm. Technol.*, *2*(4), 41 (1978).
20. V. K. Prasad, V. P. Shah, H. Hunt, E. Purich, P. Knight, and B. E. Cabana, *J. Pharm. Sci.*, *72*(1), 42 (1983).
21. V. K. Prasad, R. S. Rapaka, P. W. Knight, and B. E. Cabana, *Int. J. Pharm.*, *11*, 81 (1982).
22. H. Takahashi, Y. Watanabe, H. Shimamura, and K. Sugito, *J. Pharm. Sci.*, *74*(8), 862 (1985).
23. H. Ogata, N. Aoyagi, K. Kaniwa, T. Shibazaki, A. Ejima, N. Takasugi, E. Mafune, T. Hayashi, and K. Suwa, *Int. J. Clin. Pharmacol. Ther. Toxicol.*, 22(4), 175 (1984).
24. N. Aoyagi, H. Ogata, N. Kaniwa, and A. Ejima, *Int. J. Clin. Pharmacol. Ther. Toxicol.* *23*(10), 529 (1985).
25. V. P. Shah, J. P. Hunt, W. R. Fairweather, V. K. Prasad, and G. Knapp, *Biopharm. Drug Dispos.*, *7*, 27 (1986).
26. A. Karim, T. Burns, W. Lorraine, J. Streicher, and M. Palmer, *38*(1), 77 (1985).
27. R. B. Patel, M. C. Rogge, A. Selen, T. J. Goehl, V. P. Shah, V. K. Prasad, and P. G. Welling, *J. Pharm. Sci.*, *73*(7), 964 (1984).
28. J. P. Hunt, V. P. Shah, V. K. Prasad, D. J. Schuirmann, and B. E. Cabana, *J. Pharm. Sci.*, *70*(7), 796 (1981).
29. V. K. Prasad, V. P. Shah, P. Knight, H. Malinowski, B. E. Cabana, and M. C. Meyer, *Int. J. Pharm.*, *13*, 1 (1983).
30. G. E. Francisco, I. L. Honigberg, J. T. Stewart, J. A. Kotzan, and W. J. Brown, *Biopharm. Drug. Dispos.*, *5*, 335 (1984).
31. R. Zaman, I. L. Honigberg, G. E. Francisco, J. A. Kotzan, J. T. Stewart, W. J. Brown, V. P. Shah, and F. R. Pelsor, *Biopharm. Drug Dispos.* *7*, 281 (1986).
32. T. J. Goehl, G. M. Sundaresan, and V. K. Prasad, *Int. J. Pharm.*, *15*, 115 (1983).
33. P. J. Pentikainen, *Int. J. Clin. Pharmacol. Ther. Toxicol.*, *24*(4), 213 (1986).
34. E. D. B. Johansson, P. B. Johansen, and S. N. Rasmusen, *Acta Pharmacol. Toxicol.*, *58*, 311 (1986).

ADDITIONAL READING

Alkaysi, H. N., M. A. Salem, A. M. Gharaibeh, et al., *J. Clin. Pharm. Ther.*, *14*, 111 (1989).

el-Arini, S. K., G. K. Shui, and J. P. Skelly, *Pharm. Res.*, *7*(11), 1134 (1990).

Blake, M. I., *Drug Top*, *132*, 84 (1988).

Bramanti, G., P. Mura, A. Liquori, et al., *Int. J. Pharm.*, *49*, 241 (1989).

Blume, H., *Pharm. Ztq.*, *134*, 24 (1989).

Cunha, B. A., *Adv. Thera.*, *5*, 54 (1988).

Falamarzian, M., A. Raisi, A. Jafarian, et al., *Pharm. Acta. Helv.*, *63*, 227 (1988).

Fassihi, A. R. and D. L. Munday, *J. Pharm. Pharmacol.*, *41*(6), 369 (1989).

Gorecki, D. K., C. J. Richardson, P. Pavlakidis, et al., *Can. Pharm. J.*, *122*, 484 (1989).

Hussain, M. A., R. C. DiLuccio, and E. Shefter, *Pharm. Res.*, *6*(1), 49 (1989).

Kanazawa, H., E. Okano, M. Hasegawa, et al., *Jap. J. Hosp. Pharm.*, *15*, 351 (1989).

Kaniwa, N., H. Ogata, N. Aoyagi, et al., *J. Pharm. Sci.*, *78*, 1020 (1989).

Kassam, R. M., E. Friesen, and R. A. Locock, *J. Parenter. Enternal. Nutr.*, *13*(3), 272 (1989).

Keller, M., *Dtsch. Apoth. Ztg.*, *128*, 1565 (1988).

Lin, S. Y., H. N. Chang, J. C. Yang, et al., *Curr. Ther. Res.*, *44*, 585 (1988).

Lin, S. Y., Y. H. Kao, and H. N. Chang, *J. Pharm. Sci.*, *79*(4), 326 (1990).

Lin, L. and P. Bernando, *J. Pharm. Sci.*, *79*(2), 124 (1990).

Maublant, J. C., M. Sournac, J. M. Aiache, and A. Veyre, *Eur. J. Clin. Med.*, *15*(3), 143 (1989).

McClelland, G. A., S. C. Sutton, K. Engle, and G. M. Zentner, *Pharm. Res.*, *8*(1), 88 (1991).

Menke, G., M. Kausch, and N. Rietbrock, *Arzneim Forsch*, *38*, 300 (1988).

Meyer, M. C., G. C. Wood, and A. B. Straughn, *Biopharm. Drug Dispos.*, *10*(3), 321 (1989).

Midha, K. K., B. S. Chakraborty, R. Schwede, et al., *J. Pharm. Sci.*, *79*, 3 (1990).

Paton, D. M. and D. R. Webster, *Int. J. Clin. Pharmacol. Res.*, *8*, 227 (1988).

Pfeffer, M., N. Sauerbrey, F. Windt-Hanke, and W. Krause, *Arzneimittelforschung*, *40*(11), 1191 (1990).

Raisi, A., M. Falamarzian, H. Zia, et al., *Drug Dev. Ind. Pharm.*, *15*, 1889 (1989).

Runhaar, E. A., J. P. Neijt, J. J. Holthuis, et al., *Pharm. Weekbl. Sci. Ed.*, *11*, 218 (1989).

Sabel, B. A., P. Dominiak, W. Hauser, M. J. During, and A. Freese, *J. Pharmacol. Ther.*, *255*(2), 914 (1990).

Shaheen, O., H. Mouti, M. Karmi et al., *Curr. Ther. Res.*, *45*, 517 (1989).

Sheftner, E. and A. R. Hurwitz, *Pharm. Res.*, *6*(12), 1052 (1989).

Steinigen, M., *Pharm. Ztg.*, *133*, 30 (1988).

Uchida, T., I. Fujimato, and S. Goto, *Chem. Pharm. Bull. (Tokyo)*, *37*(12), 3416 (1989).

Upton, R. A., L. Ball, R. L. Braun, E. T. Lin, W. Liang-Gee, and L. J. Leeson, *J. Pharm. Sci.*, *80*(1), 22 (1991).

Yamakawa, I., M. Kawahara, S. Watanabe, and Y. Miyake, *J. Pharm. Sci.*, *79*(6), 505 (1990).

ELEVEN

Dissolution Rediscovered

John H. Wood
Virginia Commonwealth University
Medical College of Virginia
Richmond, Virginia

INTRODUCTION

It is difficult to say whether the in vitro dissolution of a tablet actually predicts the in vivo dissolution; however, we believe that if a tablet does not dissolve properly in our in vitro tests, it certainly won't do so in in vivo tests for dissolution; it will have a much greater chance of clinical success than its less well formulated counterparts. Furthermore, any given active ingredient cannot be expected to produce the same therapeutic effects when administered in different formulations of the same dosage form.*

It is now 20 years since Lloyd Miller of the *United States Pharmacopeia* and Edward Feldman of the *National Formulary* established in 1967 the Joint Panel on Physiological Availability, chaired by Rudolf Blyth and including many of the pharmaceutical scientists then most active in the development of dosage form dissolution-rate technology and its correlation to in vivo observations.

Miller told the first meeting of this panel that during World War II the disintegration tester was introduced as a military procurement tool to seek to minimize repeated observations of the passage of intact tablets, particularly

*From Yen (1).

enteric, through the full gastrointestinal system and their elimination in the feces. Since the pharmaceutical industry was familiar with the test, he simply carried it into the upcoming USP XV. Its degree of success in improving the general bioavailability of drugs can now never be known. However, subsequently, Canadian government drug officials did feel, based on bioavailability of some vitamin preparation components, that there was a general tendency to a loss in bioavailability with longer times for disintegration (2,3). However, by the middle 1960s a few cases of therapeutic failure with readily disintegrating tablets began to be recognized. In several of these, dissolution testing appeared to be predictive (4–6). In addition, political and other special-interest groups began to sense that there might soon develop an area of compendial inadequacy.

In the short time available to meet the deadline for USP XVIII and NF XIII, the committee adopted the first official dissolution procedures. These were a modified rotating basket as method I and the use of the disintegration testing assembly as method II. The latter was adopted with reluctance on the part of some of the committee, although the greatest body of private and government data existed for that apparatus. None of the recent authors of dissolution monographs seem to have been aware of enough of the background history of this period to have recognized the critical role assumed by Blythe in reconciling the divergent beliefs and perceived problems in the methods available to reach this first milestone.

PURPOSE FOR COMPENDIAL DISSOLUTION TESTING

The manner in which compendial dissolution testing had to come into existence virtually assured that inadequacies would be quickly perceived by those seeking precision in results, by those who had other preferred procedures, and by those who were adverse to the concept. In the final analysis, dissolution testing as a compendial procedure could be justified only if it provided an assurance of improved drug quality as perceived in pharmacotherapeutics. The ultimate need was a quality control method that assured uniform (and preferably complete) biological delivery from all lots of any given manufacturer and from all potential sources of the dosage form.

In this, it is ironic to remember the history of disintegration testing. The adoption of a 30-min time limit did not foresee that later human studies would tend to indicate that gastrointestinal disintegration was at least threefold longer in time. Some products had masked observed times because of hydration gumming of excipients. Quality control standards were easily tightened when the disks were introduced. These forced material through a mesh and thus allowed 30-min standards to be met with good precision but with no apparent physiologic relevance.

The first years after dissolution testing became official in 1970 there was an emphasis in publications on three factors: correlations of slow and high speed to effect more rapid completion of data, failings of the apparatus in precision, and a lack of in vivo correlative background for the test variables adopted. Each impinges critically on the justification for the official standards. However, it is essential to view each topic in its relation to, and implications for, the other topics.

SLOW- VERSUS HIGH-SPEED STIRRING

During the 1960s a few critical studies were available that indicated that the degree of agitation could mask or create differences in products (5,6). When this author prepared for Gerhard Levy a fast- and a slow-releasing aspirin preparation of identical chemical composition, he knew from prior work what the relative rates of absorption for the average of a panel of 30 test subjects would be (7,8). Levy, using the procedure that had demonstrated an in vitro–in vivo correlation for absorption of buffered and unbuffered aspirin (9), found that the fast tablet should be the slowest of the two. The difference in test method was in the relative degree of agitation. In the Levy low-agitation procedure, the excipients fell away from the larger crystals, allowing the aspirin to dissolve in the medium, while the fine mesh aspirin was so intermixed that in the pile formed by the disintegrated tablet the aspirin was not exposed. In the higher agitation of the Wood procedure, the dispersion of the pile permitted the enhanced solubility rate of the fine mesh to be dominant. Levy demonstrated that these two formulations had completely different dissolution rates as a function of agitation profiles, and that indeed these profiles crossed. From a human volunteer panel, he selected a group of habitually slow absorbers and another of fast absorbers. With the slow absorbers the slow dissolution profile correlated. These subjects absorbed aspirin from the large mesh crystal faster than from the fine mesh. The results with the rapid absorbers were as expected from higher agitation measurements. Thus the effect of variable gastrointestinal motility cannot be replicated by a single-test agitation rate. The implications of these aspirin studies carry over to the bioavailability of many drugs for which the potential for effective absorption is not uniform through the entire tract. In addition, where hydration of excipients under low agitation may create a gummy mass, under higher agitation dispersion is absolutely analogous to that in the Levy study. Regardless of the human agitation rate–dissolution rate profile, for a given formulation a tight statistical correlation many be established between dissolution and agitation rates, and the temptation to obtain faster data recording in quality control becomes very strong. However, can the higher dissolution rate remain predictive of absorption profiles from manufacturing variants not recognized when the faster quality control began? Thus, is dissolution becoming merely a tool to demonstrate uniformity even if it does not exist?

When formulation or processing changes are contemplated, it is critically necessary to assure that each has an identical profile to agitation and pH if interchangeability is to be sought. When a compendial dissolution standard is for a multisource drug for which human bioavailability has not been determined, it will be coincidental if the agitation dissolution dependency is at all similar for each. Hence an arbitrary test speed may minimize or accentuate real or trivial differences. Would, could, or should an existing product be removed from a USP grade on the basis of a dissolution test alone when no in vivo correlation exists for that product?

CHOICE OF DISSOLUTION MEDIA

In the first choice between physiological mimicking test conditions and "clean" laboratory tests, the known variability and difficulty resulting from the use of pepsin and mucin was considered (8). It was finally agreed that only reagent chemical components would be used for dissolution media. Despite the fact that Kuna (10) had clearly demonstrated that the resting stomach was close to neutral in pH, in contrast to the strong acid present in stimulation or testing trauma, the choice of acid (0.01 to 0.1 *N* HCl) was the choice of the advisory panel.

It was not until the FDA began their extensive comparisons of in vivo–in vitro release that the implications of the possible importance of the Kuna work began to be recognized despite the dogma of the acid stomach. Indeed, in many test conditions the protocol forced the acid stomach on the test participants. Normally in a bioavailability study, the subjects have been fasting overnight. To initiate the study, a heparin lock is inserted for blood sampling. Even the most hardened volunteer subject must have a tinge of apprehension as this occurs. Physiologically, the fear mechanism results in an acid gastric secretion. The test product is then taken in the presence of this acid. The chronic use of medication in a normal subject not otherwise traumatized is not in the presence of acid. In a later section we will see that conditions are now recognized where higher test pH values are obligatory.

CHOICE OF DISSOLUTION VESSEL AND VOLUME

The committee felt that a geometrically defined vessel with appropriate ports for stirring, sampling, and so on, was essential. A conventional round-bottomed flask had severe geometrical limitations on what could be inserted into the flask. The standard glass resin kettle was readily available commercially and since it had a ground glass lid containing entry ports, it seemed to meet initial requirements. The bottom dimple was perceived to be as advantageous to those doing dissolution as to those in synthetic chemical studies. The bottle could stand free on a lab bench.

The volume readily held, 900 mL, met the standard of those who felt that dissolution should only be performed under "sink" conditions, ignoring the fact that the real volume for dissolution in vivo probably rarely can be claimed to meet that standard. Most of the committee felt that this volume was a reasonable compromise and that one volume should be reasonably predictive of phenomena at a different volume.

INADEQUACY OF INITIAL COMPENDIAL TEST SPECIFICATIONS

Not unexpectedly, when the 1970 test methods became the subject of widespread use, weaknesses or flaws rapidly were recognized and publicized. In the basket method the paddles above and below the basket were removed from the original Pernarowski design to reduce fabrication costs. Salicylic acid test tablets, later utilized as dissolution-test calibrators, did not demonstrate the need for paddles later found for some disintegratable tablets. The sampling site did prove to be a problem at very slow basket speeds, such as 25 rpm. However, the panel majority preferred faster speeds to minimize the total time required, even though predictability might be sacrificed.

New single-spindle systems tended to be free of the wobble that developed later as shafts and baskets lost concentric geometry with repeated handling. The vibration induced in multispindle assemblies was not foreseen. However, more careful engineering soon minimized these problems.

With speeds over 100 rpm, the mesh of the rotating basket tended to create an effective wall internally to higher degrees of agitation inside the basket. Thus the basket produced a limited range of useful agitation intensity. On the other hand, the disintegration tester was too severe in its agitation and was thus sensitive only to gross differences. It did average the result of six tablets rather than producing individual tablet data. It was clearly a shock to many involved in tablet production to be confronted from basket dissolution with evidence of tablet variability too often ignored previously. Tablet variability became recognized as an inescapable concern in bioavailability studies.

Soon the inadequacies of the disintegration tester system as a dissolution method became recognized and its popularity waned. However, several alternative procedures rapidly appeared on the scene. One, in particular, the FDA paddle, quickly assumed prominence because agitation rates were readily obtainable over an extremely wide range. Equally important, federal regulations began to appear utilizing it as the test vehicle for in vivo bioavailability correlations.

With the lack of adequate agitation of fines falling from the basket for a few products, there was a tendency for these to accumulate in the dimple torus of the bottom. This led to the suggestion of commissioned round-bottomed flasks. With the advent of the FDA paddle and an emphasis on geometric symmetry, the round-bottomed flask became essential for that mode, and convenience dictated a transition to its use for the rotating basket as well.

IN VIVO JUSTIFICATION OF DISSOLUTION TESTS

By 1973 the FDA had begun to recognize that a number of drug products had bioavailability differences between brands. An intensive screen of dissolution profiles between brands demonstrated clear product differences. A series of careful bioavailability studies were commissioned using products selected from a dissolution-rate screen. For each product the FDA set performance limits on dissolution in terms of a specific percentage that was required to be dissolved in an arbitrarily chosen time. Correlating with the bioavailability studies, these dissolution specifications were intended to ensure that at least 80% of the label quantity of drug was bioavailable This 80% value resulted from the statistical confidence limits on the reality of observed differences. Thus initially for digoxin, digitoxin, prednisone, tetracycline, and oxytetracycline, and later for others, a dissolution specification assured bioavailability across a spectrum of sources.

To the extent that bioavailability is thus capable of in vitro monitoring, the use of similar dissolution conditions provides a degree of assurance for the many products for which bioavailability testing has not been done because there is no evidence of the existence of a problem. Failing information to the contrary, this presumptive assurance has a degree of validity.

However, in the last few years the FDA has found special cases, as new generic products became available, that somewhat unanticipated dissolution conditions were necessary. Thus only by using a pH 4.0 to 5.0 medium could bioinequivalent furosemide tablets be clearly distinguished (11). In a more recent study with quinidine gluconate controlled-release tablets, no one pH could be definitive in distinguishing products (12). Rather, the profile of dissolution-rate dependency on pH for the range pH 1.0 to 7.4 was essential to differentiate formulations.

DISSOLUTIONAL STANDARDS FOR NEW DRUGS

As a new drug is brought from concept to finished product within a product development group, dissolution testing serves an evolving need. Initially, dissolution parameters may permit the best selection of test products for in vivo testing. As in vivo testing proceeds, the dissolution testing serves as a reference parameter to characterize the product in test, particularly when polishing of the formulation and processing details continues concurrently. The dissolution parameters serve as the only possible continuing reference in this period.

With recognition of the imminence of a new product introduction, this quantification of product continuity becomes the responsibility of the quality assurance personnel. At this point the formulation is essentially inviolate and dissolution rates may be correlated to the permissible variations in processing variables. Major changes in formulation and processing are no longer options. Quality assurance develops a dissolution standard that is suitable to the variants open, and at the same time is like all existing compendial procedures. In particular, total elapsed time is relevant to expeditious handling. This is the standard communicated to the FDA for quality assurance. In due time, this information is also given to the compendial authorities and eventually results as the USP monograph.

As the years progress, patent protection ceases in some countries. Most of these countries do not have the U.S. standards of bioequivalence. Hence for many it is sufficient that the product meet the compendial specifications where documented. The USP is a recognized international reference standard, and here the problems begin. A new formulation made by completely different procedures and with different excipients cannot be expected to exhibit the same sensitivity to agitation intensity and solvent pH. One cannot guess a priori whether the new formulation is superior, inferior, or comparable based merely on one arbitrary dissolution standard.

Although some might question whether our compendial specifications need to be written to assure that foreign generics are adequate in quality before they may legally be used in this country, there is a moral question relating to incomplete information. For countries that cannot, for economic reasons, support the level of drug quality enforced in the United States by the FDA, our policies and laws may have to compromise between the needs of our drug industry for an adequate return on research investment and our obligations to improve world health standards. In the United States the approval of generic equivalents still tends to require, when possible, a satisfactory bioequivalence study. However, for multisourced and less-than-critical drugs, there are many exceptions based on physicochemical drug attributes for perceived potential dissolution problems. However, there are many people in authority in drug selection positions who still do not realize that equivalence of interchangeability in long-acting or controlled-release preparations is still largely a dream. Such products are approved only in their demonstrated function of extended release. If there is an optimum release profile, it is almost coincidental if several products are therapeutically equivalent even though equally bioavailable.

THE UNIVERSAL REFERENCE DISSOLUTIONAL TEST

The universal test has been sought for almost every branch of science, and our dissolution needs are no different. Slowly the dream is being equated with the universal solvent and the perpetual motion machine. We now recognize many of the components creating inter- and intrasubject variability even for absolutely identical administered dosage. We began to suspect the source of some of the subject–product interaction terms, which might confound some of our present assumptions.

How, then, can we examine the spectrum of products in the marketplace for possible candidates for full examination as to their possible bioinequivalencies? This author believes that our present dissolution methodology, properly used, can screen for the most probable problems. It has already been shown that in humans and in the beaker, product differences can exist due to agitation intensity and pH as the major variables. Minor effects due to variations in endogenous mucin (8) can be neglected in a primary screen.

Specifically, within the development of a product and in the marketplace, screen dissolution testing should determine any possible relevance of pH and agitation intensity. In pH, if only two tests can be considered, they should be pH 1.0 to 2.5 and pH 5.5 to 6.0. Agitation intensity should be at the slowest practical for adequate sampling and at an arbitrary "normal" rate. This results, minimally, in four test conditions. The contrast between slow and fast demonstrates whether any hydration or agglomeration may occur under low-intensity conditions which might impede subsequent release of drug at an adequate rate for complete absorption. This may, in turn, also correspond to differences in "fast" and "slow" absorbers due to gastric motility, food bolus, and so on. The pH dependency relates to changes occurring in the gums and other necessary excipients and whether these result in a pH dependency in those properties reflecting release of drug from its matrix.

All new products should be optimized by these in vitro criteria. In the screen of the marketplace, if there are products that behave differently from each other as a function of pH or agitation, there probably is a subgroup of the population for which these may not be equivalent and interchangeable in therapeutic effect. Unfortunately, in normal bioequivalence studies, subgroups must be large and present in normal healthy test subjects to be recognized. It is of no help to the individual who represents the tail of a distribution that the great majority were therapeutic successes if this tail represents adverse reaction or therapeutic failure that is formulation dependent. This author feels that this is the next stage in the application of our present knowledge.

The problem is: Who should perform such market screens? Obviously, at present this can only be done by a government agency or by a subcontractor such as a university laboratory or contract laboratory. Who should pay the costs? When the need becomes recognized, this will be answerable by consensus. Until then, pharmaceutical scientists have an obligation to find a medium to disseminate any limited information that is developed. An accumulation of such information will demonstrate the need for full studies. The work will then be funded by necessity.

REFERENCES

1. J. K. C. Yen, *Can. Pharm. J.*, *97*, 493 (1964).
2. D. G. Chapman, R. Crisafio, and J. A. Campbell, *J. Am. Pharm. Assoc. Sci. Ed.*, *43*, 297 (1954).
3. D. G. Chapman, R. Crisafio, and J. A. Campbell, *J. Am. Pharm. Assoc. Sci. Ed.*, *45*, 374 (1956).
4. G. Levy, *Can. Med. Assoc. J.*, *90*, 978 (1964).
5. W. E. Hamlin, E. Nelson, B. E. Ballard, and J. G. Wagner, *J. Pharm. Sci.*, *51*, 432 (1962).
6. G. Levy and J. A. Procknal, *J. Pharm. Sci.*, *53*, 656 (1964).
7. S. V. Lieberman and J. H. Wood, *J. Pharm. Sci.*, *53*, 1492 (1964).
8. J. H. Wood, *Pharm. Acta Helv.*, *42*, 129 (1967).
9. G. Levy and B. A. Hayes, *N. Engl. J. Med.*, *262*, 1053 (1960).
10. S. Kuna, *Arch. Int. Pharmcodyn. Ther.*, *152*, 79 (1964).
11. V. K. Prasad, R. S. Rapaka, P. W. Knight, and B. E. Cabana, *Int. J. Pharm.*, *11*, 81 (1982).
12. J. P. Skelly, L. A. Yamamoto, V. P. Shah, M. K. Yan, and W. H. Barr, *Drug Dev. Ind. Pharm.*, *12*, 1189 (1986).

APPENDIX

USP/NF Dissolution Test

This test is provided to determine compliance with the dissolution requirements where stated in the individual monograph for a tablet or capsule dosage form. Three types of apparatus are described herein, and the one that is to be used is indicated in the individual monograph. Unless otherwise stated in the individual monograph, Apparatus 1 is to be used.

Apparatus 1. The assembly[1] consists of the following: a covered, 1000-ml vessel made of glass or other inert, transparent material[2]; a variable-speed drive; and a cylindrical basket. The vessels are immersed in a suitable water bath of any convenient size that permits holding the temperature at 37 ±0.5° during the test and keeping the bath fluid in constant, smooth motion. No part of the assembly, including the environment in which the assembly is placed, contributes significant motion, agitation, or vibration beyond that due to the smoothly rotating stirring element. Apparatus that permits observation of the specimen and stirring element during the test is preferable. The vessel is cylindrical, with a spherical bottom. It is 16 cm to 17.5 cm high, its inside diameter is 10.0 cm to 10.5 cm, and its nominal capacity is 1000 ml. Its sides

---

[1] A suitable vessel is available commercially as Kimble Glass No. 33730, from laboratory supply houses, or as Elanco Products Division No. EQ-1900, from Eli Lilly and Co., P.O. Box 1750, Indianapolis, IN 46206. A suitable basket is available commercially from Hanson Research Corp., P.O. Box 35, Northridge, CA 91324, and from Van-Kel Industries, P. O. Box 311, Chatham, NJ 07928.

[2] The materials should not sorb, react, or interfere with the specimen being tested.

are flanged near the top. A fitted cover may be used to retard evaporation.[3] The shaft is positioned so that its axis is not more than 0.2 cm at any point from the vertical axis of the vessel. A speed-regulating device is used that allows the shaft rotation speed to be selected and maintained at the rate specified in the individual monograph, within $\pm 4\%$.

The metallic shaft is 6 mm to 10.5 mm in diameter, and rotates smoothly and without significant wobble. The basket consists of two parts, one of which, the top, is attached to the shaft. It is of solid metal except for a 2-mm vent, and it is fitted with three spring clips that allow removal of the lower part to admit the test specimen, and that firmly hold the lower part of the basket concentric to the axis of the vessel during rotation. The detachable part of the basket is fabricated of welded-seam, stainless-steel cloth, formed into a cylinder 3.66 cm high and 2.5 cm in diameter, with a narrow rim of sheet metal around the top. Shaft and basket components are fabricated of stainless steel, usually type 316. Unless otherwise specified in the monograph, use 40-mesh cloth. A basket having a gold coating 0.0001 inch (2.5 μm) thick may be used for tests carried out in dilute acid media. The dosage unit is placed in a dry basket at the beginning of each test. The basket is lowered into position before the rotation is started. The distance between the inside bottom of the vessel and the basket is maintained at 2.5 ± 0.2 cm during the test.

Apparatus 2. Use the assembly from *Apparatus 1*, except that a paddle formed from a blade and a shaft is used as the stirring element.[4] The shaft, 10 ± 0.5 mm in diameter, is positioned so that its axis is not more than 0.2 cm at any point from the vertical axis of the vessel, and rotates smoothly without significant wobble. The stirring blade, 3.0 mm to 5.0 mm thick, forms a section of a circle having a diameter of 83 mm, and is subtended by parallel chords of 42 ± 1 mm and 75 ± 1 mm. The blade passes through the diameter of the shaft so that the bottom of the blade is flush with the bottom of the shaft, and the blade is positioned horizontally at the end of the rotating shaft so that the 42-mm edge is nearest the lowest inner surface of the vessel. The distance of 2.5 ± 0.2 cm between the blade and the inside bottom of the vessel is maintained during the test. The metallic blade and shaft comprise a single entity that may be coated with a suitable fluorocarbon polymer. The dosage unit is allowed to sink to the bottom of the vessel before rotation of the blade

---

[3] If a cover is used, it provides sufficient openings to allow ready insertion of the thermometer and withdrawal of specimens.

[4] A suitable paddle is available commercially from Hanson Research Corp. and from Van-Kel Industries.

is started. A small, loose piece of nonreactive material such as wire or glass helix may be attached to dosage units that would otherwise float.

Apparatus 3. Use the apparatus described under *Disintegration (701),* with these exceptions: (a) the disks are not used; (b) the apparatus is adjusted so that the bottom of the basket-rack assembly descends to 1.0 ±0.1 cm from the inside bottom surface of the vessel on the downward stroke; (c) the 10-mesh stainless-steel cloth in the basket-rack assembly is replaced with 40-mesh stainless-steel cloth; and (d) 40-mesh stainless-steel cloth is fitted to the top of the basket-rack assembly if necessary to prevent any dosage unit from floating out of the tubes of the assembly.

Apparatus suitability test. Individually test 1 tablet of the *USP Dissolution Calibrator, Disintegrating Type* and 1 tablet of *USP Dissolution Calibrator, Non-disintegrating Type*, according to the operating conditions specified. The apparatus is suitable if the results obtained with each tablet are within the stated acceptable range for that calibrator in the apparatus tested.

Dissolution medium. Use the solvent specified in the individual monograph. If the *Dissolution Medium* is a buffered solution, adjust the solution so that its pH is within 0.05 unit of the pH specified in the monograph. [NOTE—Dissolved gases can change the results of the test. In such cases, dissolved gases should be removed prior to testing.]

Procedure. Place the stated volume of the *Dissolution Medium* in the vessel of the apparatus specified in the monograph, assemble the apparatus, warm the *Dissolution Medium* to 37 ±0.5°, and remove the thermometer. Place 1 tablet or 1 capsule in the apparatus, taking care to exclude air bubbles from the surface of the dosage-form unit, and immediately operate the apparatus at the rate specified in the individual monograph. At the times stated, withdraw the specimens from a zone midway between the surface of the *Dissolution Medium* and the top of the rotating basket or blade, not less than 1 cm from the vessel wall. Unless otherwise directed in the individual monograph, add a volume of *Dissolution Medium* equal to the volume of the specimens withdrawn. Filter the specimens, and proceed as directed in the individual monograph. Repeat the test with additional dosage-form units.

Interpretation. Unless otherwise specified in the individual monograph, the requirements are met of the quantities of active ingredient dissolved from the units tested conform to the accompanying acceptance table. Continue testing through the three stages unless the results conform at either S_1 or S_2. The quantity, *Q,* is the amount of dissolved active ingredient specified in the individual monograph, expressed as a percentage of the labeled content; both the 5% and 15% values in the acceptance table are percentages of the labeled content so that these value and *Q* are in the same terms.

Acceptance Table

Stage	Number tested	Acceptance criteria
S_1	6	Each unit is not less than $Q + 5\%$.
S_2	6	Average of 12 units ($S_1 + S_2$) is equal to or greater than Q, and no unit is less than $Q - 15\%$.
S_3	12	Average of 24 units ($S_1 + S_2 + S_3$) is equal to or greater than Q, and not more than 2 units are less than $Q - 15\%$.

Author Index

Subject Index